Making Medicines

Making Medicines

A brief history of pharmacy and pharmaceuticals

Edited by

Stuart Anderson

MA, PhD, MRPharmS, MCCP

Senior Lecturer
London School of Hygiene and Tropical Medicine
University of London, UK

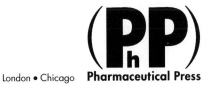

London • Chicago   **Pharmaceutical Press**

Published by Pharmaceutical Press

1 Lambeth High Street, London SE1 7JN, UK

University City Science Center, Suite 5E, 3624 Market Street, Philadelphia, PA 19104, USA

© 2005 Royal Pharmaceutical Society of Great Britain

 is a trademark of Pharmaceutical Press

Pharmaceutical Press is the publishing division of the Royal Pharmaceutical Society

Typeset by Mathematical Composition Setters Ltd, Salisbury, Wiltshire

Printed and bound by CPI Group (UK) Ltd, Croydon, CR0 4YY

ISBN 978 0 85711 099 2

A catalogue record for this book is available from the British Library

Contents

Preface xi
Acknowledgements xiii
About the editor xv
Contributors xvii

Part 1: Introduction   1

1   Researching and writing the history of pharmacy   3

The nature of the history of pharmacy   4
Approaches to the history of pharmacy   5
Uses of the history of pharmacy   6
Sources in the history of pharmacy   8
Previous histories of pharmacy   10
Plan of the book   13
References   16

Part 2: The development of pharmacy   19

2   Pharmacy from the ancient world to 1100 AD   21

The origins of medicine-making   21
Mesopotamian civilisations, 3000 BC to 539 BC   22
Egyptian civilisations, 3000 BC to 1200 BC   23
Greek civilisations, 1250 BC to 285 BC   25
Roman civilisations, 275 BC to 476 AD   29
Arabian civilisations, 400 AD to 1100 AD   32
References   36

3   Pharmacy in the medieval world, 1100 to 1617 AD   37

Developments in Europe from 1100 AD   37
The situation in England   40
The medieval hospital   43
Herbals   46
Changing medical ideas   51
Foundation of the Society of Apothecaries, 1617   53
References   54

4   Pharmacy in the early modern world, 1617 to 1841 AD   57

England after 1600   57
The Society of Apothecaries after 1617   63
Apothecaries and physicians, 1617 to 1701   64
The rise of the chemists and druggists, 1701 to 1815   67
Divergence of apothecaries, chemists and druggists, 1815 to 1841   70
The formation of the Pharmaceutical Society, 1841   72
References   75

5   Pharmacy in the modern world, 1841 to 1986 AD   77

Professional boundaries   77
Early years, 1841 to 1911   78
The Poisons and Pharmacy Act 1908   83
The rise of welfare   84
The scheme in practice   89
The National Health Service Act 1946   91
References   92

Part 3: The practice of pharmacy   95

6   The development of pharmaceutical education   97

Pharmacy education in Britain, 1841 to 1887   97
Statutory qualification   101
Pharmacy education in Britain, 1887 to 1911   104
Pharmacy education in Britain, 1911 to 1946   107
Pharmacy education in Britain, 1946 to 1986   108
Pharmacy education in Britain after 1986   111
References   112

7   The development of community pharmacy   115

Early development of community pharmacy   115
Developments in Britain   117
Chemist multiples   119
Opposition to the multiples   122
The Dickson Judgement   127
Mergers of multiples   128
Community practice   129
The National Health Service Act 1948   131
The Nuffield Report, 1986   132

Community pharmacy present and future   133
References   133

8   The development of pharmacy in hospitals   135

Hospital pharmacy before 1911   135
Hospital pharmacy, 1911 to 1948   137
Hospital pharmacy, 1948 to 1970   140
Hospital pharmacy, 1970 to 1980   143
Hospital pharmacy, 1980 to 1990   148
Hospital pharmacy since 1990   151
References   152

9   The development of the pharmaceutical industry   155

The business of making medicines   156
Origins in the 19th century   157
Developments from 1890 to 1939   162
Developments from 1939 to 1980   168
Developments from 1980 to 2000   170
Challenges and opportunities   172
References   172

Part 4: The products of pharmacy   175

**10   From alkaloids to gene therapy: a brief history of drug
       discovery in the 20th century**   177

The changing nature of drug discovery   177
Drug discovery before 1914: from alkaloids to Salvarsan   180
Drug discovery from 1914 to 1939: from Salvarsan to the
sulphonamides   183
Drug discovery from 1939 to 1945: synthetic anti-malarials,
compound E and penicillin   187
Drug discovery from 1945 to 1995: from cortisone to gene therapy   190
Beyond the 20th century   197
References   198

**11   From electuaries to enteric coating: a brief history of dosage
       forms**   203

Greek and Roman medicines   203
Arab medicines   204

Medieval medicines 205
Early modern medicines 205
Modern medicines 208
Changes in practice 218
References 219

**12 From secret remedies to prescription medicines:
a brief history of medicine quality** 223

Early medicines 223
Quack remedies and patent medicines 224
The development of quality standards 226
Patent medicines 230
Medicine Stamp Duty 234
Counter prescribing 236
Dispensed medicines 237
Quality of medicines today 239
References 240

13 From arsenic to thalidomide: a brief history of medicine safety 243

Medicines and safety 243
Development of medicines legislation in Britain 244
Development of medicines legislation in the USA 249
Adverse reactions to drugs 251
The thalidomide disaster, 1961 253
The aftermath of thalidomide 255
Post-thalidomide developments 257
Missed opportunities 258
References 259

Part 5: Pharmacy today and tomorrow 261

**14 Representation, regulation and recognition:
pharmacy in Britain, 1986 to 2004** 263

External influences 263
Internal influences 266
The changing role of the pharmacist 269
The changing nature of pharmacy employment 270
Pharmacy education 272
Continuing Professional Development 274

Role of the Royal Pharmaceutical Society of Great Britain   275
Professional regulation   277
References   280

15   The apothecary's return? A brief look at pharmacy's future   283

Unresolved issues   283
Pharmacy in the context of the public's health   285
A vision for pharmacy?   287
Glimpses of the future   289
European and North American experience   293
Choosing the future   296
Conclusion   298
References   299

Index   301

The colour plate sections are between pages 78 and 79, and 174 and 175

Preface

The history of pharmacy encompasses a wide range of subjects, from the emergence of the pharmaceutical profession and the identification of the skills and knowledge peculiar to it, to the development of medicines and ways of making and presenting them. It is a large and complex story, which has often taken different routes in different countries. The teaching of it is sadly neglected, not only in Great Britain but also in many countries throughout the world, with the result that many pharmacists working today have little idea of their professional origins and heritage.

There has been a small number of enthusiasts researching and writing about the history of pharmacy for many years. The British Society for the History of Pharmacy began life as a committee of the Pharmaceutical Society of Great Britain in 1950 and the International Society for the History of Pharmacy was founded in 1926. The tradition of writing about the history of pharmacy extends over hundreds of years. It has nevertheless been a neglected and under-researched field within the broader history of medicine for far too long.

With much already written about the history of pharmacy, is there a need for yet another book? The answer is an emphatic 'yes'. There are three key reasons why. Firstly, history needs to be re-interpreted by each new generation, in the light of further research and new insights; secondly, there is simply a need to update history in the light of developments since the last publication to the present day; and thirdly, there is a need to update the language, style and presentation of history to make it fully accessible to a contemporary audience.

Almost all the earlier histories of pharmacy have been the work of single authors. The task is now simply too big for one person working alone to tackle. In this volume, we have invited contributors to write in an accessible and involving style about an area of pharmacy's history about which they have considerable knowledge and expertise.

We hope that this book will contain something that will be of interest to a very wide audience. We hope that students about to start a career in pharmacy will find a great deal to illuminate their studies, and help them understand just why things are the way they are in pharmacy. We hope that pharmacists who have been qualified for some time will find much of interest here, but we also hope that a wider general audience will find interest in the story that is told.

My thanks go to all those who have contributed so generously to this volume, as writers, reviewers and readers. Producing it has been a mammoth task and inevitably, the odd error may have crept in. Any comments or suggestions from readers will be most welcome.

Stuart Anderson
President, British Society for the History of Pharmacy
May 2005

Acknowledgements

The writing of this book has been a collaborative effort, and a wide range of individuals has contributed to its successful completion. Above all, it would not have been possible without the ready willingness of busy people to contribute chapters in their areas of interest and expertise.

Some authors have called upon the assistance of others in the writing of their chapters to a greater or lesser extent. Stuart Anderson gratefully acknowledges the help given with Chapter 2, which is based largely on material kindly provided by Dr Juanita Burnby. Gordon Appelbe acknowledges the fact that Chapter 12 is largely based on original research by Marion Hodges MSc, BPharm, FRPharmS, MCCP, undertaken at the University of London in 1970.

Four pharmaceutical historians, John Hunt, Bill Jackson, Ainley Wade and Peter Worling, kindly undertook the substantial task of reading the entire manuscript and providing detailed comments on the whole book, as well as drawing the editor's attention to split infinitives and unnecessary commas. A particular debt of gratitude is owed to them. Virginia Berridge kindly commented on Chapter 1, and others read and commented on one or more of the remaining chapters.

Thanks to all those owners of copyright for permission to reproduce photographs and illustrations. The inclusion of these helps to bring history to life, and greatly enhances the value of the book. Their sources are indicated separately. Picture research was carried out by Simon Dunton and Briony Hudson at the Royal Pharmaceutical Society and the following organisations are thanked for making material available from their collections: the American Institute of the History of Pharmacy, AstraZeneca PLC, Bayer AG, Boots Group Archives, the British Museum, Eton College, GlaxoSmithKline, the History of Advertising Trust Archive, Österreichische Nationalbibliothek, Pfizer Limited, *The Pharmaceutical Journal*, the Royal College of Physicians, the Society of Apothecaries, Universitätsbibliothek Leipzig, US Food and Drug Administration, Victoria & Albert Museum and the Wellcome Library. Every effort was made to trace the copyright holders of the illustrations used. However, any errors will be corrected in future editions. Special thanks go to Briony Hudson and Peter Homan at the museum of the Royal Pharmaceutical Society of Great Britain for assistance in tracing appropriate illustrations for the book.

Finally, thanks are due to all those who have been involved in the development and delivery of this project, particularly Louise McIndoe of the Pharmaceutical Press for managing the project, and to Richard Anderson for editorial assistance.

About the editor

Stuart Anderson BSc (Hons), MA, PhD, MRPharmS, MCCP obtained his degree in pharmacy from the University of Manchester, taking honours in pharmaceutics. His early career was spent in the pharmaceutical industry in research and development. He then switched to hospital pharmacy, working initially in hospitals in North Wales. Subsequent posts included those of principal pharmacist at Alder Hey Children's Hospital, Liverpool, chief pharmacist at Westminster Hospital, London, and Director of Pharmaceutical Services at St George's Hospital, London. He is a former chair of the Association of Teaching Hospital Pharmacists, and was awarded the Evans Gold Medal by the Guild of Healthcare Pharmacists in 1994.

In 1993 he became a lecturer in pharmacy practice at the School of Pharmacy, University of London. He moved to the London School of Hygiene and Tropical Medicine to undertake an oral history of community pharmacy in Great Britain under the direction of Professor Virginia Berridge. He is on the staff of the Centre for History in Public Health at the School. He is president of the British Society for the History of Pharmacy, chair of the Society for the Social History of Medicine, and vice-president of the International Academy for the History of Pharmacy.

Whilst at the London School of Hygiene and Tropical Medicine he has also been closely involved in pharmaceutical policy in developing countries. He is the co-author of *Managing Pharmaceuticals in International Health* (Basel: Birkhäuser, 2004), and his report on 'The State of the World's Pharmacy' was published in the *Journal of Interprofessional Care* (2002, 16(4): 405–418). He is a former teaching programme director at the School, and is president of tropEd, the European Network for Education in International Health.

He completed a masters degree in organisational behaviour and a PhD in organisational theory at the University of London. He is the joint editor of *Studying the Organisation and Delivery of Health Services: A Reader* (London: Routledge, 2004). He is currently senior lecturer in organisational behaviour in health care at the London School of

Hygiene and Tropical Medicine, and academic director of the National Coordinating Centre for NHS Service Delivery and Organisation Research and Development.

Contributors

Stuart Anderson BSc(Hons), MA, PhD, MRPharmS, MCCP is a senior lecturer at the London School of Hygiene and Tropical Medicine. He is president of the British Society for the History of Pharmacy, chair of the Society for the Social History of Medicine, and vice-president of the International Academy for the History of Pharmacy.

Gordon E Appelbe LLB, PhD, MSc, BSc(Pharm), FRPharmS, Hon MPS(Aus), FCCP is an independent pharmaceutical/legal consultant. He is a former head of the law department and chief inspector at the Royal Pharmaceutical Society of Great Britain, and is co-author of Dale and Appelbe's *Pharmacy Law and Ethics*.

William E Court BPharm, PhD(Lond), MPharm(Nott), FRPharmS, FLS was a former president and secretary of the British Society for the History of Pharmacy. He was a former reader in pharmacognosy and lecturer in the history of pharmacy at the School of Pharmacy of the University of Bradford. He died in July 2004.

Melvin Earles BPharm, MSc, PhD, FRPharmS is a former president of the British Society for the History of Pharmacy, and a member of the International Academy for the History of Pharmacy. He studied the history and philosophy of science at University College, London, and was senior tutor for pharmacy at Chelsea College, University of London.

Shirley Ellis BPharm, PhD, FRPharmS is vice-president of the British Society for the History of Pharmacy. She retired from a career in the managed service, most recently as regional pharmaceutical officer to the Anglia Regional Health Authority, in 1999.

Peter G Homan FRPharmS, MCPP is a retired community pharmacist, and honorary secretary of the British Society for the History of Pharmacy. Since his retirement, he has worked closely with the staff of the museum of the Royal Pharmaceutical Society of Great Britain.

John A Hunt PhD, FRPharmS is a retired industrial pharmacist and a former president of the British Society for the History of Pharmacy. He is a member of the International Academy for the History of Pharmacy, and a member of the Faculty of the History of Medicine and Pharmacy of the Society of Apothecaries.

William A Jackson BSc(Pharm), MSc, FRPharmS is a former president of the British Society for the History of Pharmacy, and a member of the International Academy for the History of Pharmacy. After more than forty years in manufacturing and community pharmacy, he spent six years as Keeper of Collections in the Manchester Medical School Museum.

Michael H Jepson BPharm, MSc, PhD, FRPharmS, MCPP, MInstPkg (Dip), FIPharmM, DHMSA, MTOPRA(Hon) was formerly head of pharmacy practice at Aston University. He is a Charter Silver Medallist, a committee member of the British Society for the History of Pharmacy, and a member of the Faculty for the History of Medicine and Pharmacy at the Society of Apothecaries.

Viviane Quirke PhD is Wellcome Trust Post-Doctoral Research Fellow in the Centre for Health, Medicine and Society, at Oxford Brookes University, Oxford. She has researched and written extensively on the development of medicines during the 20th century.

Judy Slinn MA is a business historian and research fellow in the Business Organisation, Strategy and Skills (BOSS) Department of the Business School at Oxford Brookes University. She has written the commissioned histories of a number of pharmaceutical companies including May and Baker, Glaxo and Abbott Laboratories Limited.

David Taylor BSc is Professor of Pharmaceutical and Public Health Policy at the School of Pharmacy, University of London. He is also chair of the Camden and Islington Mental Health and Social Care Trust, and a member of the Department of Health's Medicines Management Advisory Group.

Nicholas Wood BPharm, FRPharmS is president of the Royal Pharmaceutical Society of Great Britain. He is also a member of the Court of Assistants of the Worshipful Society of Apothecaries of London and Deputy Visitor to the Society's Faculty of the History and Philosophy of Medicine and Pharmacy.

Peter M Worling PhD, FRPharmS is a retired wholesale pharmacist and a former president of the British Society for the History of Pharmacy. He is an honorary member of the British Association of Pharmaceutical Wholesalers.

Part One

Introduction

1

Researching and writing the history of pharmacy

Stuart Anderson

Pharmacy is concerned with all aspects of the preparation and use of medicines, from the discovery of their active ingredients to how they are used. Today, pharmacy is firmly grounded in science, and entrants to the profession undertake a four-year degree course covering not only the science but also the social and behavioural skills needed to understand people's beliefs and attitudes to the taking of medicines. The pharmacist is society's expert on medicines, and in recent decades, the focus of the pharmacist's role has shifted from the compounding of medicines to ensuring their safe and effective use by providing information and advice.

There has been a recent trend in several countries toward the deregulation of many medicines that were until recently only available on the prescription of a registered medical practitioner, and in some countries, there have been moves to allow pharmacists to prescribe prescription-only medicines in their own right, within carefully defined limits. These extended roles for the pharmacist (in diagnosing minor conditions, as independent prescribers, and as advisor on healthy lifestyles) echo the historic role of the apothecary, which has evolved over hundreds of years. Indeed, pharmacy can trace its origins and progress over thousands of years, during which there have been great shifts in the definition of what constitutes a medicine, and in the boundaries between various professional groups. To understand fully the shifting nature of the pharmacist's role in society requires knowledge of its historical context. This brief history of pharmacy aims to provide that context.

This introductory chapter aims to provide a better understanding of how the chapters that follow fit together. It begins by describing the nature of the history of pharmacy and what it encompasses. It describes different approaches to history, how these have been applied to the history of pharmacy, and the different uses that are made of history.

The chapter includes a description of the main sources available to the historian of pharmacy, and provides a brief overview of previously published histories in this area. Finally, it provides an outline plan of the rest of the book.

The nature of the history of pharmacy

The history of pharmacy encompasses the entire history of medicines and those who make them. Substances were taken by primitive man for medicinal purposes long before the start of recorded history. Slowly, individuals within communities began to specialise in the making of medicines, although in early civilisations the roles of physician, pharmacist and priest were often combined in one person. Indeed, for most of recorded history the history of pharmacy has been inseparable from the history of medicine.

An important theme in the history of pharmacy is its relationship to medicine, and how the boundaries between the professions came to be negotiated and defined. These processes occurred in different countries at different times and help to explain why the practice of pharmacy in Great Britain is rather different from that elsewhere. Throughout history, pharmacy has been shaped by the social, political and economic context in which it has existed and these factors have largely shaped what pharmacy is and how it is practised.

At the centre of the history of pharmacy are its practitioners. Who became pharmacists and why? What activities did they carry out? What skills did they need to perform their duties? How were they trained? Questions such as these lead us to an examination of pharmacy's legal and institutional framework, the educational institutions that emerged to train them, and the professional organisations that were established to protect the interests of pharmacy practitioners.

Since the beginning of the 19th century, pharmacy has been firmly grounded in science, and so the history of pharmacy includes the history of its underpinning sciences. The most notable of these are pharmacology (the study of the actions and uses of drugs), pharmacognosy (the study of drugs of natural origin), pharmaceutical chemistry (concerned primarily with the analysis and synthesis of drugs), and pharmaceutics (the science of converting active ingredients into usable pharmaceutical products). The products themselves, and the tools used to make them, are key features of the history of pharmacy, but it also encompasses the history of the pharmaceutical industry.

Pharmaceuticals, medicines and drugs

The products of the pharmacist and the pharmaceutical industry have been described by many names, the meanings of which have changed frequently over time. These names include 'pharmaceutical', 'medicine', 'medicinal product', 'therapeutic drug' and just 'drug'. However these words are not entirely interchangeable, and some clarification is necessary.

Because of the changes that have occurred in the use and meaning of these words, the preferred term for these products today is 'medicine' rather than 'drug'. Over the last 20 years, the term 'drug' has increasingly become understood as referring to illicit substances. It has become too inclusive and too imprecise. However, substitution of the word 'medicine' is not always appropriate, and the word 'drug' continues to appear in many phrases concerned with medicines, such as 'drug resistance', 'adverse drug reactions', 'drug utilisation studies' and 'drug interactions'.

In a book describing the history of these products and of those who made and sold them, it makes more sense to use the terms that were in use at the time. Pharmacists generally used the word 'drug' to describe the active ingredient (for example aspirin). The word 'medicine' was usually used to describe the product in a finished form, ready for the patient to take (for example aspirin tablets).

The word 'pharmaceuticals' is generally considered to have a broader meaning than 'medicines'. It refers not only to finished medicines but also to active ingredients and vaccines. For most practical purposes, however, these two terms are interchangeable. Nevertheless, 'pharmaceutical' is the term usually used to describe the industry, whose products can be very wide-ranging: they include not only bulk ingredients, finished products, vaccines and other biological products, but also over-the-counter (OTC) medicines, veterinary medicines, diagnostic products and medical devices.

Approaches to the history of pharmacy

Our knowledge of the early history of pharmacy has largely been defined by the written texts that were left by the practitioners of the time, although artefacts, paintings and woodcuts have also survived. The focus of these early histories tended to be the 'great men' of pharmacy, such as Galen, Avicenna and Paracelsus. This tendency has been perpetuated by later generations, anxious to identify the 'great men' of their own time. Early histories of pharmacy also tended to focus on the institutions of pharmacy, such as the founding of great societies and associations. As a result we know much more about these bodies than we do about the ordinary practitioners who joined them.

This traditional approach to the history of pharmacy reflected very closely the wider history of medicine, which emphasised the role of 'great men' (and precious few women). The founding of great institutions like the Royal Colleges, and the incremental progress of medicine, with one discovery or invention following neatly on from another, always gave a distorted picture of history. The ordinary practitioner, quietly getting on with the business of making a living and providing a useful service to the local community, was rarely seen – the patient even less so. The great institutions often had little impact on the day-to-day work of the ordinary practitioner, and the tales of discovery often disguised a chaotic process whereby obvious clues were missed or great discoveries were made by pure chance.

This approach to the history of medicine was increasingly questioned by social historians of medicine, particularly from the 1960s onwards. Following the emergence of social history in its own right in the post-war years, social historians of medicine were anxious to place the patient at the centre of discussion, to place medicine in a wider social and cultural context and to demonstrate that the true nature of progress was rather more chaotic and dynamic than linear and incremental. Until the 1960s, the history of pharmacy followed a similar route to that of the history of medicine, but the great strides that have been made in the social history of medicine in recent decades have not generally been reflected in the history of pharmacy.

Uses of the history of pharmacy

These shifts in the nature and focus of the history of medicine have highlighted debates about the nature of history itself. Interested readers should refer to key texts such as Carr's *What is History?* [1] and *Rethinking History* by Jenkins [2]. There has also been a great change in the uses to which history is put. No longer is it simply a passive subject exploring great names and events of the past. Perhaps the most common function of history has been to tell the story of the past ('narrative history'), although when we read such histories we must always be asking 'whose history?' and 'for what purpose has this history been written?'.

It is clear that some history of pharmacy, in common with the history of other professions, has been written to emphasise the great contribution that pharmacy has made to civilisation, or to encourage readers to reflect on the glorious heritage of the profession ('history as heritage'). There is often an implicit assumption that new entrants will be inspired by the achievements of their forebears. This may have had some purpose when the activities of each new generation of pharmacists were essentially the same as the generation before, but the pace of change is today so great that this is no longer the case. Retired pharmacists waxing lyrical about 'secundum artem' and the joys of pill-making have little more than curiosity value for today's generation of clinical pharmacists; what matters is knowledge about how medicines work rather than how to make aesthetically pleasing products.

History is finding important new uses, and is increasingly being used to inform current debates ('the lessons of history'). In the health field this was powerfully demonstrated by Roy Porter in his famous editorial on possible responses to the AIDS epidemic, published in the *British Medical Journal* [3]. In arguing against the use of legal sanctions such as notification, isolation and prosecution through public health agencies, he demonstrated how such approaches had failed when applied previously to sexually transmitted diseases, most notably the Contagious Diseases Act passed in mid-Victorian times in the hope of preventing the armed forces being brought down by syphilis. In this it was woefully unsuccessful.

More recently, Virginia Berridge, among others, has shown historical analysis to be a powerful and active force in policy development [4]. Contemporary history has been particularly important in this area. Fields of health policy where history has made an impact include tobacco control, the use of illicit drugs and responses to foot and mouth disease. The importance of a historical dimension is now such that the Economic and Social Research Council (ESRC) requires many of its funded research initiatives to have some historical input. There is a history and policy website where historians can post discussion papers on issues of contemporary policy interest (www.historyandpolicy.org), so in the widest health policy context the voice of history is increasingly heard.

For the history of pharmacy the challenge is to recognise the different ways in which history can be used, and to ensure that its voice is heard wherever it might be relevant and appropriate. For pharmacy's policy-makers the challenge is to recognise that history has an important contribution to make.

Sources in the history of pharmacy

There is now a vast range of material available to the historian of pharmacy. A search of 'pharmacy' and 'history' in the Wellcome Library index generates reference to over 4800 publications. Published sources are normally divided into primary sources (original documents, illustrations, artefacts or recordings) and secondary sources (such as books). A useful guide to sources in pharmaceutical history has been published by the British Society for the History of Pharmacy [5].

Documentary material includes the archives of professional institutions, like the Society of Apothecaries and the Royal Pharmaceutical Society of Great Britain (RPSGB); Acts of Parliament and documents issued by government departments; the archives of pharmaceutical companies; and prescription records and account books from community pharmacies. Other sources include wills, letters, papers and even references appearing in fiction. Pharmaceutical histories have been published based on the works of Shakespeare and Agatha Christie, amongst many others.

Prescription books

Another important source available to pharmaceutical historians is prescription record books. Large runs of prescription books survive, and provide a rich source of data, about both the medicines being used and the social strictures of the time. They can be used for many different purposes, such as plotting social trends in the use of medicines over time, and monitoring shifting patterns of medicine use [6]. Many such records are lodged in local record offices, although extensive runs are also to be found in the archives of the RPSGB and the Wellcome Library for the History and Understanding of Medicine.

Oral history

Although documents have been the major source of information available to historians of pharmacy they are by no means the only one. Increasingly, oral history has been developed, in which interviews with both ordinary practitioners and those involved in shaping policy are recorded [7]. A series of interviews with senior figures in the world of pharmacy has been recorded and is lodged with the RPSGB museum [8]. Separate programmes of interviews with both community and hospital pharmacists have been completed, and these are available as part of the

National Life Stories Collection in the National Sound Archives at the British Library in London [9].

For those interested in this area, a useful introduction to the use of oral history in the history of medicine has been published by the National Sound Archive at the British Library [10].

Pharmacy illustrations

From an early stage there was a need to pass on the skills and knowledge of the maker of medicines from one generation to the next. This task was often undertaken by monks, whose literacy skills were often supplemented by their ability to produce lavish illustrations. As a result, many of the early works, including those of Avicenna and Galen, contained illustrations that provide a unique insight into the life and work of the apothecaries of the time.

Hermann Peters began another tradition within the history of pharmacy in 1889, by producing *A Pictorial History of Ancient Pharmacy* [11]. This brought together for the first time a wide range of illustrations relating to pharmacy. These were mostly of woodcarvings, hand-painted illustrations from books, and some larger paintings. The topic of pharmacy in art has been the subject of a number of publications, most notably Wittop-Koning's book in 1952 [12].

Another source of pharmacy illustration has been reference to it in cartoons. Many of the images of pharmaceutical references in the political cartoons of the 18th and 19th centuries are well known, not least through the 1989 publication *The Bruising Apothecary: Images of Pharmacy and Medicine in Caricature* [13]. Perhaps less well known are pharmacy cartoons from later periods, such as those that appeared in *Punch*, and those that continue to appear in the medical, pharmaceutical and popular press. These frequently provide the historian with important insights into changing perceptions, trends, activities and status in relation to the pharmacist.

In more recent years, since the invention of photography, photographs have provided a rich source of material. They provide information not only about the inside and outside of pharmacies, but also about the people involved with pharmacy, both as its workforce and as its customers. They also extend to the range of products available, and how they were made, and the great variety of medicinal forms and ways to make them, both on an individual and industrial scale. A pictorial record of photographs in the RPSGB's collection was published in 1991 [14].

One of the intentions of this book is to reflect the diversity of the illustrations available to us in the history of pharmacy. Today, the choice is vast. To those mentioned above have to be added collections relating to pharmacy artefacts, the equipment used by the pharmacist, and the products of the industry. In recent decades there have been a number of lavishly illustrated histories of pharmacy, including Mez-Mangold's *A History of Drugs* [15] and Cowen and Helfand's *Pharmacy: An Illustrated History* [16].

Pharmacy artefacts

The final source of evidence for the history of pharmacy is its artefacts – those physical things that have survived the ravages of time. Again, there is great diversity in these. Perhaps the earliest surviving examples are Egyptian medicine containers dating from the time of the Pharaohs. There are medicine pots dating from the 15th century, and large numbers of early pestles and mortars survive.

Many books have been published that illustrate pharmaceutical artefacts, most notably Leslie Matthews' *Antiques of the Pharmacy* [17] and John Crellin's *Glass and British Pharmacy 1600 to 1900* [18]. The artefacts themselves are now held at the Science Museum in London. Those interested in pharmaceutical artefacts will find Bill Jackson's many publications illuminating, with his book *The Victorian Chemist and Druggist* providing a valuable starting point [19]. There has likewise been a wide range of publications describing the vast number of pharmaceutical inventions that were developed and promoted by their inventors, particularly those dating from the early 19th century [20].

Previous histories of pharmacy

The history of pharmacy has been a neglected and under-researched field within the broader history of medicine for far too long, yet there is a tradition of writing about it that extends over 200 years. The earliest written history, at least of British pharmacy, is usually credited to John Mason Good. He wrote *The History of Medicine, so far as it relates to the Profession of the Apothecary*, which was published in 1795 [21]. This was, however, more of a political treatise than a history, produced on behalf of one of the predecessors of the RPSGB, the General Pharmaceutic Association of Great Britain.

After the foundation of the RPSGB in 1841, one of its founders, Jacob Bell, wrote an account of its formation and development. This was turned into a book, *An Historical Sketch of the Progress of Pharmacy in Great Britain*, which he produced in conjunction with Theophilus Redwood [22]. The book became the first on the history of pharmacy published by the RPSGB itself, in 1880.

These two publications came to define both chronology and narrative for the history of pharmacy for many of the histories that followed. However, these accounts were highly partisan, based on 18th and 19th century medical politics. Patrick Wallis notes that these early histories have three tendencies: to take London as the sole arena for the history of pharmacy; to follow a legalistic and scientific narrative, thus avoiding the blurring of social and economic complexities; and to assume precise boundaries between the different categories of practitioner operating at the time [23]. Wallis reminds us of the constant need to examine and question the assumptions underpinning historical narratives.

The Bell and Redwood account laid the foundation for a number of further histories of pharmacy in the early decades of the 20th century. These included the two volumes of *Chronicles of Pharmacy* by A C Wootton [24], edited by Peter McEwan, a former editor of the *Chemist & Druggist*, in 1910. In America, La Wall published a comprehensive work in 1927 entitled *Four Thousand Years of Pharmacy: An Outline History of Pharmacy and the Allied Sciences* [25]. Several other accounts of the history of pharmacy followed, including Thomson's *The Mystery and Art of the Apothecary* in 1929 [26].

The next milestone was James Grier's slim volume, *A History of Pharmacy*, published by Pharmaceutical Press in 1937 [27]. Although over the following decades a number of useful articles were written on the history of pharmacy, there were no further general books on the subject until the 1960s, when three important volumes were published: Leslie Matthew's major work, *History of Pharmacy in Britain*, in 1962 [28]; George Trease's *Pharmacy in History* in 1964 [29]; and Poynter's edited volume, *The Evolution of Pharmacy in Britain*, in 1965 [30].

Further significant contributions have subsequently appeared elsewhere, particularly in other European countries and the USA. Notable amongst these is *Kremers and Urdang's History of Pharmacy*, published by The American Institute of the History of Pharmacy [31]. This ran to third and fourth editions, which were extensively revised by Glenn Sonnedecker, and contained an extensive chapter on the history of pharmacy in Britain by Leslie Matthews. Finally, of course, there has been Sydney Holloway's comprehensive *Royal Pharmaceutical Society of Great Britain 1841 to 1991: A Political and Social History*, published in 1991 by Pharmaceutical Press [32].

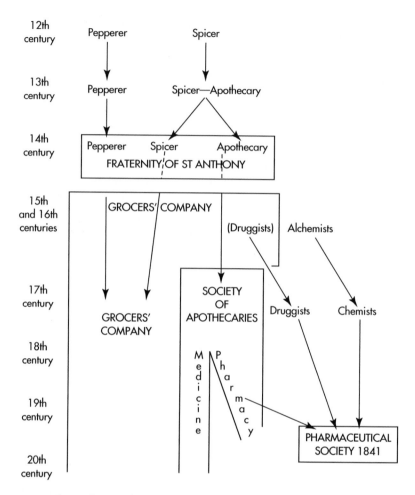

Figure 1.1 The evolution of English pharmacy (with special reference to London). Modified from [29], p. 32.

To these general histories must be added countless individual contributions to the history of pharmacy. The British journal *Pharmaceutical Historian* has been publishing papers on the history of pharmacy since 1967. The American Institute for the History of Pharmacy has been publishing *Pharmacy in History* since 1954. Papers on the history of pharmacy also appear periodically in history of medicine journals such as *Social History of Medicine* and *Medical History*. Indeed, *Medical History* published a special supplement on the English Apothecary in 1983 [33].

Plan of the book

This book is divided into four main parts, the first of which contains this introductory chapter. Part 2 has four chapters and provides a brief chronological account of the main features in the development of pharmacy from antiquity to the present day. In Chapter 2 we explore the origins of pharmacy around the world, from the ancient world to around 1100 AD. We examine the spread of pharmacy westwards to Europe and eventually to Great Britain and North America, and highlight how and why practice in different parts of the world, and indeed in the various countries of Europe, came to be different.

Chapter 3 takes the story of pharmacy forward during the medieval period from 1100 to around 1617, when the Worshipful Society of Apothecaries was formed in Great Britain. Chapter 4 describes key events in Britain during the early modern period, leading up to the foundation of the Pharmaceutical Society of Great Britain in 1841. It includes an account of the Rose Case, which played a major part in defining the role of the apothecary. Finally in this part, Chapter 5 takes the story up to the publication of the Nuffield Report on pharmacy in 1986, with a focus on developments around the turn of the 20th century.

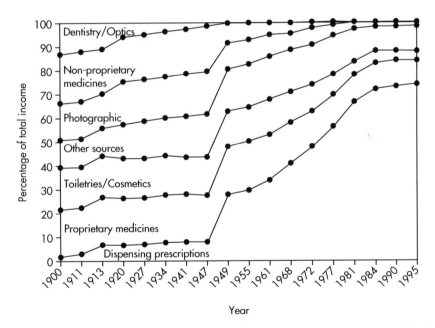

Figure 1.2 Sources of income of community pharmacists, 1900 to 1995. From [34]; English version of graph reproduced by permission from [9], p. 50.

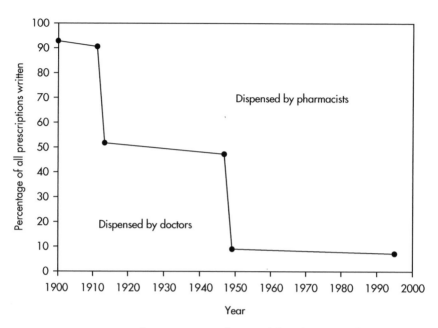

Figure 1.3 Proportion of prescriptions dispensed by doctors and pharmacists, 1900–1995. Based on [34], p. 335 English version of graph reproduced by permission from [35], p. 14.

Some of the themes that emerge from the first part are explored in more detail in later sections. In Part 3 we focus on the practice of pharmacy, on what pharmacists actually did, and where they practised. In Chapter 6 we consider how pharmacists were educated and trained, and how this has changed over time. Chapter 7 examines how pharmacy practice in the community has evolved, including the origin of the multiple companies and the negotiations under National Health Insurance that led to pharmacists becoming contractors. Chapter 8 looks at the evolution of pharmacy practice in hospitals, and Chapter 9 provides a brief account of the origins of the pharmaceutical industry, and its emergence as one of today's great global industrial sectors.

Part 4 focuses on pharmacy's products, beginning in Chapter 10 with a very brief account of the history of therapeutics, and the various eras of drug development, from the isolation of alkaloids in the early 19th century to the development of beta-blockers and H_2 antagonists in the late 20th century. Chapter 11 provides a history of dosage form, from electuaries and draughts to pills and tablets. In Chapter 12 we explore the issue of drug quality. This chapter catalogues the diversity of products available to the public in earlier centuries; the rise of patent and proprietary medicines; the place of nostrums and quack remedies and the role of counter prescribing. The last chapter in this section considers the history of drug safety.

Finally, in Part 5, we link our history to both the present and the future. In Chapter 14 we consider the rapidly increasing pace of change over the last 10 or 20 years and explore the emergence and impact of pharmacogenomics, and the rise of subdisciplines such as pharmaco-economics, pharmacovigilance and pharmacoepidemiology. We consider the role of the global pharmaceutical industry, and its impact on the practice of pharmacy. We look at the continuities as well as the changes that have taken place, and we relate the past firmly to the present.

In Chapter 15, we reflect on what the future might hold for the profession of pharmacy. This chapter considers a range of possible directions in which pharmacy might go in the future, providing some international comparisons and placing pharmacy in a wider social, political and economic context. What have been the attitudes of governments and international bodies to pharmacy, and how have other health professions, such as doctors and nurses, reacted to this? And what does the future hold for pharmacy?

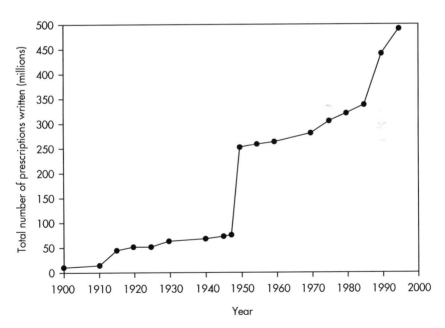

Figure 1.4 Number of prescriptions dispensed, 1900–1995. Based on [34], p. 336; reproduced by permission of the Fondation Mérieux.

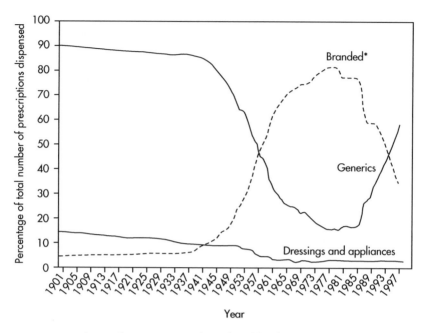

Figure 1.5 Change from generic to brand and back, 1900–1997. Data from the *Compendium of Health Statistics,* 11th edn; published by the Office of Health Economics, 1999, p. 76; graph reproduced by permission from [35], p. 17. * Includes generic brands (where a generic drug has been given a brand name).

While there inevitably remains uncertainty as to the exact direction pharmacy will take, we hope that readers of this book will at least have a clearer idea of where pharmacy came from, and how it reached the stage at which it is now.

References

1. Carr E H. *What is History?* London: Penguin Books, 1990.
2. Jenkins K. *Rethinking History.* London: Routledge, 1991.
3. Porter R. History says no to the policeman's response to AIDS [editorial]. *British Medical Journal* 1986; 293: 1589–1590.
4. Berridge V. Public or policy understanding of history? *Social History of Medicine* 2003; 16: 513–523.
5. Burnby J G L, Hutton D A. *A Guide to Sources in Pharmaceutical History.* London: British Society for the History of Pharmacy, 1990.
6. Anderson S C, Homan C. Prescription books as historical sources. *Pharmaceutical Historian (London)* 1999; 29: 51–54.
7. Anderson S C. I remember it well: oral history in the history of pharmacy. *Social History of Medicine* 1997; 10: 331–343.

8. Hunt J A. Recording 20th century pharmacy. *The Pharmaceutical Journal* 2000; 265: 942–943.

9. Anderson S C, Berridge V S. The role of the community pharmacist in health and welfare, 1911–1986. In: Bornat J, Perks R B, Thompson P, Walmsley J, eds. *Oral History, Health and Welfare*. London: Routledge, 2000: 48–74.

10. Thompson P, Perks R. *An Introduction to the Use of Oral History in the History of Medicine*. London: National Life Stories Collection, National Sound Archive, British Library, 1993.

11. Peters H. *A Pictorial History of Ancient Pharmacy*. Translated from German by William Netter. Chicago: Engelhand, 1889.

12. Wittop-Koning D A. *Art and Pharmacy*, 2nd edn. Deventer, Holland: The Ysel Press Ltd, 1952.

13. Arnold-Forster K, Tallis N. *The Bruising Apothecary: Images of Pharmacy and Medicine in Caricature*. London: Pharmaceutical Press, 1989.

14. Tallis N, Arnold-Forster K. *Pharmacy History: A Pictorial Record*. London: Pharmaceutical Press, 1991.

15. Mez-Mangold L. *A History of Drugs*. Basle, Switzerland: F Hoffmann-La Roche and Co. Ltd, 1971.

16. Cowen D L, Helfand D L. *Pharmacy: An Illustrated History*. New York: Abrams, 1991.

17. Matthews L G. *Antiques of the Pharmacy*. London: G Bell & Sons, 1971.

18. Crellin J K, Scott J R. *Glass and British Pharmacy 1600 to 1900*. London: The Wellcome Institute for the History of Medicine, 1972.

19. Jackson W A. *The Victorian Chemist and Druggist*. Princes Risborough: Shire Publications Ltd, 1981.

20. Anderson S C. The golden age of pharmaceutical invention 1830 to 1890. *Pharmacy History Australia* 2003; 2(20): 5–7.

21. Good J M. *The History of Medicine, so far as it relates to the Profession of the Apothecary*. London: General Pharmaceutic Association of Great Britain, 1795.

22. Bell J, Redwood T. *An Historical Sketch of the Progress of Pharmacy in Great Britain*. London: The Pharmaceutical Society of Great Britain, 1880.

23. Wallis P. The first English histories of pharmacy: their origins and influence. *Pharmacy in History* 2000; 42(1–2): 36–46.

24. Wootton A C. *Chronicles of Pharmacy*, Vols I and II. London: Chemist and Druggist, 1910.

25. La Wall C H. *Four Thousand Years of Pharmacy: An Outline History of Pharmacy and the Allied Sciences*. Philadelphia: J B Lippincott & Co., 1927.

26. Thompson C J S. *The Mystery and Art of the Apothecary*. London: Lane, 1929.

27. Grier J. *A History of Pharmacy*. London: Pharmaceutical Press, 1937.

28. Matthews L G. *History of Pharmacy in Britain*. Edinburgh: E & S Livingstone, 1962.

29. Trease G E. *Pharmacy in History*. London: Baillière, Tindall and Cox, 1964.

30. Poynter F N L (ed.). *The Evolution of Pharmacy in Britain*. London: Pitman Medical, 1965.

31. Sonnedecker G. *Kremers and Urdang's History of Pharmacy*, 4th edn. Madison, WI: The American Institute of the History of Pharmacy, 1976.

32. Holloway S W F. *Royal Pharmaceutical Society of Great Britain 1841 to 1991: A Political and Social History.* London: Pharmaceutical Press, 1991.
33. Burnby J G L. A study of the English apothecary from 1660 to 1760. *Medical History Supplement* 1983; 3: 1–128.
34. Anderson S C, Berridge V S. L'héritage perdu du pharmacien: professionalisation, spécialisation et accroissment de la protection sociale. In: Fouré O, Opinel A, eds. *Les Thérapeutiques: Savoirs et Usages.* Saint Julien en Beaujolais: Collection Fondation Marcel Mérieux, 1999.
35. Anderson S C. The historical context of pharmacy. In: Taylor K M G, Harding G, eds. *Pharmacy Practice.* London: Taylor and Francis, 2001.

Part Two

The development of pharmacy

2

Pharmacy from the ancient world to 1100 AD

William E Court

Over a period of half a million years the human species developed from hunter-gatherers to food producers. The availability of surplus food permitted the setting up of ordered societies. Primitive people discovered tools such as the lever, the wedge and the wheel, yet it is only in the last 5000 years that organised societies have proliferated. Early civilisations appeared in Iraq, Iran and Egypt, although great societies also evolved in India, China and South America. Travel and inter-tribal communication was difficult and occurred only slowly. Later European and North American cultures were largely derived from those in the Middle East.

This chapter provides a brief introduction to the origins of the occupation of pharmacist and to the making of medicines. Their antecedents are to be found in most of the early civilisations of the ancient world, and occurred largely independently of each other. The early history of pharmacy is practically inseparable from the early history of medicine, yet as we shall see, separation between the diagnosis and treatment of disease on the one hand, and the making of medicines on the other, can be traced back over 4000 years. The chapter takes the story from the mists of time up to about the year 1100 AD, and from consideration of the entire known world to a focus on western Europe.

The origins of medicine-making

Humans have been subjected to disease, illness and accident since the beginning of time. The early practice of treating symptoms resulted in the emergence of a specialist in most primitive societies, although the causes of disease states were not understood. Whether called witch doctor, wise woman, medicine man, priest, hakim or physician, these people – by trial, error and careful observation – soon learned the value of the plants growing around them. Thus, from a confusion of magic, superstition and instinct, early communities developed a knowledge of the food plants necessary for bodily development, the poisonous plants detrimental to health and, somewhere in between, medicinal plants that alleviated symptoms of illness. Some minerals and animal products were also used in early folk medicine.

This chapter considers key events and individuals in the five civilisations that have most influenced developments in Europe – Mesopotamia, Egypt, Greece, Rome and Arabia. However, similar developments were occurring in other civilisations: Chinese pharmacy, for example, traces its origins to the emperor Shen Nung in about 2000 BC. He investigated the medicinal value of several hundred herbs, and wrote the first *Pen T'sao*, or native herbal, containing 365 drugs [1].

Mesopotamian civilisations, 3000 BC to 539 BC

The Sumerians (3000–2400 BC), a non-Semitic people who inhabited Lower Mesopotamia (the area between the rivers Tigris and Euphrates in modern Iraq), are believed to have developed the world's first urban civilisation around 4000 BC. They are known to have used plant drugs, wound washing, plasters and bandaging. Babylon (2200–1300 BC), on the banks of the Euphrates, was the centre of two extensive but short-lived empires. The earlier empire comprised the whole of Mesopotamia, and flourished in the reign of King Hammurabi (1795–1750 BC). Although destroyed by the Hittites in 1595 BC, Babylonian civilisation re-emerged, and for centuries influenced scholarship throughout the known world. The early Babylonians studied mathematics, geology and metallurgy, as well as astrology and astronomy. They also developed early systems of weights and measures.

Although they understood the methods of manufacture of soap, leather, vinegar, beer, wine and glass and could extract natural plant aromas and animal products, they were not true chemists or technologists, because their comprehension was based on trial and error. Their drugs included balm of Gilead, colocynth, hellebore, liquorice, mustard, myrrh, oleander, opium, opopanax and storax. During King Hammurabi's reign a system of laws, known as Hammurabi's Code, was established. Medical and surgical practice was regulated, and it was not necessarily associated with magic or superstition. Diagnosis and treatment became separated from the preparation of medicines, which was carried out by assistants called apothecaries [2–4].

Druggists' shops, 1900 BC

Biblical records suggest that the apothecary was synonymous with the perfumer, who prepared volatile oils and unguents [5]. In Sippara, a town on the Euphrates river, druggists' stalls or shops were known to be operating in about 1900 BC. There is also evidence that the Babylonians traded with Asia, Arabia and Egypt via caravan trains bringing non-indigenous spices essential for the preservation of fish and meats in the winter season.

The Assyrians (1900–612 BC), a warlike Semitic race from northern Mesopotamia, overran Babylon. The city of Nineveh, lying to the east of the River Tigris, had royal libraries in which the last monarch, Assur-Bani-Pal (668–627 BC), established a vast library of clay tablets in the 7th century BC. Many of these clay tablets have survived, and some 800 fragments reveal information on mainly Babylonian medical matters.

A primitive understanding of drugs and pharmaceutical processes enabled the formulation of draughts, mixtures, infusions, decoctions, medicinal wines, enemas, poultices and ointments (see Chapter 11). Of the 250 vegetable drugs and 120 minerals recorded, many are still in use today. Examples include myrrh, poppy, thyme, castor seed, liquorice, storax, peppermint, cannabis, mandragora, fats, oils, waxes, milks, honey and livers. Animal excreta were also listed, and were used to disgust the evil spirits [2,3]. The characteristic symbol of the medical profession, the rod and intertwined serpents (known as the *caduceus*), has been found on Babylonian pottery.

The second Babylonian empire, which emerged when the Babylonians overran Assyria in 612 BC, reached its peak under King Nebuchadnezzar (605–562 BC) and ended when Cyrus the Persian invaded in about 539–538 BC. The subsequent Persian era, lasting over 200 years (538–330 BC), made no significant contribution to the advancement of pharmacy.

Egyptian civilisations, 3000 BC to 1200 BC

At the same time as the Mesopotamian civilisations developed, another great empire was developing in north-east Africa. Its history is well documented in inscriptions on tombs, ceramics and papyri. Communities inhabited the Nile valley from at least the 4th millennium BC and civilisation progressed in cycles interrupted by periods of stagnation and decadence. The Egyptians discovered that wet strips of the pithy stems of

Cyperus papyrus reeds, when pressed together, yielded a form of paper that scribes could write on using a picture language. Papyrus scrolls, often found preserved in caves or tombs, have provided much information on Egyptian medicine and surgery. The papyri record the years 1900–1100 BC, and further detail is presented in the works of later authors, including Herodotus the Greek (5th century BC), Manetho the Egyptian (3rd century BC) and Pliny the Roman (1st century AD).

Papyrus Ebers, 1500 BC

The *Papyrus Ebers* is a medico-pharmaceutical treatise some 4.5 metres in length, which was produced in about 1500 BC. It records about 875 prescriptions and some 700 drugs derived from vegetable, animal and mineral sources. Amongst the vegetable drugs are spices, castor seed, poppy and acacia; the animal sources include milks, livers, waxes and excreta. The minerals include alum, stibnite (antimony), salt and copper carbonate. The papyrus is named after George Ebers, a German Egyptologist who bought it in a Luxor bazaar in 1875 and translated it. Other papyri, some eight in all, deal with gynaecological, surgical and veterinary matters.

Having mastered the art of fermentation, the Egyptians used wines and beers, together with milk, as vehicles for their liquid medicines. They also used honey as an excipient for the incorporation of solids in pills, and waxes were used in ointments. The range of formulations included infusions, decoctions, teas, gargles, inhalations, snuffs, fumigations, troches (lozenges), pills, enemas, suppositories, poultices, lotions and plasters (Chapter 11) [3,6,7]. Primitive chemical technology was developed by the Egyptians, who understood the practice but not the theory of enamelling, glass tinting, ceramics and dyeing. Indigo blue from the indigo plant and alizarin red from the madder root were used to dye textiles and were probably used for the coat of many colours that Israel gave to his young son Jacob [8].

Egyptian medicine advanced beyond that of the Assyrian culture. The recipes were stated quantitatively and fresh and dried plants were used. The Egyptians knew whether to dry these materials in sunlight or in shade. They also comminuted (ground up) drugs in mortars or hand-mills and employed sieves and balances. The use of non-indigenous drugs suggests both trade and horticulture. The cultivation of introduced plants was important because the flora of Egypt was limited by the country's geography – a flooding river hemmed in by the Arabian and Libyan deserts.

Early Egyptian medicine embraced demon possession, magic and superstition, but later medical practice was more rational because the emerging physicians made use of plant drugs and chemicals. Evidence from tombs and papyri reveals the development of the physicians as a middle class, between the aristocracy and the farmers and craftsmen. Egyptian physicians generally specialised in one part of the body; for example there were eye physicians, teeth physicians and intestinal physicians. Often they had priestly titles, although they were not really priests.

In Egyptian society, diagnosing and treating disease and making medicines were separate and distinct roles, although they could be combined in one person. The *pastophor*, or preparer of medicines, was a member of the priestly profession, and the physician-pharmacist was a highly respected member of society, pharmacy being a special branch of medicine [3].

Egyptian mythology relates that Isis, the wife of the god Osiris, revealed the secrets of pharmacy to her son Horus. Thoth, the scribe among the gods, was known as *ph-ar-imki*, which translates as 'warrant of security'. This is the origin of the word 'pharmacy'. The Graeco-Latin *pharmakon* meant 'drug' [9].

Up to 1600 BC there was a trend towards scientific method in Egypt, but magic and sorcery were ever present, and many formulae in the papyri are accompanied by spells and incantations. The general scientific value of Egyptian medicine was low and methods based on custom and practice held sway. Although Egyptian influence waned, the effect of Babylonian culture continued for a further millennium under Assyrian, Persian and then Macedonian Greek rule, which was contemporary with, and at times rivalled, Greek culture.

Greek civilisations, 1250 BC to 285 BC

There is little doubt that Mesopotamian and Egyptian experience influenced Greek culture, but other societies also produced new ideas and methods. In Crete, a Bronze Age culture had prospered, art had blossomed and a script for writing was developed. Temple medicine was practised and the importance of hygiene was understood. In the region now called Anatolia (in Turkey), the Hittites, who thrived in the 2nd millennium BC, developed iron smelting; this was a remarkable advance for the time. Further south, in southern Syria, around the ports of Tyre and Sidon, lived the Phoenicians, who were great navigators and traded widely in the Mediterranean. Their greatest contribution to society was a consonantal alphabet, which facilitated writing of their Semitic language. This replaced the cuneiform and hieroglyphic systems, and in Greece, with the addition of vowels, became the basis of Western alphabet systems.

The Babylonians and Egyptians made empirical observations, developed arithmetical systems of weights and measures, advanced surgery and medicine, and mastered technologies such as glass making, smelting and dyeing. However, understanding of science made little progress during the 3000 years between 1500 BC and 1500 AD. Francis Bacon (1561–1626 AD) observed that technology preceded the intellectual arts, and fell into disgrace when man had time to think of them. It was this attitude that led to the decline of interest in physical, chemical and mechanical sciences.

Greek influence spanned some 900 years; the first phase (600–300 BC) was the most original and creative, and was contemporary with and influenced by the Persian Empire that spread from the Punjab in the east to Macedonia in the west. Ionia, a region of Anatolia, was a centre of the flourishing Greek empire, trading with its Mediterranean neighbours by land and sea.

Early medical theories

The early philosophers congregated in Miletus in southern Ionia and debated the nature of matter. Anaximenes, in the 6th century BC, considered the four elements from which all matter was made to be fire, air, water and earth. Later, Heraclitus of Ephesus, in about 460 BC, added to this theory by stating that all things were composed of two types of opposites – wet/dry and hot/cold. These, he believed, were always in conflict, and so all things were in a state of perpetual change, a phenomenon controlled by *logos*, a principle of order and intelligibility [10].

Around the 6th century BC, the spread of Persian power caused the Ionian scholars, including Pythagoras of Samos, to flee westwards. Followers of Pythagoras stressed the importance of an experimental approach, and around the same time, Alemaeon of Crotone, a Greek physician and philosopher, used dissection and vivisection to study animals, and so established experimental physiology and, by studying the senses, empirical psychology. A Sicilian, Empedocles (490–430 BC), further developed the concept that everything was made up of the four elements (fire, air, water and earth), and it became well established in Western medical thought for the next 2000 years.

The philosopher Democritus (460–370 BC) developed a primitive atomic theory, and observed that 'nothing is created out of nothing'.

However, a plausible atomic theory, and modern chemistry, would develop only some 2200 years later, from John Dalton's explanation in 1807 AD [10].

Hippocrates and Greek medicine

Greek medicine involved the use of three sources of knowledge and practice: the temple practice of Asclepius or healing by the gods; the physiological opinions of the philosophers; and the practice of the superintendents of the gymnasia. For medicine, undoubtedly the most revered Greek philosopher was Hippocrates, although doubts have been expressed about whether such a man existed. Nevertheless, the *Hippocratean Corpus*, some 70 volumes, was found in the library at Cos, where Hippocrates (460–377 BC) reputedly lived. The books, which were probably produced by a group of scholars, were later studied in the library of Alexandria (3rd century AD), where copying, correction and preservation took place.

The Hippocratean group developed the theory of the four liquid humours – blood, phlegm, bile and black bile. Disease was the result of an excess of one of these liquid humours, and treatment was to eliminate the excess from the body. Purgatives, emetics and enemas were used to cleanse and purify the body of disease, and *pharmakon* thus became the purifying remedy. Hippocratic medicine used some 300–400 drugs, fewer than employed by the Egyptians.

The Hippocratean group also enunciated four main principles for the practice of medicine. These were that:

- medicine cannot be based on postulates;
- disease cannot be pinned to three or four causes only, but to many causes;
- experimental evidence is essential; and
- the patient must not suffer.

The directors of the gymnasium (where the gladiators were trained) contributed much to diet, hygiene and systems of exercise. Hippocratic medicine regarded man in relation to his environment, although medicine was a luxury for the leisured classes. Nevertheless, the major limitation of Greek science was the absence of instruments for exact measurement and analysis.

Aristotle and Theophrastus

Greek scholarship declined as scientific study moved from the experimenters to the moralist thinkers such as Socrates (469–399 BC) and

Plato (427–347 BC), although the latter fostered mathematics. Aristotle (384–322 BC) joined the Academy in Athens and made a great contribution to biology, classifying animals into genera and species. He cited 500 species, of which he had personally dissected 50. He left the Academy and founded the Lyceum.

A true polymath, on his death he left for his followers detailed treatises on botany, physics, anatomy, physiology, mathematics, astronomy, geography, mechanics, music and grammar. His works are considered by many to be the starting point of modern science. However, Aristotle failed to advance and apply science in his own declining world. The Greeks did not acclimatise plants and animals and did not advance agriculture, metallurgy or textiles, and so Greece declined. After Plato, the Academy also declined but the Lyceum, using Aristotle's teamwork strategy, prospered.

Theophrastus (372–287 BC), a pupil of Plato, joined Aristotle and eventually became head of the Lyceum, a post he held for 35 years. He was assigned natural philosophy, and established the discipline of botany, clearly differentiating plants from animals. Attacking the theory of the four elements, he stressed the value of the empirical approach and experimental evidence. His successor, Strato (328–270/268 BC), established the true course of research by observation and subsequent experimental proof. His works included the prophetic statement 'chemical combination is a union of several bodies capable of such combination involving the transformation of the properties of the bodies combined'. Theophrastus understood contemporary folk medicine and was evidently familiar with the *rhizotomoi* (pharmacobotanists) who collected and sold indigenous vegetable roots.

At about this time the Macedonian, Alexander the Great (356–323 BC) was spreading his empire widely throughout Asia Minor, as far as India and into Egypt, where he built a new city named Alexandria. Alexander, a pupil of Aristotle, realised the value of science and invited the Lyceum to move to the Museum of Alexandria. Under the patronage of the Ptolemys, Greek learning thrived. However, science was not put to the service of man: only a fusion of Egyptian and Greek religious practice was offered to the paid slaves.

Nevertheless, the miracles performed in the temples were often skilful applications of science. In pious frauds, for example, the expansive power of hot air was used to open doors, move statues and rustle drapes. The museum permitted advances in medicine: Herophilus (335–280 BC) founded the medical school, dissected the human body and wrote a handbook for midwives. It also promoted mathematics, astronomy, geography and architecture. The museum prospered until Ptolemy IX (146–117 BC) promoted Egyptian institutions over others and drove out most of the Greek scholars.

Roman civilisations, 275 BC to 476 AD

Greek society and culture declined because of a lack of interest in practical matters and the overwhelming desire to reason and theorise without evidence. The Romans were very different. From about 300 BC onwards they began the expansion of their empire, first overrunning two literate nations, the Hebrews and the Greeks. The Graeco-Roman era began in 275 BC. Greek and Latin became the languages of the upper classes and grammar consciousness stimulated the encyclopaedists and translators, such as Cicero (106–43 BC) and Lucretius (1st century BC). In the Museum of Alexandria, Hebrew literature was translated into Greek and by 100 BC, there was a Greek Bible, or *Septuagint*, which played an important part in the development of Christianity.

Sadly, as the all-conquering Romans overran Syracuse in Sicily in 212 BC, the Greek scientist Archimedes (287–212 BC) perished. His work on mechanics and hydrostatics had enabled the Roman advances in engineering. In a period of about 800 years (300 BC to 500 AD) the Romans built many major civil engineering projects, including sewage disposal systems, aqueducts, defensive walls, and central heating. At the same time they created impressive cities across Europe, including Chester, York and Bath in Britain. The Romans also laid the foundations of law and government.

Greek medicine was adopted by the wealthy Romans. It took hold as a result of the efforts of a number of powerful men. Mithradates IV, King of Pontus (115–63 BC), was a Greek ruler of Persian origin who studied the effects of drugs on his unfortunate prisoners. He was helped by Krateus, his physician and the compiler of the first known illustrated herbal (a list of plants having medicinal uses). Although Mithradates was defeated by Pompey in 66 BC, Krateus' work was reproduced by many subsequent Roman authors.

Celsus and Scribonius Largus

Aurelius Cornelius Celsus (20–50 AD) collated and edited volumes of Greek medicine and although apparently a medical practitioner, he was really a translator and editor of other people's work, including the eight-volume *De Medicina*, which refers to 250 drugs and 100 surgical instruments. Another translator, Pliny the Elder (23–79 AD), was the author of an encyclopaedia of natural history. Both books would become widely read in printed form from 1487 AD onwards.

As the Roman legions spread throughout Europe they took their way of life, including medical treatment, with them. Thus Scribonius Largus (1–50 AD) accompanied the Emperor Claudius to Britain in 43 AD and brought with him his book *De Compositione Medicamentorum*. Probably devised for the expedition, it was a collection of prescriptions and treatments: it referred to opium as a painkiller, ginger, costus, cedar wood oil and minerals such as alum, copper and silver salts, sulphur and soda. In all there were 242 vegetable drugs, 36 minerals and 27 animal drugs [11].

Dioscorides, 50–100 AD

Two great men in particular came to dominate Roman medicine. The first was Pedanius Dioscorides (50–100 AD), who was a surgeon to the armies of the emperors Tiberius and Nero. He produced a famous *Materia Medica* (a list of materials of animal, vegetable and mineral origin having medicinal uses) in inferior Greek. Dioscorides probably borrowed from the earlier writings of Theophrastus and Krateus. An illustrated version of Dioscorides' Herbal, *Codex Aniciae Julianae*, was produced by a Byzantine copyist in 512 AD. The herbal referred to some 600 plants and gave instructions on drying, extraction and adulteration. There was also reference to the Doctrine of Signatures, in which it was believed that for every ailment there was a specific plant remedy, and that God had left a clue for the expert to find in the plant's colour, shape or other physical feature [12].

Galen, 129–199 AD

The second of the great Roman medical men was Galen, or Claudius Galenus to give him his full name. He was born in 129 AD at Pergamum in north-western Asia Minor. He was Greek trained and, after 12 years of study, became a physician and surgeon to the gladiators. Apart from a successful career as a medical practitioner, Galen was an experimenter who dissected animals of many species. His works comprised 22 volumes.

He developed the humoral pathology scheme, which combined earlier ideas with his own idea of the four temperaments of man. Galen's scheme united the Hippocratic theory of the four liquid humours (blood, phlegm, bile and black bile) with the Pythagorean four elements (fire = hot + dry; air = hot + moist; earth = cold + dry; water = cold +

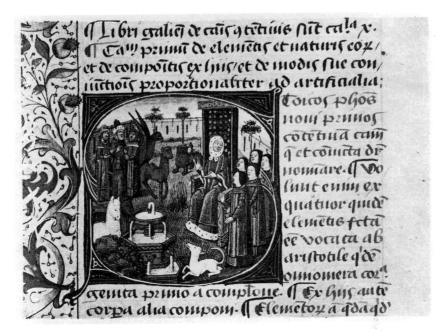

Figure 2.1 Galen lecturing on the elements; a 15th-century miniature. Source: Leersum *et al.*, *Miniaturen der lateinischen Galenos-Handschrift*; published by Sijthoff, 1910. Reproduced by permission of the Wellcome Library, London.

moist) and the four temperaments of man (choleric, sanguine, melancholic and phlegmatic). All illness was judged to be the result of imbalance between these various elements, and treatment was based on attempts to restore the balance.

Although erroneous, Galen's hypothesis held sway until at least 1600 AD and was reproduced in many later books. Galen referred to the drugs that he kept in his *apotheca* or storeroom. He described some 473 vegetable, animal and mineral drugs including hyoscyamus (henbane), colocynth (bitter apple), opium and turpentine. He was famed for theriaca (black treacle) and hiera picra (holy bitter or aloes and canella) but his best formulations were cold creams and ointments, which were referred to as galenicals, although this term would eventually become much more widely applied [3,11].

Practitioners of medicine

Medicine in the Roman era involved many people; the *servi medici* were slaves, the *rhizotomi* root gatherers, the *pharmacopolae* drug peddlers, the *unguentarii* sellers of salves and the *sagae* wise women, but the better educated became physicians and rose in esteem, joining the *equites*, or upper classes [3]. Medicines were stored in the *apotheca* and prepared in the *iatreion*, names giving us 'apothecary' and 'iatro-' as in iatrochemistry (medicinal chemistry).

By 364 AD the Christian Roman Empire had divided into two: Rome controlled the west, Constantinople the east. The Romans contributed little to science, but they did organise and collate knowledge and were severely practical in applying science and medicine for the public good. As Vandals and Goths swept south in 476 AD the Roman Empire in the west fell.

The Christian religion arose in Judea at the start of the first millennium. It spread worldwide as a compassionate code of ethics that placed little value on earthly things. Consideration of Christ's compassion and love of humanity dominated many of the subsequent great achievements of mankind. The churches enforced belief and obedience; the questioning of dogma and natural philosophy was heresy, and heretics were suppressed and often slaughtered. As a result, science went underground during the Dark Ages (735–1150 AD). Increasingly, medicines were prepared by the monks, although the powers of saints and holy relics were also employed.

Arabian civilisations, 400 AD to 1100 AD

In the east the city of Byzantium, renamed Constantinople by Constantine in 330 AD and now Istanbul, developed a flourishing drug trade. Byzantium prospered especially during the period 400–900 AD, and here many of the Greek and Roman works were translated into Arabic, copied and preserved, complete with inevitable additions (both good and bad), omissions and errors. Religious oppression of the scholars in Byzantium caused a migration of scholars to Jundi-Shapur in south-west Persia, where the Nestorian Christians continued to carry out translations into Syrian and Arabic.

It thus fell to the Arab nations to preserve the Graeco-Roman culture. The Arabs, a group of Semitic nations, had overrun the ancient civilised world by conquering Syria, Persia and Egypt. Tragically the great library of Alexandria was destroyed in 643 AD, not by the Arabs but by fanatical non-Christian pagans fighting equally fanatical Christians.

The Prophet Mohammed (570–632 AD) founded Islam in what is now Saudi Arabia. It is a religion that shares a common heritage with Judaism and Christianity. In the 100 years following Mohammed's death the Arab empire continued to expand, from the Indian border to Spain. Arabic was the language of scholars in Islam, yet the main figures in science at the time were not Arabs. Alchemy, a feature of the late Alexandrian school, flourished under the Arabs, who sought the Elixir of Life and the Philosopher's Stone that transmutes base metals to gold [13,14]. Their unsuccessful efforts did, however, lay the foundations of chemistry. From Alexandria to Persia Greek knowledge spread amongst the Arabs, and Baghdad once again became a centre of culture and learning.

Under enlightened rulers in the 6th to 9th centuries AD a remarkable collation of knowledge occurred. Jabir (Geber) ibn Hayyan (born in 776 AD) was considered the greatest chemist in Islam and his work was published in the 10th century. Johann Mesue the Senior (777–857 AD), a Nestorian Christian from Damascus in Syria, was Harun-al-Raschid's court physician and an authority on Galen. He probably founded Baghdad's medical school, and he reputedly introduced the milder purgatives, senna and tamarind, into medicine. His formulary *Selecta Artis Medicinae* has not survived.

Apothecary shops, 850 AD

The shops of drug sellers appeared in Persia about 750 AD, and apothecary shops (a specific Arab creation) appeared later, around 850 AD. These had a number of characteristics: firstly, there was a separation of medicine from pharmacy; secondly, they were shops run by educated men with a high code of ethics; thirdly, a precise education was established for apothecaries, and finally they prepared a wide range of medicines including classical, Persian and Indian drugs and chemicals.

To the north, other nations compiled their own indigenous materia medica, encouraged by the earlier Roman influence. Lists of indigenous medicines are known to have existed and included instructions for medical usage. In southern France an edict was promulgated by Louis the Pious in 794/5 AD ordering the planting of herbs and medicinal plants in all the Royal gardens in Aquitania. This is the first known recognition of the importance of the cultivation of such plants in Western Europe. Many herbals that influenced European pharmacy survive from this period.

Rhazes, 865–925 AD

Al Razi or Rhazes (865–925 AD), 'the Persian Galen', was physician-in-charge at Baghdad's great hospital and oversaw its rebuilding [14].

Rhazes was a prolific writer, teacher, chemist and planner. He published a comprehensive review of medical knowledge at the time. It was an encyclopaedia derived from Greek, Syriac, Arabic, Persian and Indian sources, modified by his own experience. He encouraged the use of pills and mentioned brandy and arrack-type preparations (arrack was an alcoholic spirit distilled from toddy or palm wine). He also pioneered systematic practical chemistry in a well-equipped laboratory.

Avicenna, 980–1037 AD

One of the most important Arabs from a European perspective was the scholar Avicenna, or Ibn Sina (980–1037 AD) [15]. He was born at Afaana, a small town near Bukhara, now in Uzbekistan. When aged only seven he could recite the whole of the Koran, and when ten he began to study logic, the philosophy of the Greeks, geometry and the sciences. Subsequently, when only fifteen, he decided to study medicine. Avicenna's father was a tax collector for the Emir, and he was allowed to study in the Emir's extensive library until it was destroyed by fire. He then found it necessary to move to Bokhara.

Later he was to lead a roaming life and become an influential writer. He began to write *al-Qanum* (or the *Canon of Medicine* as it

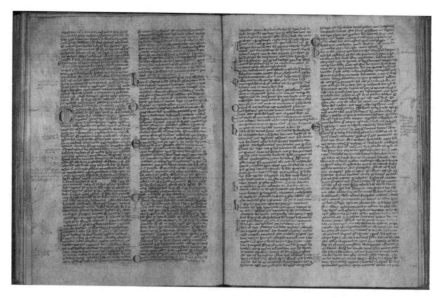

Figure 2.2 Avicenna's *Canon of Medicine*. Pages from the copy owned and annotated by Dr John Dee, alchemist and astrologer to Queen Elizabeth I; Reproduced by permission of the Royal College of Physicians.

became known in the West), which sought to link the teachings of Hippocrates and Galen with the biology of Aristotle. Avicenna then moved to Jaij, a well-known centre for study that had a large library. Once again he was forced to move, this time to Hamadhan. There he continued with his writing, but he became involved in politics and was forced to go into hiding in the house of a druggist. He moved to Isfahan where he acted as the Emir's personal physician. He accompanied the Emir on military expeditions and it was then that he learnt Arabic. However, he became very sick, and he died before the army reached Hamadhan.

Avicenna has been called 'the Hippocrates of the Arab world'. The *Canon of Medicine* was translated into Latin in the 12th century by Gerarde of Cremona and became the basis of medical study for centuries. Another of his books was a formulary that dealt with the materia medica of the day. It included some 760 drugs and their antidotes, and advocated the silvering of pills [3]. In all he wrote some 200 books. Together with Galen he appears on the coat of arms of the Royal Pharmaceutical Society of Great Britain.

The migration westwards, 700–1100 AD

Increasing religious oppression resulted in the continuing movement of scholars from Persia to the west. Centres of learning that were already flourishing in Italy (in Salerno and Padua) from the 8th century were joined by Cordova and Toledo in Moorish Spain in the 10th century, and by Montpellier and Paris in France in the 11th century, quickly followed by Naples and Bologna in Italy.

Further westward, migration of scholars occurred after disagreements in Paris, leading to scholars settling in England. This eventually resulted in the founding of universities at Oxford (1190 AD) and Cambridge (1209 AD). Great libraries were developed and scholars translated, commented on and added new knowledge and ideas to the Latin and Greek scrolls that had been saved in monasteries.

By the end of the 11th century, therefore, the basic conditions for the development of a separate profession were in place: natural materials having medicinal uses had been identified; the means of preserving and passing on this knowledge, through a common language and the written word, existed; basic technologies for the processing of raw materials had been developed; and first steps in the specialisation of occupations had already taken place. Despite church opposition to science in the Dark Ages, monastic medicine across Europe had preserved knowledge, and this spread to England. It was only a matter of time before the separation of the professions of medicine and pharmacy was formally recognised in Europe.

References

1. Anderson S C. The historical context of pharmacy. In: Taylor K, Harding G, eds. *Pharmacy Practice*. London: Taylor and Francis, 2001: 4.
2. Oppenheimer A L. Mesopotamian medicine. *Bulletin of the History of Medicine* 1962; 36: 97–108.
3. Trease G E. *Pharmacy in History*. London: Baillière, Tindall and Cox, 1964: 1–18.
4. McGrew R E. *Encyclopaedia of Medical History*. London: Macmillan Press, 1985.
5. The Holy Bible. Exodus 30: 22, 34; Exodus 37: 29; Ecclesiastes 10: 1; Ecclesiasticus 38: 1–8.
6. Sigerist H E. *A History of Medicine*. New York: Oxford University Press, 1951: 1, 3.
7. Mann J. *Murder, Magic and Medicine*. Oxford: Oxford University Press, 1992.
8. The Holy Bible. Genesis 37: 3.
9. Schmitz R. *Geschichte Der Pharmazie*. Eschborn: Govi-Verlag, 1998: Band 1: 352–353.
10. Partington J R. *A History of Chemistry, Vol. 1*. London: Macmillan and Co., 1997; 1.
11. Matthews L G. *History of Pharmacy in Britain*. Edinburgh: E & S Livingstone, 1962: 1–28.
12. Court W E. The ancient doctrine of signatures or similitudes. *Pharmaceutical Historian* 1999; 29(3): 41–48.
13. Holmyard E J (ed.). *Alchemy*. Harmondsworth: Penguin Books, 1957 (reprinted 1968): 25–32; 43–59; 60–104.
14. Burland C A. *The Arts of the Alchemists*. London: Weidenfeld and Nicolson, 1967.
15. Shellard E J. Avicenna 980–1037. *Pharmacy International* 1980; 3: 176–177.

3

Pharmacy in the medieval world, 1100 to 1617 AD

Stuart Anderson

The early centuries of the second millennium were a wretched time for those who lived in them. There were constant wars and frequent epidemics of devastating diseases, and the lives of the great majority of people were short and miserable. No sooner had the Normans conquered England in 1066 than Pope Urban II called for a crusade; the crusades were to last over 200 years. The Black Death cast its shadow over the whole of Europe for centuries. However, the five centuries from around 1100 to 1600 were not without progress, not least in the fields of medicine and pharmacy.

In this chapter, the focus shifts from continental Europe to England, where developments in several areas of medieval life helped shape the practice of pharmacy at this time. These included the growing importance of the craft guilds; the role of the monasteries in preserving medical scholarship and knowledge; the development of the medieval hospital, and the continuing production of herbals as a means of disseminating knowledge. The chapter begins with a discussion of developments in Europe, leading to the separation of pharmacy from medicine in Italy in 1231. Later, in Britain, tensions between different groups within the guilds led ultimately to the foundation of the Society of Apothecaries in 1617, where this chapter ends.

Developments in Europe from 1100 AD

The continuing migration of scholars from Persia to the west from the 8th century onwards led to the creation of important centres of learning in Italy, Spain and France, and later England. The medical school at Salerno, for example, was a remarkable centre of scholarship where Islamic and Christian cultures met and prospered. It was the leading school of medicine and pharmacy in Europe. Its greatest period lasted from the conquest of Salerno by the Normans in 1076 to about 1224, after which it began to decline. At least 100 texts by more than 30 authors have survived, including translations from Arabic to Latin by Constantinus Africanus, and the *Antidotarium* of Nicolaus Salernitanus, which contains 139 complex prescriptions in alphabetical order [1].

Another important manuscript resulting from the Salerno school is the *Antidotarium* of Matthæus Platearius. This is usually known as the *Circa instans*, which are its opening words. It was a medical text based on the work of Dioscorides, which had been translated into Latin in the 6th century. It introduced distillation to European pharmacy and broke away from monastic interpretations by stressing the value of chemistry in medicine. These early texts were extremely influential on the way pharmacy was practised over the next few hundred years.

A School of Medicine was founded at Montpellier in France as early as the 8th century, but it reached the peak of its fame in the 13th and 14th centuries. It had a significant impact on English pharmacy and medicine, because of the trade contacts between the town and Gascony, which was in English hands. Celebrated teachers and students of Montpellier from this period include Gilbert the Englishman, who died in 1250, and John of Arderne of Newark near Nottingham, a famous English surgeon who lived from 1306 to 1390.

In Spain, a number of Arab scholars were active during this time. Albucassis (or Abu-l-Qasim al-Zahrawi) of Cordova produced a manual for apothecaries called the *Liber servitoris*; he also prepared and distilled chemicals. Averroes or Ibn Rushed (1149–1198), a Spanish Moslem, compiled *The General Rules of Medicine*. Ibn-al-Baitar (1197–1248) of Malaga wrote the *Jami or Corpus of Simples*, describing some 1400 drugs, including 300 from Arab medicine. These included nutmeg, clove, rhubarb and musk.

At the end of the 11th century, the fragile European political order was to be seriously disturbed. The world of western Christendom, which was emerging from the barbarism of the Dark Ages, collided with the highly civilised world of Byzantium, which by this stage had passed its political prime. Both were opposed by the world of Islam, whose Arabic culture was as different to that of the Turks in Asia as it was to the Christians in Europe [2]. For both medicine and pharmacy, the consequences were to be great.

Impact of the Crusades, 1095 to 1291 AD

On 27 November 1095, Pope Urban II was visiting France when he became concerned with the reform of the French church. He took the opportunity to suggest that a Crusade should liberate the Holy Land from the grip of Islam. For a generation the Moors had been strengthening their hold on the Iberian Peninsula; they had captured Baghdad in 1055, and were making forays into Syria and Palestine. The Pope appealed to Christians for both a Spanish expedition and a relief of the pressure on the Holy Land. He also hoped to heal the schism that had occurred between the Holy See and the Byzantine world. Christians who joined the Crusade were to be given absolution.

The First Crusade lasted until July 1099: there were to be four more lasting until the end of the 13th century. During these years in the East, Christians not only married into local families, but also developed the tastes and flavours of the Levant, including spices from the Orient. One consequence was that the spice trade with England boomed. The Crusaders were also exposed to many new ideas, some of which related to the practice of medicine and pharmacy. They included the separation of pharmacy from medicine, and the fact that the compounding of drugs was often undertaken on a grand scale, as it was in the great al-Manuri hospital of Cairo. Furthermore, it was noted that in Middle Eastern countries, government officers were appointed to inspect the shops and markets run by pharmacists and herbalists.

The Crusades had other unforeseen results. In England, King Richard I pledged himself to a Crusade, but he needed money, so he borrowed in Italy on his way to the Holy Land, and again in Syria and Palestine. Later, in 1271, Edward I also decided to join a Crusade, and he borrowed money from the Italians. Italian companies later financed Edward III's wars in Flanders and France. Eventually many of these companies ran into financial difficulties, and the bankers were ruined because Edward III reneged on his loans [3].

European trade moved gradually westwards. This resulted in the introduction into England of all the requirements of a commercial centre, such as accurate weights and measures, coins for trading, and the collection of taxes and tolls. It was into this emerging commercial environment that the sellers of drugs and spices slowly established themselves.

The Edict of Palermo, 1231 AD

The Arabs introduced into Sicily the concept of a separation of pharmacy from medicine in Europe. The idea received its first formal recognition in 1231 as a result of an edict of Frederick II of Hohenstaufen, who was Emperor of Germany and King of Sicily. Frederick spent many formative years in Sicily. He was highly intelligent: he spoke fluent French, German, Italian, Latin, Greek and Arabic, and he had a good knowledge of many subjects, from philosophy to medicine.

Frederick had been a significant figure in the Crusades. Despite having been excommunicated by the Pope, he set off to the Holy Land, arriving in 1228. Through careful diplomacy, he was able to regain Jerusalem for the Christians. It was with this triumph still ringing in his ears that he returned to his palace in Palermo. There he presented his edict creating a clear distinction between the responsibilities of physicians and those of apothecaries, and he laid down regulations for their professional practice [4].

The main features of the Edict of Palermo were that medicine and pharmacy were separate professions requiring particular skills and responsibilities; that physicians and apothecaries could not enter into a business relationship; the law sought to prevent exploitation of the sick, and there was government supervision of pharmacy. A set dispensatory (list of drugs) had to be used, and the government attempted to limit the number of premises and control prices. Finally, the druggists (*confectionarii*) and apothecaries (*stationarii*) had to stock certain drugs and keep them no longer than 1 year.

The edict initially related only to Sicily and southern Italy. However, the idea that the diagnosis and treatment of disease should be separated from the preparation of medicines soon spread across continental Europe, and Frederick's decree provided the basis for similar legislation elsewhere. For example, in Basle in Switzerland an Apothecaries Oath was drawn up in 1271. It spelled out the relationship between physicians and apothecaries; it stated that 'no physician who cares for or has cared for the sick shall ever own an apothecary's business in Basle, nor shall he ever become an apothecary'. In Germany, pharmacists formed themselves into a society in 1632. However, the idea of separation did not reach Britain or Ireland until several centuries later.

The situation in England

At the time of the Norman Conquest in 1066, the population in Britain remained sparse, particularly in the north, and had only reached about 1,250,000 in the whole of England [5]. Soon after the first invasions of the Angles and Saxons of northern Europe from across the North Sea in 440 AD, the Romans departed Britain. They left behind outstanding remnants of their civilisation, but little is known about pharmacy in the intervening period. However, monks such as Saint Aldhelm, Saint Boniface and Saint Augustine built libraries in their great abbeys, and the works of Hippocrates, Galen and Dioscorides, amongst others, were available to the monks. An Anglo-Saxon monk, the Venerable Bede (673–735 AD) wrote a treatise on medicine entitled *De natura rerum*.

In Wessex, King Alfred (849–899 AD) defeated the Danes, reorganised government and encouraged scholarship. One important outcome was the *Leech Book of Bald*, written between 900 and 950 AD [6]. This was a compendium of therapeutics and pharmaceutical remedies, encompassing a wide range of plant and animal materials, and especially indigenous drugs. However, generally in Britain there was little development in either medicine or pharmacy during the six centuries from the Anglo-Saxon invasion to the Norman Conquest.

The Guilds

The invading Normans brought to England a system of law and order, known as the feudal system, and traders were soon organising themselves into craft and merchant guilds. Pharmacy in England at the time was essentially a trading activity, and the Guild of Pepperers (founded in about 1180) and the Guild of Spicers (about 1184) included traders in drugs among their members. Many indigenous and foreign drugs appeared in the herbals and were regularly traded. A surprising number had therapeutic effects: of 119 such drugs still in use today, 74% have actions consistent with their traditional use [7]. As pharmacy organised and developed in Britain in the second millennium the quality and understanding of these drugs steadily improved [8].

Guilds (or 'Gilds') originated during the Anglo-Saxon period, before the Norman Conquest. The earliest guilds were the 'Frith Gilds', which seem to have been mostly concerned with feasting, although they later came to have religious overtones and trading purposes. These had their origins in the days of King Athelstan, who reigned from 924 to 939. The Frith Guilds were followed by 'the Knights' gilds, which conducted trade on behalf of the King. Two such gilds were established in Canterbury and Dover. The Domesday Book records the existence of two storehouses rented for the king, two for Queen Edith, and even the houses and stalls of the burgesses and moneyers [9].

Following the Norman Conquest many other towns set up what came to be called the 'Gild-Merchant', the primary aim of which was to further the mercantile interests of its members, and at the same time exclude strangers from its benefits [10]. For example, in Leicester (a town whose wealth, as with many other towns, was based on the wool trade) all the wool packers and wool washers were excluded unless they belonged to the Leicester Gild-Merchant. Furthermore, only Leicester gildsmen could buy goods from non-gildsmen. The Gild-Merchant was indeed powerful [11]. Towns were usually most busy at the time of the weekly market, as it drew large crowds from the surrounding districts [12]. Of even greater importance were the fairs [13]. It was through fairs that the long-distance trade of medieval England was carried on.

The registration of craftsmen, 1363

We do not know precisely when the situation changed from there being a single 'gild-merchant' for all merchants in the town, to there being individual gilds for each craft or trade. A town might at first have only two or three separate gilds, but by a decree of King Edward III in 1363 every craftsman, whether master or apprentice, had to be enrolled in a gild [14]. This was re-enforced during the reign of Philip and Mary (1553–58), when no cloth, haberdashery wares, groceries or mercers' wares could be sold unless the proprietor was a member of a gild of a city, borough or market town; however, this did not include fairs.

There were some important exceptions to the rule. The first was if the person named was living in and belonged to the Duchy of Lancaster, a large and dispersed area throughout the kingdom. Such persons could claim exemption from all tolls on their wares as late as the time of King George III (1760–1820) [15]. Another exception was that of the Hanseatic League, a group of foreigners and merchants who already controlled most of the trade in Scandinavia and the Baltic, as well as northern Germany. They were unpopular because the English merchants did not have equally good concessions in Germany [16,17].

In the later Middle Ages, merchants could become very wealthy, and could even rank with the great landowners. In due course they accumulated enough money to be able to lend it to the king. London was by far the largest city in Britain and by 1430 it had over 100 gilds. These gradually merged and by the end of the 15th century there were twelve Great Companies: the Mercers, the Grocers, the Drapers, the Fishmongers, the Goldsmiths, the Skinners, the Merchant Taylors, the Haberdashers, the Vintners and the Clothworkers. Those who traded in drugs and spices were included with the Grocers. All of these companies still exist today. A struggle for ascendancy between the Great Companies was only settled in 1515 by an Act of the Court of Aldermen.

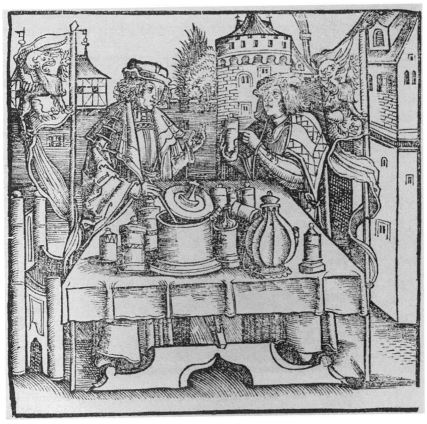

Figure 3.1 Preparation of theriac, a cure-all medicinal treacle with many and varied ingredients. A 16th-century woodcut from Hieronymus Brunschwig, *Liber de arte distillandi. De simplicibus*, 1500.

The medieval hospital

It would be wrong to imagine that drugs were only prepared and sold in shops and markets during this period. There was another important location for pharmaceutical knowledge, and that was the hospitals. Probably the first hospitals in Britain at which pharmacy was practised were the Roman military hospitals known as *valetudinaria* [18]. St Giles Hospital in Beverley and St Nicholas in Pontefract were both founded before the Norman Conquest. Hospices were originally established as refuges for travellers. At least two Yorkshire hospices, one in Holderness and the other in York, are thought to have been founded in the 10th century. The one in York was so busy that the Saxon king Athelstan recognised that urgent help was needed by the canons who ran it: he was instrumental in the founding of St Peter's hospital [19]. In another case, Flixton was considered 'so desolate that it was established as a house of refuge in order to protect travellers from being devoured by the wolves'.

About 1148, St Bartholomew's in Smithfield, London, was besieged by those who hoped to obtain relief from an aching head, and yet another from 'ryngyng of his erys'. There were many others who had attacks of epilepsy, or suffered from dropsy and fevers [20]. Another not uncommon feature of the times was ergotism, known as 'Saint Anthony's Fire' because of the blackening and shrivelling of the skin caused by gangrene. Ergotism is the effect of long-term ergot poisoning, usually resulting from ingestion of alkaloids produced by the *Claviceps purpurea* fungus that invades rye and other grains [21].

Early infirmaries

It was in 1170 that St Thomas of Canterbury became a focal point for pilgrimage in England; other hospitals and hospices sprang up in the Channel ports and along the Pilgrims' Way, at Dover, Maidstone, Strood, and further inland at Salisbury [22]. The hospital at this time was both guesthouse and infirmary. For example, in about 1194 a 'herbergia' was founded on the outskirts of Oxford, so that 'therein infirm people and strangers might receive remedy of their health and necessity'.

The 14th century was probably the greatest time for pilgrimages, but as with many other things, it encouraged vagrancy. The Statute of Labourers, enacted in 1350, attempted to restrain idleness and begging. A tendency grew to reserve beds for chronic invalids, and in particular beggars were to be moved on within a day and a night [23]. At about this time one form of relief became prevalent, namely the assistance of women in childbirth. The foundation of Holy Trinity in Salisbury specifically mentioned that it was for lying-in women until they were delivered, recovered and churched.

In 1414 there was a further attempt to reduce the use of hospitals by laypersons who were able-bodied, both by the patrons of the hospital and by the warden who ran it. The first patrons were nearly always men of probity, even if they were mostly concerned about their standing in the next world, but their descendants frequently used the hospital as a hostelry for themselves and their retinue. In some cases the privilege of board and lodging was even given away by patrons as a 'reward' for services, particularly if it was royal service. Abuse by wardens and officials could be even greater. One warden of St John and St Thomas' at Stamford defrauded the poor of their alms and locked the rooms where strangers and sick should have been accommodated. In other cases the buildings were in such a poor state of repair that they had almost fallen into ruin.

Leprosy and lazar houses

There were, however, other types of institutions providing care for the sick. These included the leprosy hospitals or lazar houses. Although leprosy was frequently misdiagnosed, it nevertheless seems to have been quite a common illness. The two earliest leper houses were established in Rochester and at Harbledown. It has been suggested that the appearance of leprosy was probably the result of the Saracen invasions into Spain, which then moved into northern Europe [24]. Leprosy is caused by *Mycobacterium leprae* and infection spreads by means of nasal droplets and skin lesions in immune-deficient people. The incidence of leprosy rapidly increased, as did the number of leper houses or lazars. Lepers had to announce their presence by means of clappers or bells, were not allowed into towns, and had to huddle in leper houses on the outskirts [25].

The Black Death and pest houses

One disease above all others played havoc in England during the 14th and 15th centuries. The illness commonly known as the 'Black Death' is thought to have been Bubonic plague, named after the buboes or painful swellings of the lymph nodes that result, although there remains some dispute about this. In most cases death was swift. Plague is caused by the bacterium *Yersinia pestis*, which is spread by fleas with the help of animals such as the black rat [26].

Plague probably originated in the steppes of Central Asia, from where it was carried west by Mongol armies. The Mongols besieged the Genoese colony of Kaffa on the Crimea, and it was spread from the Crimea by Genoese ships returning to Sicily. The disease first manifested itself in October 1347, spreading clockwise from Italy, the nearby islands of Sardinia, Corsica and the Balearics, and thence to mainland Europe [27].

The Black Death probably arrived in England at Melcombe Regis (Weymouth) in June 1348, and it had reached London by November. Four further outbreaks occurred between 1361 and 1391. It continued into the 15th century, with outbreaks occurring in 1406, 1464, 1479 and 1500. Between these major outbreaks there were lesser ones [28]. Towns and cities established special institutions outside their boundaries for the treatment of these patients, known as pest houses. There was one on the Scottish island of Inchkeith in 1475, and in 1594 one was opened on 3 acres of land adjoining St Bartholomew's Hospital in London [29].

Subsequently plague became endemic, with the Great Plague occurring in 1665. This was to play a decisive part in determining the respective roles of physicians and apothecaries in the years that followed. It is the first epidemic in England that can be identified with certainty. Once the Black Death finally subsided it was estimated that about one-third of the population of Europe had died.

Herbals

Whether practising in retail premises or in public institutions, the maker of medicines required access to knowledge about them. Before the days of the printed word this was a problem, and the spread of knowledge required laborious copying by hand of extensive manuscripts. This was invariably done by monks, and usually involved copying Latin texts. When Arabic and Greek medicine began to penetrate the European universities in the 13th century, however, medicine had to master a new literature and therapeutics [30].

The earliest known herbal is the *Alexipharma* by Nikander, who lived about 200 BC. The term 'herbal' itself did not come into use until the beginning of the 16th century; herbals sometimes include references to animals, such as scorpions. A herbal is said to have been written in Greece by Diclos of Carystus, but no evidence of it has survived. Crateus (or Krateuas), physician to the king of Pontus, Mithridates, from 120 to 63 BC, also produced a herbal, but only a few fragments are now known. Of much greater importance was the *De Materia Medica* of Dioscorides (50–100 AD).

A later important herbal was the *Herbal of Apuleius*. This is now in Leiden, and dates from about 600 AD, or possibly earlier. It was first translated into Anglo-Saxon in about 1000 AD. One of the Apuleius manuscripts was copied at the Abbey of Bury St Edmunds in about 1120. The *Herbal of Apuleius* retained its popularity for many years, until the arrival of *De Viribus Herbarum* by Macer Floridus. This was probably composed by Odo, Bishop of Meung. It was presented in Latin verses, which largely accounted for its popularity.

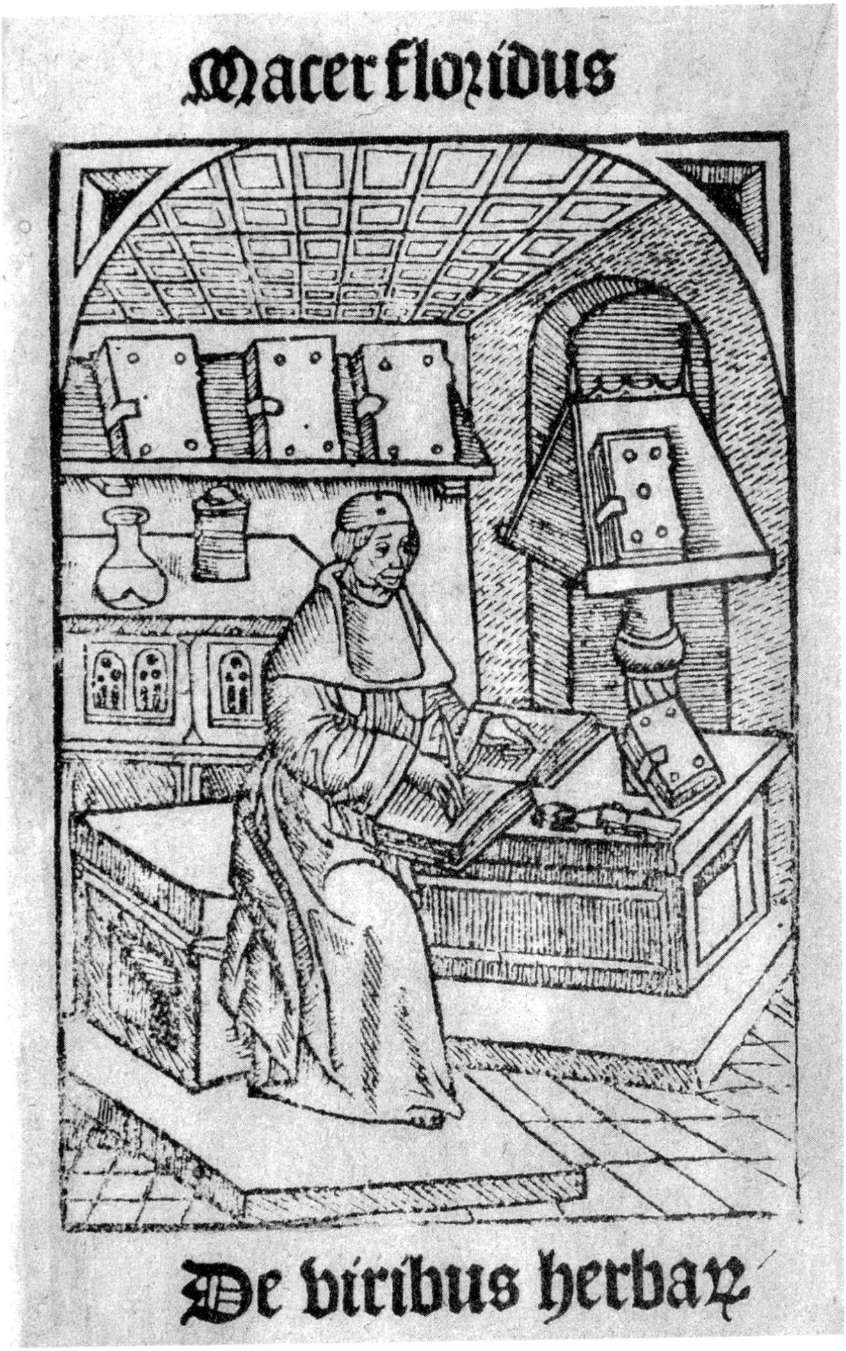

Figure 3.2 Frontispiece of Macer Floridus, *De Viribus Herbarum*, 1477, first printed in Geneva, 1500. Reproduced by permission of the Wellcome Library, London.

It was sometime before 1250 that Gilbertus Anglicus produced the *Compendium of Medicine*, now regarded as an important text. In the early 15th century this work was translated from Latin into Middle English. This was not only a measure of its success but also a reflection of a new desire to learn 'secrets', as medieval medicine was often called. In fact the book could be more legitimately called an encyclopaedia because of the subjects it covered. It included a herbal of some 144 species, starting with *Amigdalus* and continuing to *Zuchara* or sugar cane. It proved to be immensely popular and was translated into French, English, Dutch and Spanish.

Woodcuts and printing

Despite the popularity of herbals, illustrations at this time were usually poor and the plants depicted difficult to identify, whether in the ground or illustrated. A better means for the reproduction of illustrations was required. This came with the introduction of woodcuts in Europe at the beginning of the 15th century, thought to be an independent European invention. Soon afterwards the first printed herbals were published following the introduction of moveable type. The first of these was probably that of Macer Floridus, *De Viribus Herbarum*, published in 1477.

The incunabulae (or early printed books) were all published in Mainz. The first were the *Latin Herbarius* and the *German Herbarius*, both by Schoffer, and the *Hortus Sanitatis* by Jacob Meydenbach. Schoffer had been an associate of Gutenberg, who was renowned for this use of moveable type. Schoffer was to become his successor and inheritor of his press and type. This was undoubtedly the most important discovery of the later Middle Ages, but plagiarism of these early herbals was soon rife. The invention of printing led to a rapid expansion in the production of herbals.

English herbals

Two of the earliest printed herbals were in English: the *Herball* of Richard Banckes in 1525, and *The Grete Herball*, which was largely taken from an earlier publication, *Le Grand Herbier*. William Turner (1500–1568) also wrote a useful book in English, called *The Names of Herbes in Greke, Latin, Englishe, Duche and Frenche with the Commune Names that Herberies and Apotecaries Use*. One of the most influential English herbalists was John Gerarde (1545–1612). There have been suggestions that Gerarde took much of his material from that of Rembert Dodoens, although this remains a matter of controversy [31].

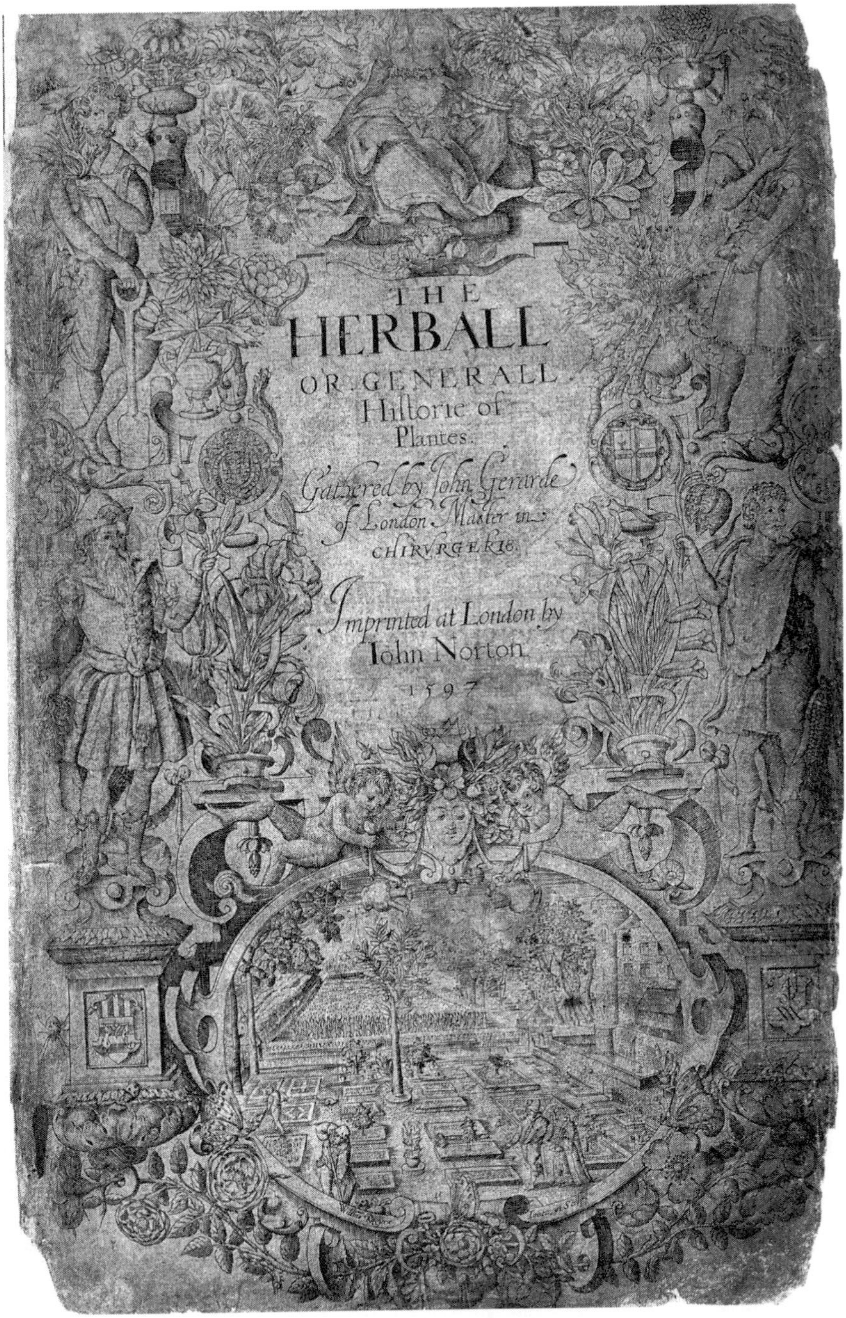

Figure 3.3 Frontispiece of *The Herball or, Generall Historie of Plantes* by John Gerarde, published in 1597. Reproduced by permission of the Wellcome Library, London.

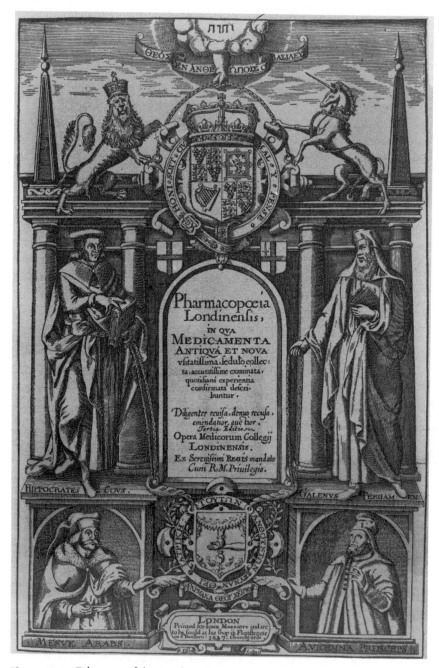

Figure 3.4   Title page of the *London Pharmacopoeia*. This 1627 version is one of a succession of revisions that appeared soon after the 1618 'first' edition.

Another English herbal was the *Theatrum Botanicum* by John Parkinson (1567–1640), who is better known for his *Paradisi in Sole Paradisus Terrestris*, with its main emphasis on horticulture. The work includes 109 woodcuts of about 780 plants. He was a practising apothecary with a fine garden in Long Acre, London, and was known to both John Tradescant and Thomas Johnson [32]. Finally, there were the so-called 'outlandish herbals' (describing plants indigenous to other countries), such as Garcia Da Orta's *Colloquies on the Simples and Drugs of India*, and the *Rerum Medicarum* of Francis Hernandez, one to the east and the other to the west.

Herbals were a vital source of information for those preparing medicines, but one of their features was their diversity and inconsistency. State authorities in several countries began to recognise the need for a degree of standardisation, and the idea of official formularies or pharmacopoeias gained support. The first official pharmacopoeia, to be followed by all apothecaries, originated in Florence in Italy [33]. The *Nuovo Receptario*, published in 1498, was the result of collaboration between the Guild of Apothecaries and the Medical Society, an early example of the two professions working constructively together.

In England, the need for a formulary or pharmacopoeia that would provide a standard for the whole of the country was first recognised during the reign of Elizabeth I (1558–1603). The College of Physicians had previously considered such a publication, but it was not until 1589 that a group of members was nominated to be responsible for preparing each of the sections [34]. Salts, chemicals and metals were included, although there was still some argument regarding their use in medicine. At that time extracts and impure vegetable salts were also included with chemicals.

A committee was formed in 1594 to examine the draft text. Progress was slow and it was only due to the interest of Henry Atkins and Theodore de Mayerne, the King's physicians, that the pharmacopoeia was finally published. A Royal Proclamation was issued on 26 April 1618 commanding all apothecaries to follow its instructions. However, this edition was judged to be flawed, and a second edition was published in December [35]. It is this volume that is recognised as the first *London Pharmacopoeia*.

Changing medical ideas

The early centuries of the second millennium were not an easy time for the emergence of a distinct pharmacy profession. The guilds were often over-bearing in their attitudes, the monasteries with their infirmaries led to little progress in the use of medicines, and the plants referred to in the herbals were on the whole difficult to identify. Political upheaval due to wars and Crusades, and epidemics like the Black Death that drastically reduced the population, did not help. However, towards the end of the period one man had the courage to think differently, and his ideas were destined to change the practice of medicine forever. That man was Paracelsus.

Paracelsus, 1493 to 1541

Theophrastus Bombastus von Hohenheim was born on 17 December 1493 at Maria-Einsiedeln near Zurich, which at that time was part of Germany rather than Switzerland. The title 'Paracelsus' was self-bestowed, and resulted from his own inflated opinion, as he believed himself to be greater than Celsus, the writer who lived in the first century. His father, Wilhelm von Hohenheim, was also a doctor, and he taught his son the elements of medicine and alchemy.

Paracelsus went to work in the Tyrol, and became familiar with the properties of semi-precious metals. Later he gained an MD at the University of Ferrara and was invited by the city authorities of Basel to become the town's physician and professor of medicine. He held this post for only two years, during which he extolled the great medicinal powers of minerals, and publicly burned the books of Avicenna and Galen with sulphur and nitre. This did nothing to endear him to his fellow professors. Eventually he was invited to Salzburg by the Prince Palatine, but he died not long after he arrived in April 1541, aged only 48 [36]. It was to be 40 years before Paracelsus's works were collected and edited: it was another 400 years before they were published in modern German.

Paracelsus's great contribution was his questioning of the works of Avicenna and Galen, and his belief in chemical remedies, such as mercury, lead and sulphur. He urged the study of chemistry, although he did not deny the possibility of transforming one metal into another. He also had great faith in his 'secret remedies' and believed in the Doctrine of Signatures. One of his favourite remedies was opium in the form of a pill or tincture, to which he gave the name 'laudanum'. He also introduced new dosage forms for the administration of medicines, including extracts and tinctures. However, his contribution took many years to be recognised and taken up, and his impact on English pharmacy during his own lifetime was negligible [37].

Foundation of the Society of Apothecaries, 1617

For practitioners of pharmacy in England during the 16th century it was very much business as usual. Since its foundation the London apothecaries had been members of the Grocers' Company, which had a monopoly on the importation of drugs. Nevertheless, they retained their identity as pharmaceutical practitioners [38]. The apothecaries were a relatively small cluster of individuals among a large and powerful group of wholesale merchants, and they were undoubtedly overshadowed by them. The 1515 Act of the Court of Aldermen was followed by a period of relative stability and order in the Great Companies.

In 1588 the apothecaries petitioned Queen Elizabeth I to grant them a monopoly in the selling and compounding of medicines. Not surprisingly, the more influential members of the Grocers' Company opposed such a move, and the petition was unsuccessful. However, the grocers did eventually agree to make the apothecaries a separate section within their company, in 1607. The apothecaries were not content with this arrangement, and petitioned King James I, who had ascended the throne in 1603, to give them complete independence, like the physicians and the surgeons.

James I signed a new Charter in 1617. This established the London apothecaries as a corporate body, under the title 'The Worshipful Society of the Art and Mystery of the Apothecaries'. The charter listed the names of 121 apothecaries whose petition was being granted. Initially it related only to the London neighbourhood; the founders of the new Society had little interest in the development of pharmacy in the provinces. One of its most influential members, and most generous benefactors during the early years, was Gideon de Laune, who is often regarded as the founder of the Society. De Laune was one of several apothecaries to the court of James I.

Impact of the Charter

The granting of the Charter represents an important landmark in the regulation of what was to become the profession of pharmacy – it set minimum training standards, rules for practice, and introduced a system of inspection. Most importantly, it stipulated an apprenticeship lasting a minimum of 7 years. At the end of this period apprentices appeared before the master and wardens of the Society to be examined orally on their knowledge of simples and 'concerning the preparing, dispensing, handling, commixing and compounding of medicines'. Until the candidate passed he could not set up as an apothecary in or around London. However, there was nothing to stop him practising in the provinces.

The Charter granted the apothecaries a valuable monopoly, because it was unlawful for members of 'other mysteries to furnish, have, hold, or keep an apothecaries shop'. The Society was given the right to hold property, to appoint a master and two wardens, and to make rules for the practice of members within a 7-mile radius of the city of London. The master and wardens were authorised to enter the premises of 'any person whatsoever', question them, and prohibit from practice those found to be unskilled or ignorant of their profession. They also had power to examine all stock and to condemn any found to be 'corrupt, unmedicinable, pernicious or hurtful' and to burn it 'before the offender's doors' [34].

The political and legal frameworks that were a prerequisite for the development of pharmacy in England were now in place, and the scene was set for the next phase in its evolution.

References

1. Trease G E. *Pharmacy in History*. London: Baillière, Tindall and Cox, 1964: 16.
2. Bridge A. *The Crusades*. London: Granada, 1980: 110–112.
3. Thrupp S L. *The Merchant Class of Medieval London*. Chicago: University of Chicago Press, 1948: 2–7, 87.
4. Anderson S C. The historical context of pharmacy. In: Taylor K, Harding G, eds. *Pharmacy Practice*. London: Taylor and Francis, 2001: 6.
5. Trevelyan G M. *A Shortened History of England*. Harmondsworth: Pelican Books, 1967: 133.
6. Cockayne O (ed.). *Leechdoms, Wortcunning and Starcraft of Early England &c, Volume 2*. London: Longman Green, 1865.
7. Farnsworth N R, Akerele O, Bingel A S, Soejarto D D. Medicinal plants in therapy. *Bulletin of the World Health Organization* 1985; 63(6): 965–981.
8. Court W E. A matter of standards: The quest for authentic, reproducible and reliable plant drugs. *Pharmaceutical Historian* 2002; 32(4): 50–58.
9. Whitelock D. *The Beginnings of English Society*. Pelican History of England, Volume 2. London: Penguin Books, 1952; 46–47, 60.
10. Gross C. *The Gild-Merchant*. Oxford: Oxford University Press, 1890: 1, 4, 5–7.
11. Hazlitt W C. *The Livery Companies of the City of London: Their Origin, Character, Development, and Social and Political Importance*. New York: Benjamin Blom, 1969 (reissue of 1892 publication, London: Swan Sonnenschein).
12. Unwin G. *The Gilds and Companies of London*. London: Frank Cass & Co. (reprint), 1966: 245–247.

13. Stenton D M. *English Society in the Early Middle Ages 1066–1307. Pelican History of England, Volume 2.* London: Penguin Books, 1951: 178–185, 201.

14. Whittet T D. The apothecary in provincial gilds. *Medical History* 1964; 8(3): 245–273.

15. Exemption from tolls. *Manor of Enfield, Duchy of Lancaster.* British Library Acc. 549, July 1836.

16. Dollinger P. *The German Hansa* (translated by Ault D S and Steinberg S H). London: Macmillan, 1970: 62.

17. Gies J, Gies F. *Merchants and Moneymen: The Commercial Revolution 1000–1500.* London: Arthur Baker, 1972: 171.

18. Whittet T D. The history of pharmacy in British hospitals. In: Poynter F N L, ed. *The Evolution of Pharmacy in Britain.* London: Pitman Medical Publishing, 1965: 17.

19. Clay R M. *The Mediaeval Hospitals of England.* London: Methuen, 1909: 2–30.

20. Thompson C J S. The apothecary in England from the thirteenth century to the close of the sixteenth century. *Proceedings of the Royal Society of Medicine (History Section)* 1914; 8: 36.

21. Park K. Medicine and society in medieval Europe 500–1500. In: Wear A, ed. *Medicine in Society.* Cambridge: Cambridge University Press, 1992: 62.

22. Clay R M. *The Mediaeval Hospitals of England.* London: Methuen, 1909: 35–69.

23. Clay R M. *The Mediaeval Hospitals of England.* London: Methuen, 1909: 213–225.

24. Talbot C H. *Medicine in Mediaeval England.* London: Oldbourne, 1967: 24–37, 38–55, 102–163.

25. Porter R. *The Greatest Benefit to Mankind. A Medical History of Humanity from Antiquity to the Present.* London: Harper Collins, 1997: 121–122.

26. Cartwright F F, Biddiss M. *Disease and History*, 2nd edn. Stroud: Sutton Publishing, 2000: 22–40.

27. Porter R. *The Greatest Benefit to Mankind. A Medical History of Humanity from Antiquity to the Present.* London: Harper Collins, 1997: 122–127.

28. Talbot C H. *Medicine in Mediaeval England.* London: Oldbourne, 1967: 163–166.

29. Wilson F P. *The Plague in Shakespeare's London.* Oxford: Clarendon Press, 1927: 74.

30. Getz F M. *Healing and Society in Medieval England.* Madison: University of Wisconsin Press, 1991: xxxvi–xli, dustcover.

31. Burnby J. John Gerarde and his contemporaries. *Pharmaceutical Historian* 1999; 29(2): 19–23.

32. Anderson F J. *An Illustrated History of the Herbals.* New York: Columbia University Press, 1977: Introduction, 23–35, 36–50, 59–65, 73–97, 106–112, 121–155, 163–180.

33. Anderson S C. The historical context of pharmacy. In: Taylor K, Harding G, eds. *Pharmacy Practice.* London: Taylor and Francis, 2001: 6.

34. Trease G E. *Pharmacy in History.* London: Baillière, Tindall and Cox, 1964: 110.

35. Earles M P. The Pharmacopoeia Londinensis 1618: A new look at an old problem. *Pharmaceutical Historian* 1982; 12(2): 4–5.
36. Holmyard E J (ed.). *Alchemy*. Harmondsworth: Penguin Books, 1957 (reprinted 1968): 161–169.
37. Trease G E. *Pharmacy in History*. London: Baillière, Tindall and Cox, 1964: 82.
38. Trease G E. The Spicer-Apothecary of the Middle Ages. *Future Pharmacist* 1957: 54.

4

Pharmacy in the early modern world, 1617 to 1841 AD

Peter M Worling

The period from the beginning of the 17th century to the middle of the 19th century was one of transition and change for pharmacy in Great Britain. Occupational boundaries relating to the preparation and supply of medicines were constantly challenged, with successive disputes between physicians and apothecaries, and between apothecaries and chemists and druggists. Ideas about the nature of disease began to change, along with the substances used to treat them. Quality and standards continued to cause concern, and more precise herbals and formularies began to appear.

This chapter takes the story of pharmacy forward from the founding of the Society of Apothecaries in 1617 to the foundation of the Pharmaceutical Society of Great Britain in 1841. These changes took place within a complex and difficult political, social and economic context, and we begin with a brief account of the situation in England at the start of the 17th century.

England after 1600

The death of Elizabeth I in 1603 brought the first Elizabethan age to an end. James I inherited a Protestant state with many underlying conflicts that were barely being kept under control. These schisms lead to a Civil War (1642–1648), the execution of King Charles I, and a continuing deep-seated fear by the Protestant majority of being overwhelmed by the Catholic minority [1].

The population in England and Wales at this time has been estimated at about 5.5 million, with 2 million in Ireland and 1 million in Scotland. There was a vast difference between the living conditions of rich and poor. The King and his court, together with the nobility, lived in large houses surrounded by great estates, separated from the rest of the population. People in the towns, and particularly in London, lived in terrible conditions, packed together in tenements that frequently collapsed without warning. The streets were covered in sewage, which encouraged the spread of disease, and there were regular outbreaks of plague, borne by the fleas on rats. Smallpox, dysentery, typhus, typhoid and tuberculosis were rife, limiting any increase in population numbers. Infant mortality was particularly high, especially in the towns [2].

Medical practice, 1607 to 1701

Medical practice at the beginning of the 17th century was still largely based on the system of medicine introduced by Hippocrates. This had been consolidated as a comprehensive theoretical system of treatment by Galen in the 2nd century. It was believed that disease was caused by the imbalance of the body's four humours. Physicians examined their patients to determine which humour was in excess and prescribed accordingly. Many of the treatments involved bleeding, purgatives,

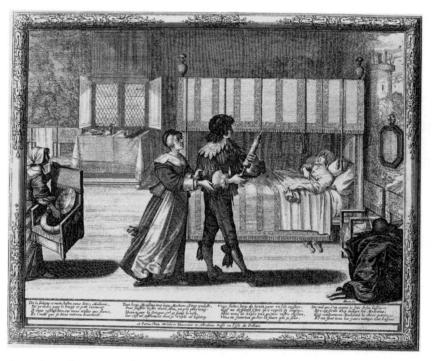

Figure 4.1 Home visit: the patient reacts sceptically when told how much better a clyster (or enema) will make her feel. Engraving by Abraham Bosse, France, 1680. Reproduced by permission of the Wellcome Library, London.

diaphoretics and clysters (enemas) to rid the body of these noxious influences. It was not unusual for heroic treatment to further weaken an already weak patient, although presumably those of a more robust constitution took such medicine in their stride [3].

Members of the public had a number of options if they needed treatment. The first was to call in a physician, but their fees were very high and they were therefore generally only used by the rich, although there are instances of them treating the poor for a reduced fee or for no charge. The case notes of Dr John Hall of Stratford (Shakespeare's son-in-law) indicate that he would see all members of the households he

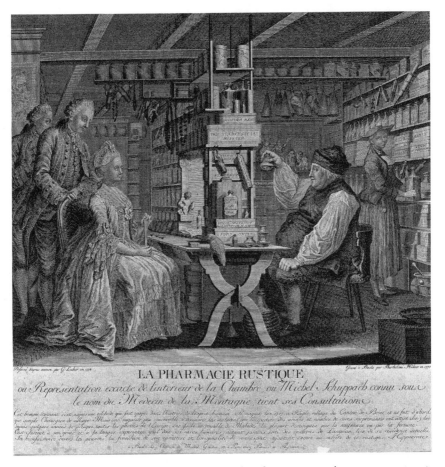

Figure 4.2 Apothecary examining a sample of urine. 'La pharmacie rustique', engraving by Barthelemi Hübner, 1775, after a drawing by G Locher showing Michel Schuppach at his pharmacy in Switzerland in 1773. Reproduced by permission of the Wellcome Library, London.

visited, including the servants, although it is likely that their masters paid their costs for them. He also treated people of different religions, and a number of ordinary citizens with whom he was acquainted [4].

The middle classes, both in London and in the country towns, usually relied on the apothecary to supply any medicines prescribed by the physician. The apothecary was also consulted for his advice on treatment, and this aspect of the apothecary's business steadily increased during this period. He understood that he was not permitted to charge for his consultation, and was quite prepared to rely on the sale of drugs and medicines for his profit.

The poor also relied on the apothecary, while those who could not afford his charges were dependent on the help they could obtain from their family, the padre or minister of religion, or perhaps the local wise woman. This was particularly the case in country districts where there was a long tradition of using plants for their medicinal properties. This practice had been refined by trial and error through the ages, although this was no guarantee of efficacy [5].

Scotland was largely free of the persecution of witches, which was rife during the 17th century in England. This allowed the traditional forms of healing, passed down through many generations, to continue. Healing using prayers, rituals and a wide range of herbs whose pharmaceutical action had been learned by practical use, was common. By the end of the 17th century the clan chiefs were consulting lowland doctors for their advice, but the traditional healers, supplemented by advice from the local minister of religion and schoolmaster, were the only medical service available to a large part of the community [6].

The poor and the credulous were also at the mercy of the many quacks and mountebanks (or travelling salesmen) operating in the cities and at the county fairs. These practitioners advertised their cure-all salves and ointments by handbills and in person. Through this publicity a number of remedies became well known, although many had little effect and did little to relieve the symptoms of the diseases they were supposed to cure [7]. These remedies were nevertheless profitable for their proprietors.

In time a number of apothecaries produced their own medicines, such as Elixir Salutis or Daffy's Elixir: this was compounded before 1680 by the Reverend Thomas Daffy, Rector of Redmile, and later by his daughter Elizabeth. It was said to consist of senna, jalap, aniseed, caraway seeds and juniper berries macerated in alcohol, to which treacle and water were added [8]. There was apparently a good demand for the elixir. John Harrison of London also started to supply an Elixir Salutis,

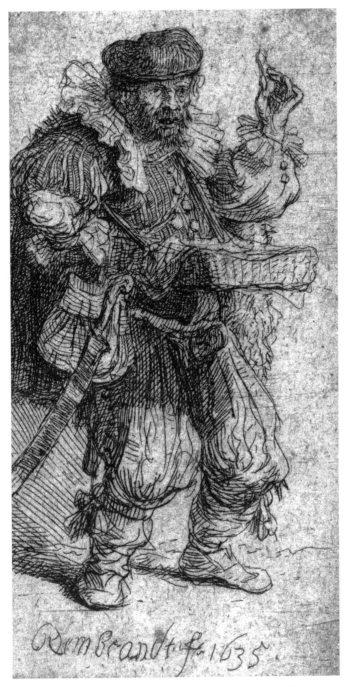

Figure 4.3   A medicine vendor. Rembrandt etching dated 1635. Reproduced by permission of the Wellcome Library, London.

and there was considerable disagreement between him and Elizabeth Daffy over the rights to the formula [9].

The apothecaries faced competition from many quarters. In London in 1600 there were 100 apothecaries, 50 physicians and 250 other medical practitioners. Many of the latter held an ecclesiastical licence to practise from the Bishop of London or the Dean of St Paul's. Some physicians as well as apothecaries kept open shop and sold medicines to their patients, but the apothecaries had the advantage that they did not charge for treatment, only the medicines supplied. Although they were not considered the equal of the physician, their standing in the community increased over time and they played an increasingly important part in the country's healthcare [10].

Formularies and pharmacopoeias

Physicians and apothecaries had a number of sources from which to obtain information about treatment. Formularies were produced locally for use in the city or municipality where they were printed. European formularies were widely used but had no national standing. Slowly there grew a realisation by the medical authorities that many of the ingredients in use were inactive. These were slowly discarded, and from 1600 onwards a number of new pharmacopoeias and dispensatories were published [11]. A revised edition of the *London Pharmacopoeia* was published, in Latin, in 1618, and further editions were published at irregular intervals thereafter. An *Edinburgh Pharmacopoeia* was published in 1699, and a *Dublin Pharmacopoeia* in 1806.

Publication of the *London Pharmacopoeia* encouraged the printing of other books of formulae. Nicholas Culpeper brought out an English translation of the *London Pharmacopoeia* in 1649, which was very critical of some of the older remedies, and greatly annoyed members of the Royal College of Physicians. Nevertheless it was well received by the public and it went into many editions. William Salmon's *New London Dispensary* was issued in 1676, and the *Dispensatory* of John Quincy appeared in 1721. Thomson's *The London Dispensatory* (1811) and Gray's *Supplement to the Pharmacopoeia* (1828) were other publications that supplemented the official pharmacopoeias, translating and helping to clarify the contents [12].

Succeeding volumes of the *London Pharmacopoeia* reflected the growing understanding of the use of medicines and the new drugs that were coming into use. Publication of the *Sceptical Chemist* by Robert

Boyle in 1661 demolished the principle of treatment based on the four humours, and introduced the concept of an 'element' as an entity that could not be further divided. Despite this, the humoral theory was still the commonest form of orthodox medicine in the first half of the 18th century. Successive editions of the *London Pharmacopoeia* introduced ever more substances: the 1667 edition added Peruvian bark and benzoic acid; in 1721 sulphurated potash and ferrous sulphate were added; and 1746 saw the inclusion of ammonium carbonate and nitrous ether, amongst others.

The 1809 edition introduced a new scientific nomenclature from the Continent developed by Morreau, Lavoisier, Berthollet and Fourcray, which led to the names of entries being changed to the Latin forms. Vegetable alkaloids were first isolated in the early 1800s, and this work was reflected in the addition of morphine, quinine, strychnine and veratrine to the 1836 edition. The 1851 edition of the *London Pharmacopoeia* was the last before it was absorbed, along with the *Edinburgh Pharmacopoeia* and *Dublin Pharmacopoeia*, into the *British Pharmacopoeia* of 1864 [13].

The Society of Apothecaries after 1617

Adulteration of imported spices and drugs was a long-standing problem. The Wardens of the Grocers' Company had originally been made responsible for the 'garbling' of food and drugs (examining and removing impurities found in them) early in the 15th century. They continued to do so, but the 1617 Charter gave the Society of Apothecaries the power to search apothecaries' shops in London and for 7 miles around it, and to inspect their drugs. The Society was concerned about the poor quality of drugs that, they said, were being supplied to them by the druggists. To combat this problem they opened their own dispensary in 1623, so that they could supply their members with preparations guaranteed to be of good quality [14].

This venture was very successful, and those apothecaries who had originally invested in the company found it to be a profitable undertaking. This encouraged other members to take shares. With the growing use of chemicals in medicine, a chemical laboratory was opened in 1671, so that the complete range of medicines and galenicals could be supplied. In 1703, the Society was granted the contract to supply the Royal Navy with medicines, and this monopoly continued until 1823. The Society also supplied the Army and the East India Company with their requirements. Their commercial ventures continued as a profitable source of income for members until 1922, when the laboratories and the associated retail shop were closed [15].

Apothecaries and physicians, 1617 to 1701

The Charter of 1617 stated that before anyone could become a freeman of the Society of Apothecaries, he had to serve an apprenticeship with a master apothecary for a period of 7 years, followed by an examination. During this time, the apprentice was thoroughly versed in all aspects of the business. He would be trained in recognising all the substances in use and the secrets of compounding these into medicines, in accordance with the physician's instructions. It was not unusual for the apothecary to visit the patient, usually alone, although sometimes they would accompany the physician.

The principal role of the Royal College of Physicians was to prevent unlicensed medical practice. The physicians had a monopoly within the City of London and for a 7-mile radius around it, and they bitterly resented the encroachment of the apothecaries. The position was complicated, because the apothecaries' charter did not specifically prevent them examining and treating patients, although it was accepted that they could not charge for their services, only for the medicines supplied.

There were other factors favouring the apothecaries' service. During the Civil War (1642–1649), the apothecaries largely supported the parliamentary cause. The physicians' patients, many of whom came from the ruling classes, left London and the physicians followed them, leaving the apothecaries to continue serving the remaining population. This position was further aggravated during the plague of 1665, when again most of the apothecaries stayed with the people. This consolidated their role in giving medical advice and supplying medicines. The final factor was the Great Fire of London in 1666, during which the Guildhall and the Apothecaries' Hall were destroyed. Because the Society of Apothecaries was in a stronger position, they were able to rebuild their premises quickly and re-establish their position in London.

There were numerous handbills and posters issued by both sides drawing attention to the shortcomings of the other. The members of the College of Physicians particularly objected to losing their dispensing business to apothecaries, who were in competition with them. In 1696, to resolve the problem, the physicians opened their own dispensary at their premises in Warwick Lane. Two other dispensaries were opened in London, both of which were staffed by apothecaries. The Society of

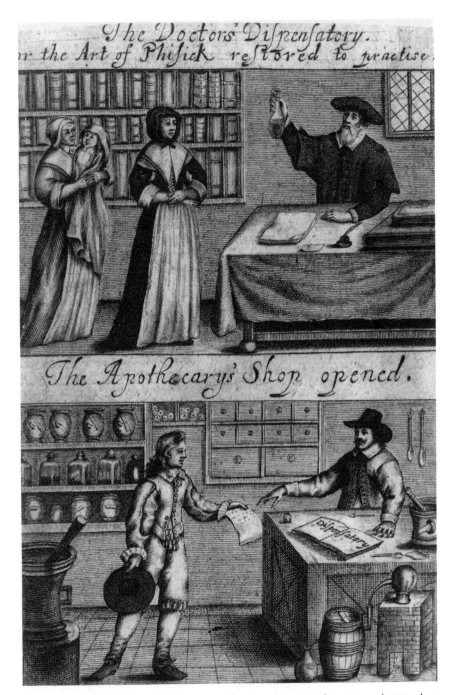

Figure 4.4 The doctor's dispersary and the apothecary's shop opened. Woodcut, about 1680, by William Faithorne. Reproduced by permission of The Trustees of the British Museum.

Apothecaries complained bitterly, although it is unlikely that it had much effect on the apothecaries' businesses and the venture was closed in 1725 [16].

The Rose Case

Matters were brought to a head in February 1701. William Rose was an apothecary with a business in Nicholas Lane, St Martin-in-the-Fields. He treated William Seale, a butcher, administering medicines to him without acting under the directions of a physician, and without asking for or taking any fee, but charging for the medicines. The Royal College of Physicians brought an action before the Court of the Queen's Bench under Lord Chief Justice Holt. The case against Rose was based on the physicians' charter, confirmed by other Acts of Parliament, which prohibited any persons, not members of the College, from practising medicine in London or for 7 miles around.

The facts were not disputed and the jury referred the question of whether Rose had practised medicine to the Court. The Court judged that the business of an apothecary was to make and compound or prepare the prescription of a physician. In this case Rose had acted as a physician by diagnosing the disease and also prescribing the best remedy to be applied for its treatment and so judgement was given in favour of the Royal College of Physicians.

The Attorney General advised the Society of Apothecaries, on behalf of Rose, to move a 'writ of error' in the House of Lords asking for a reversal of the judgement. The Society based their arguments on the 'custom and practice' of the business of the apothecary to make and compound medicines and supply these to all persons, without charging a fee for any advice given. In their opinion, the physicians were attempting to use their charter to create a monopoly of medicine, to the prejudice of the poor who could not afford their charges, and the sick, who could not always obtain the services of a physician readily in the case of sudden accidents and illness.

After hearing the evidence presented by both sides, their Lordships accepted the argument that it was contrary to custom and against the public interest to prevent the apothecaries from giving advice and treatment. They reversed the judgement of the Queen's Bench, finding in favour of the Society of Apothecaries [17]. This case had a profound influence on the activity of the apothecary. It legitimised his activity as a practitioner of medicine, and the majority of apothecaries developed in this direction, supplying medicines and giving advice on treatment. It also encouraged the chemist and druggist's role as a dispenser of medical prescriptions.

The rise of the chemists and druggists, 1701 to 1815

Once the rights of the members of the Society of Apothecaries were clearly established, their relationship with the physicians was much smoother. In due course, the apothecaries were recognised by the physicians as fellow practitioners, but with a lesser social standing. Adam Smith wrote in 1790 that they were 'the physicians of the poor at all times and of the rich when the danger is not very great'.

Apothecaries now had to contend with competition from the increasing number of chemists and druggists. Because of the growing emphasis on free trade, the control of the Guilds over who could open a business was weakened. This, coupled with the growth of credit now available from the chemist's wholesale suppliers, enabled many young men who had finished their apprenticeship with an apothecary or a chemist and druggist to start their own business [18].

There is some debate as to when the terms 'druggist' and 'chemist and druggist' were first used. It has been suggested that the first official use of the term 'druggist' was in the preliminary to the charter of the Royal College of Physicians presented to Charles II in 1663 in order to gain greater powers for their Guild. It refers to the 'frauds, abuses and deceits of diverse apothecaries, druggists and others'. This charter was not granted, but it confirms that the term was in use [19].

The term 'chemist and druggist' became the most frequently used title. The rapid increase in the number of chemists and druggists, and the relative stability of the numbers of members of the Society of Apothecaries, can be judged from the entries in succeeding issues of the London Directory and the Post Office Directory. The change was from nine apothecaries, two chemists and 38 druggists in 1738 to 24 apothecaries, and 127 chemists, druggists, or chemists and druggists in 1800. The numbers of apothecaries are probably understated, because only those keeping an open shop would wish to be listed [20].

Apothecaries and chemists and druggists

While the Rose Case of 1701 had effectively settled the dispute between the apothecaries and the physicians, disagreements between the apothecaries and the chemists and druggists emerged, each side accusing the other of supplying adulterated drugs and preparations. The apothecaries complained that the druggists were making up prescriptions and selling pharmaceutical preparations, although they had no training or classical education. This was not entirely accurate – the druggists went through a period of apprenticeship to a chemist and druggist master or in some cases to an apothecary, followed by a period as an assistant.

Opportunities for apprenticeship increased with the increasing number of chemists and druggists' shops. Although there was no restriction on who might open a chemist's shop, there is no evidence that they were opened by untrained people. When the Medicine Stamp Act was introduced in 1783, it listed any 'surgeon, apothecary, chymist or druggist who had served a regular apprenticeship as exempt to sell compounded medicines free of tax'. This was the first piece of legislation affecting the retail chemist and druggist.

The Apothecaries Bill 1748

The jurisdiction of the Society of Apothecaries applied only to their members, so they sought a monopoly over the supply of medicines in order to have control over the druggists. A petition was presented to parliament on behalf of the apothecaries of London, supported by apothecaries in other areas of the country, as well as non-members. This explained that physicians and surgeons had to be examined by the respective colleges and approved by their colleagues before they could practise. There was, however, no restraint on anyone acting as an apothecary, and they believed that the compounding and sale of medicines should be subject to similar safeguards. They asked the House of Commons to grant such remedy as they thought fit.

A committee of the House was formed to consider the petition and reported back after due deliberation, deciding that the best course of action was to revive the legislation passed in an Act of Parliament in 1724. This gave the physicians the power to search for and destroy unfit drugs on the premises of apothecaries *and* chemists and druggists. This was not the expected outcome, and the Society of Apothecaries now had the embarrassment of having to oppose their own Apothecaries Bill of 1748. Their position was saved as parliament was prorogued before the bill was heard, and it lapsed [21].

Although this attempt to introduce control over the compounding and sale of medicines did not succeed, the problems caused for apothecaries by unlicensed and untrained retailers, and the competition from chemists and druggists, continued. The next attempt to introduce control was by a private group of apothecaries, not through the Society.

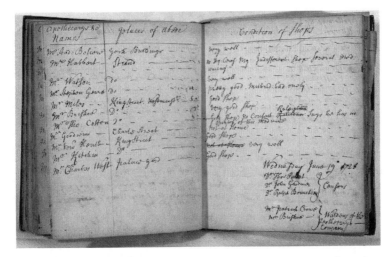

Figure 4.5 Extract from Visitation notebook recording inspections of apothecaries' shops by members of the Royal College of Physicians. Reproduced by permission of the Royal College of Physicians.

Meetings were held to discuss the situation and it was proposed to form a general association of apothecaries with the title the 'General Pharmaceutical Association of Great Britain' [22]. The elected committee decided to contact all the educated practitioners of pharmacy throughout Britain, to ask for their support. They also set out to gather information on the malpractices that were rife in the country.

Evidence was collected showing that adulterated drugs were being used, that prescriptions were being incorrectly compounded, and that some grocers in country districts were prescribing and selling medicines. This information was collated and copies given to the College of Physicians, the Corporation of Surgeons and the Society of Apothecaries. On 6 February 1795, a petition was presented on their behalf by Sir William Dolben, asking parliament to rule that all physicians' prescriptions could only be compounded by trained apothecaries after they had undergone a 5-year apprenticeship and an examination to judge their competence. This probably went too far – it did not get support and the Pharmaceutical Association broke up [23].

The Apothecaries Act 1815

In 1802 a new Medicine Act was passed, which extended the range of stamp duty to many common remedies in addition to patent medicines. Some amendments to the Act were granted after the apothecaries and the chemists joined together to oppose them, but there was still an increase in costs. A further cost increase resulted from the imposition of a tax on glass, introduced in 1812. This pressure on the apothecaries' profit added to the difficulties they were facing caused by the growing competition from chemists and druggists, and some action had to be taken [24].

At a meeting held to discuss what they could do to deal with the effects of the increase in costs, it was suggested that it would be more useful to concentrate on improving the position of the profession as a whole, not just one aspect of their problems. An Association was formed, which elected a committee to take this matter forward and drafted a bill to place before parliament. This proposed the creation of a separate body with the power to examine apothecaries, surgeon-apothecaries, midwives and dispensing chemists. They would also be given the power to grant practice licences, to regulate apprenticeships, and to found schools to train candidates in medicine and pharmacy.

The Association tried to enlist the support of the College of Physicians, the College of Surgeons and the Society of Apothecaries. The two colleges were not keen to become involved. The sponsors of the bill were members of the Society of Apothecaries, so it was placed in a difficult position, but declined to be involved. The chemists and druggists, on the other hand, responded vigorously. Their main objection was to the proposed management structure, as they were excluded from the managing committee. This would have had power to decide the appropriate qualification for compounders and dispensers of medicine [25].

The Standing Committee of chemists and druggists formed in 1802 to protect their interests now took over the action. An advertisement was placed in *The Times, Morning Herald*, and other newspapers to enlist the support of chemists and druggists nationally, and MPs were also approached. It was emphasised that chemists and druggists had long experience in making up prescriptions for medical practitioners, and were more competent at compounding than the apothecaries. Consequently it was unacceptable to give the apothecaries power over chemists and druggists. A meeting was then held with the Society of Apothecaries and they agreed to withdraw any reference to chemists and druggists in their bill.

Divergence of apothecaries, chemists and druggists, 1815 to 1841

The Apothecaries Act of 1815 was subsequently placed on the statute book, although it was unsatisfactory in many respects. It introduced some control over the practice of medicine, and anyone practising medicine without legal qualifications could be fined. However, less reputable practitioners avoided the consequences by declaring themselves bankrupt; experienced practitioners who were not members of the Society were often pursued, many thought unfairly.

These regulations did not apply to surgeons or midwives: the chemists and druggists were unaffected and continued to give advice and dispense. There was little protection for the public, who found it difficult to distinguish between the service given by the apothecaries and the chemists and druggists. The major difference between the apothecary and the dispensing chemist was that the apothecary visited the patient at home. The dispensing chemist did not leave his shop, but otherwise offered a similar service [26].

By the 1820s, the practice of both medicine and pharmacy had become unsustainable. In theory, practically anyone who wanted to enter medicine could open a shop, setting themselves up as a chemist and druggist, without any training. The trained chemists, who had served an apprenticeship, agreed that this was unsatisfactory and a solution had to be found.

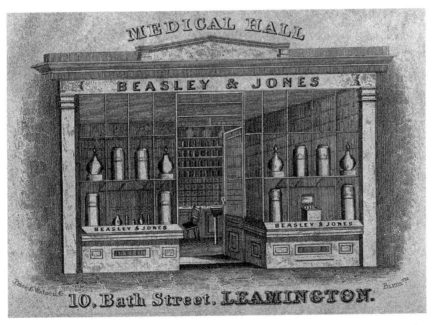

Figure 4.6 Trade card of Beasley and Jones, chemists at Leamington, showing the shop front about 1820. Reproduced by permission of the Wellcome Library, London.

There were a number of attempts to remedy the situation. Enquiries were held and draft bills proposed. Henry Warburton MP was appointed chairman of a Parliamentary Select Committee of enquiry into the medical profession. Eventually a bill was drafted proposing that a college of medicine should be established. Only those registered by the college following an examination would be allowed to practise medicine. One of the weaknesses of this measure was that there were no sanctions on those who would continue to practise even if unqualified. There were other complications, and the bill was withdrawn.

Clause 28 of the Apothecaries Act 1815 stated that nothing in the Act would in any way affect the trade or business of a chemist and druggist, in the buying, preparing, compounding, dispensing or vending of drugs, medicines and medicinal compounds, wholesale and retail. The chemists and druggists continued to recommend treatments. Some went much further, visiting their customers, diagnosing disease and supplying medicine. This created the situation where the Society of Apothecaries was prosecuting physicians who had undergone a course of medical education and examination, because they had not obtained the licence of the Society of Apothecaries; while druggists who had no medical training, but were acting as medical practitioners, were not prosecuted.

The licentiates of the apothecaries considered this very unfair and in 1814 brought a case against a chemist called Greenhough, who regularly left his shop to visit his customers, acting in every way as an apothecary. The case was heard before Mr Justice Maul. He asked the jury to rule whether Greenhough had acted as an apothecary and they ruled in his favour. The apothecaries appealed to the judges of the King's Bench, who agreed with their submission that he had acted as an apothecary. The judges were of the strong opinion that chemists and druggists could not act as apothecaries and were restricted to the trade of a chemist and druggist, selling medicines as set out in the original Act [27].

The formation of the Pharmaceutical Society, 1841

This ruling created a difficult situation that was further complicated by a bill introduced in 1841 by Benjamin Hawse MP, a member of Warburton's committee. Initially it was believed that this bill was aimed at the reform of the medical profession and did not apply to pharmacy. When the bill was published in February, however, it was clear that it did. It proposed that after 1 February 1842, no person could practise medicine without a certificate, and after December 1842, no one could carry out the business of a chemist and druggist without a certificate issued according to the provisions of the Act. This would have placed the chemists and druggists under the supervision of the apothecaries.

The bill defined 'practising medicine' as recommending, prescribing or ordering any medicine, remedy or application. The responsibility of the chemist and druggist was defined as a person who shall deal in, mix or dispense for sale any drug or medicine. If this became law the chemist and druggist would not have the right to prescribe, and he could also be prosecuted for recommending a simple medicine or instructing the patient how to take his medicine. The members of the proposed ruling council who were to administer the Act did not include a chemist and this was also unacceptable [28].

A meeting was called for 15 February 1841 at the Crown and Anchor Tavern in the Strand. Many of the leading members of the profession were present, including William Allen, Jacob Bell, Thomas Keating and J S Leischer. They formed a committee to collate the objections to the bill. This committee met with Mr Hawes, who agreed to withdraw the bill and to reword it without any reference to the chemists and druggists. It was reintroduced with some modifications, but these were also unacceptable, and the bill failed to get any support in the House of Commons.

It was obvious to the committee that if they were to have any control over the future of pharmacy, they had to take the initiative to introduce a system of education and to put their activities on a professional footing, otherwise parliament would eventually pass legislation that could put the control of pharmacy into the hands of others. Jacob Bell was keen to make progress. He was well aware that the chemists and druggists were willing to work together to oppose legislation that would affect their business, but it was considered unlikely that they would be prepared to join and support a permanent organisation.

Objectives of the Society

Many meetings were held in London before a way forward could be found, and it was not until 5 April 1841 that a proposal to form the Pharmaceutical Society of Great Britain was agreed. The Society would have the objectives of benefiting the public, elevating the profession of pharmacy by proper education, protecting the collective and individual interests of its members in the event of a hostile attack in parliament or otherwise, and establishing a club to relieve decayed or distressed members. A public meeting of chemists and druggists was held at the Crown and Anchor Tavern on 15 April 1841 at which the resolution was explained and then put to the meeting. It was unanimously accepted [29].

Much remained to be done. Regulations for the Society were drawn up and agreed at a further meeting on 1 June 1841. It was resolved that the committee would form the first Council of the Society who would hold office until May 1842, when the number would be reduced to 21 members by election. Premises were rented at 17 Bloomsbury Square, London, in December and this enabled the work of establishing a School of Pharmacy to begin, coupled with drawing up the examination regulations and the appointment of examiners.

The first anniversary meeting was held on 17 May 1842. William Allen, the president, presented a progress report. This was considered satisfactory, and there was a healthy financial position, because the money collected to oppose the 1815 Act had been passed over to the Society by its trustees. The foundation of the Society marked an important change in the control and development of the profession of pharmacy. Up until this point, the members' energies had been spent trying to protect their businesses and themselves from control by the physicians and surgeons through Acts of Parliament. Now the initiative was taken by the chemists and druggists to protect their public and their profession [30].

Charter of Incorporation

The profession was fortunate in being led by dedicated men of great ability. They understood the importance of providing for the education of the members and the need to achieve acceptable professional standards, by examination of new entrants to the profession. Their lead was supported countrywide and soon lectures on suitable subjects were being given in many provincial centres. A significant milestone was reached on 5 November 1842, when the Council presented a petition to the Queen, seeking the grant of a Royal Charter of Incorporation. This was granted on 16 February 1843 and officially recognised the efforts of the Pharmaceutical Society, indicating that its objectives were approved of by the government of the day.

A great deal was achieved in a short space of time. Despite some members of the medical profession regarding the Society with suspicion, the foundations of a professional body were laid. The education and advancement of its members was under way, and the profession could now speak with one voice. That voice belonged to the owners of businesses, for only owners could be admitted to membership of the Society.

References

1. Davies S. *A Century of Troubles, 1600 to 1700*. London: Pan Macmillan, 2001: 7–9.
2. Davies S. *A Century of Troubles, 1600 to 1700*. London: Pan Macmillan, 2001: 11.
3. Lane J, Earles M. *John Hall and His Patients, with a Medical Commentary by Melvin Earles*. Stratford upon Avon: The Shakespeare Birthplace Trust, 1996: xxxiii.
4. Lane J, Earles M. *John Hall and His Patients, with a Medical Commentary by Melvin Earles*. Stratford upon Avon: The Shakespeare Birthplace Trust, 1996: xx.
5. Bowser W. *The Medical Background of Anglo Saxon England*. London: Wellcome Historical Library, 1993.
6. Bieth M. *Healing Threads*. Edinburgh: Polygon, 1995: 84.
7. Thompson C J S. *Quacks of Old London*. New York: Barnes & Noble Inc., reprinted 1993: 43.
8. Matthews L G. *History of Pharmacy in Britain*. Edinburgh: E & S Livingstone, 1962: 291.
9. Thompson C J S. *Quacks of Old London*. New York: Barnes & Noble Inc., reprinted 1993: 255.
10. Sloan A W. *English Medicine in the Seventeenth Century*. Bishop Auckland: Durham Academic Press, 1996.
11. Thompson C J S. *The Mystery and Art of the Apothecary*. London: Lane, 1929: 143.
12. Matthews L G. *History of Pharmacy in Britain*. Edinburgh: E & S Livingstone, 1962: 86–87.
13. Grier J. *A History of Pharmacy*. London: Pharmaceutical Press, 1937: 141–145.
14. Grier J. *A History of Pharmacy*. London: Pharmaceutical Press, 1937: 111.
15. Matthews L G. *History of Pharmacy in Britain*. Edinburgh: E & S Livingstone, 1962: 190.
16. Matthews L G. *History of Pharmacy in Britain*. Edinburgh: E & S Livingstone, 1962: 113.
17. Hunt J A. Echoing down the years. *The Pharmaceutical Journal* 2001; 266: 191–195.
18. Copeman W S C. *The Worshipful Society of Apothecaries of London. 1617–1815*. Oxford: Oxford University Press, 1986: 53.
19. The closing century. *Chemist & Druggist* 1900; 56: 142.
20. The title of Chemist and Druggist. *Chemist & Druggist* 1926; 105: 90.
21. Attempted legislation in 1748. *Chemist & Druggist* 1926; 105: 198.
22. Hunt J A, Jones I F. The first Pharmaceutical Society: A history of the General Pharmaceutical Association of Great Britain. *The Pharmaceutical Journal* 1997; 259: 997–999.

23. Bell J, Redwood T. *An Historical Sketch of the Progress of Pharmacy in Great Britain.* London: The Pharmaceutical Society of Great Britain, 1880: 40.
24. Newman C. *The Evolution of Medical Practice in the Nineteenth Century.* London: Oxford University Press, 1957: 59.
25. Bell J, Redwood T. *An Historical Sketch of the Progress of Pharmacy in Great Britain.* London: The Pharmaceutical Society of Great Britain, 1880: 51.
26. Burnby J G L. A study of the English apothecary from 1660 to 1760. *Medical History Supplement* 1983; 3: 1–128.
27. The Apothecaries Company [report]. *The Lancet* 1841–42; 1: 159–162.
28. Bell J, Redwood T. *An Historical Sketch of the Progress of Pharmacy in Great Britain.* London: The Pharmaceutical Society of Great Britain, 1880: 88.
29. Holloway S W F. *Royal Pharmaceutical Society of Great Britain 1841 to 1991: A Political and Social History.* London: Pharmaceutical Press, 1991: 91–92.
30. The first annual meeting of the Pharmaceutical Society [report]. *The Pharmaceutical Journal* 1841–1842; 1: 633–639.

5

Pharmacy in the modern world, 1841 to 1986 AD

John A Hunt

The foundation of the Pharmaceutical Society of Great Britain ('the Society') in 1841 represents the beginnings of modern pharmacy in Britain. This chapter briefly explores its first 150 years. William Allen, the first president of the Society, had excellent connections with senior political figures, and this greatly helped to give the Society a firm foundation. Within a year the Society had over 2000 members, and as early as February 1843 it was granted a Royal Charter [1].

The Society's early history was often turbulent, with continuing skirmishes over professional boundaries, the formalisation of the pharmacist's education, and the outbreak of two world wars. Two themes, the rise of the multiples and the powers of the Society, are intimately tied up with the development of community pharmacy, and are considered in Chapter 6. However, one development had a much wider impact, and that was the emergence of the welfare state. This is the focus of the present chapter.

Professional boundaries

In the early Victorian period the boundaries between the healthcare professions continued to be vague and ill defined. Patients still had a confusing choice – they might consult an apothecary and receive free medical advice but pay high prices for drugs; or they could consult a physician whose medicines might be less expensive but whose advice would be costly. A prescription given by the physician could be taken to an apothecary or to a chemist and druggist, who would possibly be less expensive. Alternatively they might opt for a 'counter prescription' from the chemist and druggist, a proprietary product, or a 'nostrum' made to the chemist's own formula.

The chemists and druggists were constantly criticised by other groups for their lack of training and qualifications. For example, the father of Jacob Bell, a founder of the Society, had worked for many years in the Post Office, decided to leave, took over a chemist and druggist's business in Haymarket without significant training, and was successful [2]. From the beginning a principal aim of the Society had been to establish proper training and qualifications and to counter these criticisms.

These confusing healthcare boundaries were largely peculiar to England and Wales. In other countries in Europe and in Scotland it was usual for physicians to write prescriptions and for apothecaries to dispense them, dispensing by doctors often being forbidden. In England and Wales apothecaries had largely evolved into what we now call general medical practitioners. The consequence was that the doctors dispensed most of their prescriptions themselves. This left the emerging class of chemists and druggists, who evolved into the pharmacists of today, with little dispensing activity. At the end of the Victorian period pharmacists probably dispensed less than 10% of prescriptions written in England and Wales. The result was that pharmacists were dependent on 'over the counter' trade for much of their livelihood. The 'chemist' was regarded as a shopkeeper, selling a wide variety of medicines, toiletries and various other goods.

The situation was at the root of many problems until at least 1911. In continental Europe pharmacists were able to concentrate on dispensing prescriptions written by doctors and on giving health advice – this resulted in highly professional establishments, a difference that is still evident when pharmacies in Britain are compared with those in France and Germany. The restricted title 'pharmacist' was slow to be adopted in Britain. Even in the early years of the 21st century the term 'pharmacist' is not well understood, and the less specific term 'chemist' persists in the public mind and, equally, in reports on pharmaceutical affairs in the media.

Early years, 1841 to 1911

Following the grant of the Royal Charter the founders of the new Society set about developing a legal framework for pharmacy: this eventually resulted in the Pharmacy Act of 1852. The Act restricted certain titles, such as pharmaceutical chemist and pharmaceutist, to those who had passed the Society's major examination. It also established a register of successful candidates. It did not prevent others from practising pharmacy, and did not provide a legal definition of the practice of pharmacy. Opponents of the bill were concerned that a monopoly of trade should not

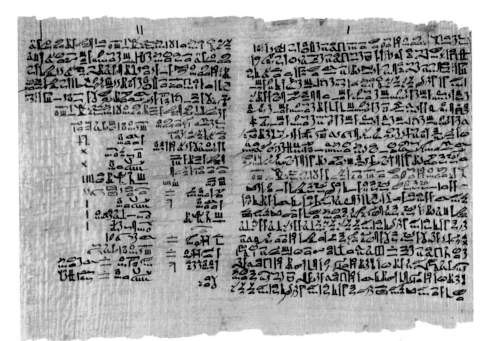

Plate 1 Papyrus Ebers, scroll dating from c. 1552 BC and discovered by Georg Ebers in 1872/1873. Reproduced by permission of Leipzig University Library (Papyrus Ebers, Cols I–II, alt. nos XXXXVII and XXXXVIII, Universitätsbibliothek Leipzig).

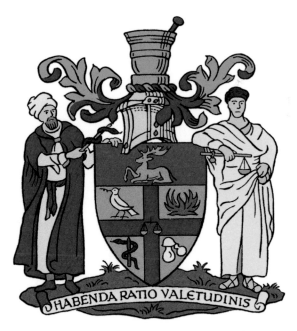

HABENDA RATIO VALETUDINIS

Plate 2 Coat of arms of the Royal Pharmaceutical Society of Great Britain, depicting Avicenna (left) and Galen (right).

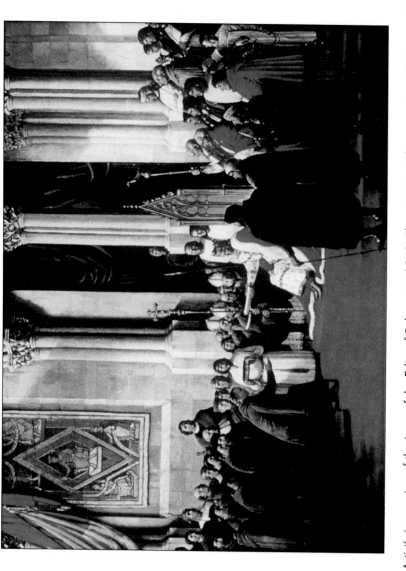

Plate 3 Artist's impression of the issue of the Edict of Palermo in 1240. The painting, 'The separation of pharmacy from medicine', is from the series 'Great Moments in Pharmacy' commissioned by Parke, Davis & Company from the artist, Robert A Thom, between 1948 and 1964. Reproductions of the series were distributed to pharmacists throughout North America as a means of promoting public knowledge of pharmacy. Reproduced by permission of Pfizer Limited.

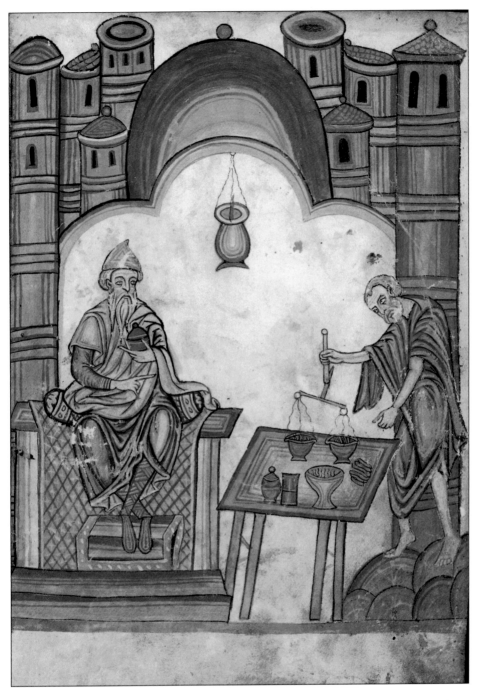

Plate 4 Pharmacy, Germany, early 13th century. Reproduced from Eton ms 204 by permission of the Provost and Fellows of Eton College.

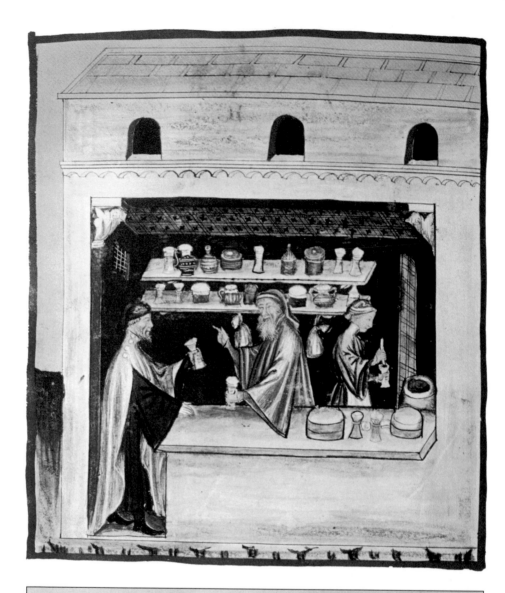

Triacha. ꝯpo. ca. ꝛ. fic. Glectꝰ que libāt gallum. auencōꝛ q̃ ꞇranfit. x̃ . annū. ymam̃. ꝯ̃ uenen̄
ꞇ egꞇuꝛices. ca. ꞇ. fri. nocum̃. p̃. x. annos. facit uigilias. Remō nocī. cū ifrigiꝛantibꝫ. uꞇ.aꝗ
oꝛꝛeū ꝯuemꞇ mag· frī. ſembꝫ. breme .ꝛ ꞇgioibꝫ. frīs. ubiꝗꝫ tn̄. cū fiūꞇ necꞇum̃ꝫ .

Plate 5 Apothecary's shop showing preparation of theriac around 1390.
Reproduced from the manuscript Tacuinum Sanitatis, probably of Veronese origin, by
permission of the Austrian National Library (Bildarchiv, ÖNB, Wien).

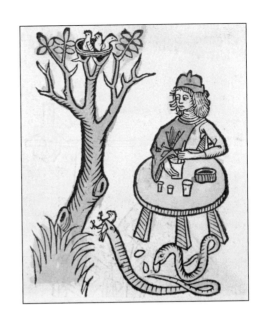

Plate 6 Apothecary preparing theriac. Hand-coloured woodcut from Ortus Sanitatis, Tractatus de animalibus, published in Mainz in 1491.

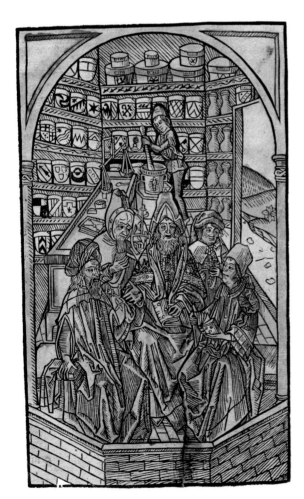

Plate 7 Five old apothecaries in an apothecary's shop; an apprentice works with a pestle and mortar in the background. Coloured woodcut from Hortus Sanitatis, published in Augsburg in 1496. Reproduced by permission of the Wellcome Library, London.

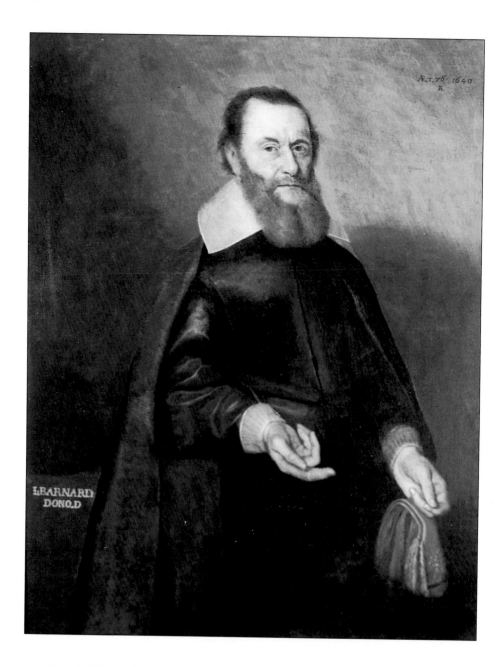

Plate 8 Gideon de Laune in 1640. Oil painting in the style of Cornelis Jonson van Ceulen. Reproduced by kind permission of the Worshipful Society of Apothecaries of London.

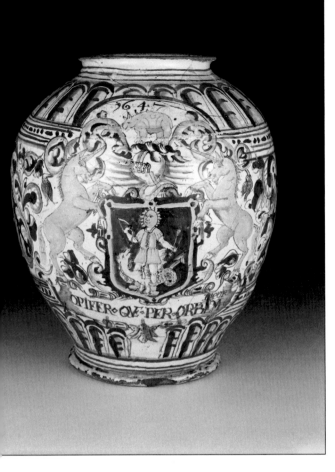

Plate 9 Delftware tin-glazed earthenware drug or display jar bearing the coat of arms of the Worshipful Society of Apothecaries; dated 1647.

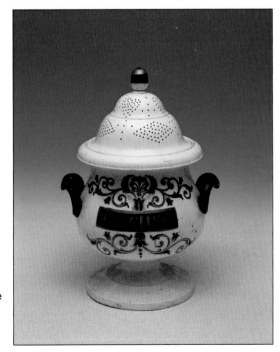

Plate 10 Decorative leech jars were a feature of pharmacies in the early 19th century and were often accompanied by matching storage jars for tamarind and honey.

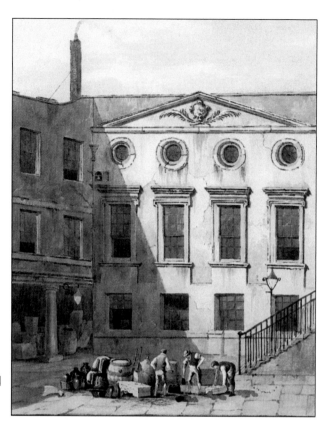

Plate 11 Courtyard of the Apothecaries' Hall painted by George Shepherd in 1814. Reproduced by the permission of the Worshipful Society of Apothecaries of London.

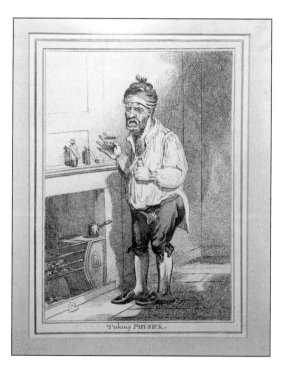

Taking PHYSICK.

Plate 12 'Taking Physick'. Cartoon by James Gillray, c. 1800.

be granted to a chartered body. These deficiencies were to pose serious threats when the National Insurance Bill was published in 1911 [3].

Later, the Pharmacy Act of 1868 gave the Society the right to examine and to set up a register of all chemists and druggists, in addition to the register of pharmaceutical chemists. It restricted further titles, such as pharmacist and chemist and druggist, to registered persons. However, the legislation was largely related to the sale of poisons, and it was public fears about the increasing problem of poisoning that had, in part, led to the enactment. The Society had hoped to restrict 'the dispensing or compounding of the prescriptions of physicians and surgeons' to registered persons, but that was a step too far for the politicians of the day. The 1868 Pharmacy Act created a register of those who might 'keep open shop for retailing, selling or compounding poisons'. In this way, the emphasis on 'trade' as opposed to dispensing activities was maintained. Again, this was to pose problems in 1911, when *The Lancet* was quick to point out that existing poisons legislation offered little protection to pharmacists, as it referred only to sales, not to the dispensing of prescriptions [4].

Threats to pharmacy

A judgement in 1880 opened the way for multiple shop ownership by corporate bodies, of which the pioneer was Jesse Boot (see Chapter 6). Others followed rapidly, both in London and the provinces. They secured business by offering medicines at reduced prices, employing their greater purchasing power to buy on beneficial terms. This was to cause considerable resentment in the ranks of independent traders [5].

One of the people who found themselves in this position was William (later Sir William) Glyn-Jones (1869–1927). Following a brief period working in the office of a mining surveyor, he served a pharmacy apprenticeship in Aberdare and then moved to London. He worked initially as a dispensing assistant to doctors in Fulham and Bermondsey, attending evening classes in pharmacy and qualifying in 1891 [6]. His thoughts turned to medicine as a career and he went so far as to register as a medical student, but in 1893 he opened a pharmacy business in the East India Dock Road.

At a time when doctors did almost all dispensing in such localities themselves, and the sale of proprietary medicines, a major part of retail pharmacy business, was beset by price-cutting by the larger stores, Glyn-Jones faced considerable problems, but in both these issues he became a leading protagonist.

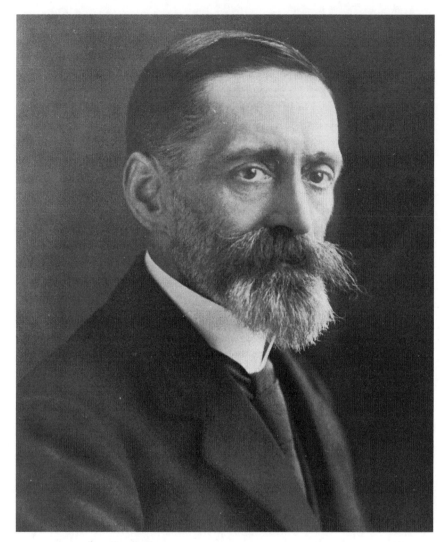

Figure 5.1 Sir William Glyn-Jones.

Proprietary Articles Trade Association

Glyn-Jones took decisive action to address the problems besetting pharmacy; he established a monthly journal, *The Anti-Cutting Record*, in 1895. This, reported *The Pharmaceutical Journal*, was to be sent to every chemist in business in the UK and was stated to be 'published in the interest of retail pharmacists, wholesale patent medicine dealers and of the proprietors who ensure a fair profit to the vendors of their articles'. It declared [7]:

> If we are satisfied that the manufacturer is taking steps to ensure a living profit on his goods, we will do everything that lies in our power to assist him, and will always discountenance the practice of substitution in connection with his article. On the other hand, we will do all in our power to facilitate the retailer being able to offer a suitable substitute which does bear a profit, in place of the article of the manufacturer who refuses to protect when the great bulk of the work and expense in connection with that protection is taken off his hand.

Pharmacists willing to support the scheme were invited to pay an annual subscription of half-a-crown. The established journals were doubtful and *The Pharmaceutical Journal* commented: 'Whether the promoters of this scheme will be able to any extent to overcome the inertia that so widely prevails is doubtful' [8]. The *Chemist & Druggist* commented similarly. In fact things moved rapidly: the Proprietary Articles Trade Association (PATA) held the first meeting of its Council in February 1896, and within a year a major new force in pricing affairs had been established.

The rapidity with which the PATA was established was largely a result of the efforts of Glyn-Jones. In the first six months of 1896 he addressed local pharmaceutical association meetings in Exeter, Nottingham, Edinburgh, Leeds, Halifax, Sheffield and Cardiff, as well as London. The *Anti-Cutting Record* became the official PATA journal and by 1908 had reached a circulation of over 10,000. So began the practice of retail price maintenance (RPM) with regard to medicines, an enterprise that served the interests of 'the pharmaceutical calling' until recently [8]. RPM for medicines was finally ended in 2001.

The Chemists' Defence Association

The name of Glyn-Jones was becoming well known in pharmaceutical politics, and he was elected to serve on the Pharmaceutical Society's council in 1899. His immediate areas of interest included doctor dispensing and support for pharmacists involved in legal action. He moved quickly, through the PATA council, to establish a chemists' defence fund, which in November 1899 was established as The Chemists' Defence Association Limited.

Its aims were to provide legal advice and defence on all matters relating to business, to watch new legislation, and to appoint a legal adviser and an analytical chemist for the purpose. A prospectus was issued setting out 20 rules. On 2 December 1899 *The Pharmaceutical Journal* reported

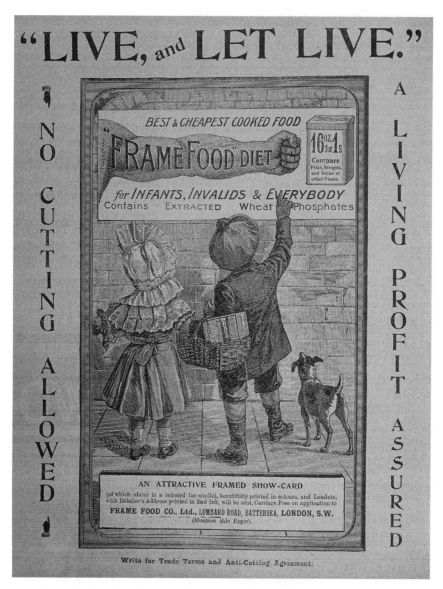

Figure 5.2 Extract from the *Anti-Cutting Record*, March 1897.

that the Association had 'fairly commenced business' and went on to say: 'Mr Glyn-Jones is a plausible speaker, and his success in securing support for his latest venture ... seems to be only second to that which attended the establishment of the Proprietary Articles Trade Association' [9]. Already Glyn-Jones was earning the reputation that later moved Lloyd George to refer to him as 'the Welsh terrier' [10].

The Drug Trade Appeal Fund

Glyn-Jones next turned his attention to the Medicine Stamp Acts, which taxed the retail sale of proprietary medicinal products. Under the Acts, a number of prosecutions were being brought by the Inland Revenue against pharmacists. In 1902 Glyn-Jones brought a test case to court in which he based his defence on a long dormant exemption that had granted chemists the right to sell 'known, admitted and approved remedies' free from stamp duty. He was successful, and the subsequent decision of the High Court in 1903 in the case of *Farmer v. Glyn-Jones* restored this right to the trade.

This action had convinced him of the need to establish a fund to support pharmacists in appeals against unsatisfactory judgements. Through a letter to *The Pharmaceutical Journal* in July 1902 [11] he established the Drug Trade Appeal Fund, and rapidly raised over £1000 for the purpose. In August 1902 a committee was established to administer the fund. At the same meeting a warning was given, which was not always heeded in the future. Glyn-Jones was not of robust constitution, and frequently allowed his intense work activities to compromise his health. He was to die at the age of 58 with his work unfinished [8].

The Poisons and Pharmacy Act 1908

The legal framework within which pharmacy was operating at the end of the 19th century was unsatisfactory. Bills were introduced to parliament on behalf of the Society in 1903, 1904 and 1905, but all failed. At the Liberal election victory in 1906 a pharmacist, Richard Winfrey, was elected to represent south-west Norfolk. He introduced further bills for the Society in 1906, 1907 and 1908, which again failed. The government introduced its own bill in 1908, and following a reconciliation of views between William Glyn-Jones and Jesse Boot, the Act became law in December 1908.

The Poisons and Pharmacy Act regularised the position of corporate bodies, and also permitted the sale of certain poisons for agricultural and horticultural use by unqualified traders authorised for the purpose by local authorities [12]. Glyn-Jones was instrumental in securing the passage of the Act. It offered advantages for pharmacy, later put to good use in the 1911 National Insurance Act. The problems encountered during the passage of the 1908 Act highlighted the need for the Society to be well prepared for securing members' interests in any proposed future legislation. At the annual general meeting of the Society in May 1908 he secured the establishment of a Parliamentary Fund to oppose certain sections of the government's bill [13]. In April 1909 *The Pharmaceutical Journal* reported that Glyn-Jones, now Parliamentary Secretary to the Society, was likely to be adopted as a parliamentary candidate [14]. He secured his seat in parliament as the Liberal member for Stepney in December that year.

The power of the medical profession grew steadily during the 19th century. The British Medical Association (BMA) was formed at a meeting in Birmingham in 1856 from members of the Provincial Medical and Surgical Association. It renamed its journal the *British Medical Journal*. By 1901 the BMA had a membership of over 18,400 and was a substantial body [15]. There were many issues, particularly the making, supply and dispensing of medicines and poisons, where the medical profession shared an interest with the pharmacy profession.

By 1910 discussions were in hand between the Society and the BMA around a range of topics, with ten delegates from each body. Points at issue included dispensing by doctors, and whether this should be transferred to pharmacists; unqualified prescribing (counter prescribing by pharmacists) and how it might be prevented; and the possibility of joint action to curb the sale of dangerous, secret or useless 'nostrums'. In December 1910 the issues remained unresolved, but they were about to be completely overtaken by unexpected events.

The rise of welfare

The election of a Liberal government in 1906, with Herbert Asquith as Prime Minister from 1908 and David Lloyd George as Chancellor of the Exchequer, saw the introduction of a mass of social legislation that collectively laid the foundations for the welfare state. Laws enacted included the Education (Provision of School Meals) Act 1906, the Medical Inspection of School Children Act 1907, the Employment of Children Outside School Hours Act 1908, the Non-Contributory Old Age Pensions Act 1908, the Housing and Town Planning Act 1909 and the National Insurance Act 1911.

This last was to have a profound effect on the practice of pharmacy and medicine in Britain. Its introduction was substantially due to the efforts and influence of David Lloyd George. Lloyd George was elected MP for Caernarfon at a by-election in 1890, beginning a parliamentary career that was to last until his death in 1945. He earned the sobriquet 'The Peoples' Champion' as a result of the Liberal reforms of 1906 to 1912 [16].

The National Insurance Bill

Events in the spring of 1911 took the medical and pharmaceutical bodies by surprise. At the time, many employed people paid small amounts each week to the numerous 'friendly societies', either national societies or small local groups. In return, the societies contracted with local doctors to provide free consultation and medicines to their members in time of need. This was a form of medical insurance in the absence of a national scheme. Lloyd George introduced the National Insurance Bill to parliament on 4 May 1911, in his capacity as Chancellor of the Exchequer. It proposed changes that would fundamentally alter the practice of pharmacy and medicine in primary healthcare. Part I of the bill referred to medical services to be made available to those insured under the provisions of the Act.

The bill covered employed persons only, and was limited to those earning less than £160 per annum and up to 70 years of age, the pensionable age at the time. The figure of £160 per annum was the base level for income tax liability. Benefits were to include unemployment pay in certain trades only, but all the insured would be entitled to medical attendance: 'Free doctoring for everybody who is a contributor to the scheme', as Lloyd George put it.

The medical benefit did not initially cover dependents. Sick pay would be initially at the rate of 10 shillings a week for men and 7s 6d (seven shillings and six pence) for women, reducing after 13 weeks and ceasing after 26 weeks. Benefits were to be financed by compulsory deduction from weekly wages of 4d for men and 3d for women, with the employer contributing a further 3d for all insured employees and the state contributing 2d similarly. Proposed contributions thus totalled 9d for males and 8d for females. 'Nine pence for four pence!' claimed Lloyd George in speeches to the electorate [17].

Doctors and drugs

For the pharmacy profession one of the most significant features of the bill was that for the first time there was state recognition of the need to 'separate the drugs from the doctors', a phrase that appeared early in the Chancellor's speech to parliament [18]:

> The first thing I think that ought to be done is to separate the drugs from the doctors, because the patient, as long as he gets something that is coloured and thoroughly nasty is perfectly convinced that it must be very good medicine. Therefore there ought to be no inducement for an underpaid doctor to take it

out in drugs. I suggest there should be a separation of drugs and doctors, the doctors' business being confined to prescribing; it should be for the chemist to dispense. I have no doubt that the friendly societies will make as good a bargain with the chemists as they did with the doctors. I believe that in Scotland, where they do most things well, that is the practice at the present moment. Wherever there is a chemist available, there should be separation.

The matter was not quite as simple as might have been hoped. The friendly societies played a major part in health provision for the employed classes. A feature of the bill was that approved friendly societies, which were regulated under the terms of the Friendly Society Act 1896, were to carry out much of the administration under the proposed scheme. Contributions were to be made by means of stamps purchased from post offices and stuck to employees' cards, covering the cost of the employer and employee contributions; an activity that was to become a feature of wage offices throughout the country. This feature of the bill brought about a good deal of protest and grumbling about 'stamp licking' and provided abundant material for political cartoonists.

Medical benefits were to be administered by the approved friendly societies, which would contract with doctors to provide consultation and necessary treatment, and with 'chemists' to provide dispensed medicines [19]. The bill did not attempt to change the available systems of hospital treatment, still based on voluntary (charitably supported) hospitals and the old Poor Law infirmaries. It did provide for the construction of new sanatoria for the treatment of tuberculosis, for which insured persons were to pay 1s a year and the state 4d. There was also to be a maternity benefit of 30s.

Friendly society control

The response of The Pharmaceutical Journal was unambiguous: 'Chemists and druggists do not want to bargain with friendly societies; if there is any bargaining to do it should be done with the government, and the result of the bargaining should be inserted in the bill.' The most satisfactory outcome, it suggested, would be to adopt the German system of a schedule of prices and allow any registered pharmacy to supply medicines at those prices. The writer raised the spectre of perhaps 12 million insured people obtaining medicines from depots chosen by friendly societies. If so, what would become of the pharmacist who was not chosen by a friendly society? Should doctors and pharmacists unite to obtain equitable terms from the government? asked a leading article in The Pharmaceutical Journal [20].

They did not do so. Each group had its own important battles to fight. *The Lancet* commented [21]:

> It is significant to note the statement that, as far as possible, the field of work of the physician is to be demarcated from that of the pharmacist, in that the latter would be entrusted with the supply of medicines. Any step of this nature can only be welcome to the practitioner, and *The Lancet* has already expressed an opinion on this point. At the present moment, outside Great Britain, it is practically only in the United States and some Swiss cantons that the doctors fulfil the double functions of physician and dispenser. In all other countries dispensing by doctors is strictly prohibited.

The general practitioner rank and file were less enthusiastic about the loss of earnings from dispensing, as were the BMA negotiators. A week later, *The Lancet* was commenting that the anomalous state of pharmacy law was inadequate to ensure that dispensing would be done by pharmacists. Existing law referred only to sales, and dispensing under the new scheme would not necessarily entail a sale, prescriptions being free to insured persons. The friendly societies had already indicated that they might set up dispensaries for the purpose and establish a central drug depot. Existing law would not require them to employ pharmacists for the purpose. This could be disastrous for many pharmacists in business, particularly those in working class districts [22].

It was evident that the Society was facing unprecedented opportunities and real threats: the opportunity to take over the majority of dispensing activities from the doctors, but the threat of losing these activities to unqualified friendly society employees. The doctors were also objecting to control by the friendly societies, whom they believed had underpaid them for medical services in the past.

Negotiations with government

Pharmacy was fortunate in having Glyn-Jones as its Parliamentary Secretary and as an MP. He and Lloyd George had a Welsh background and a political party in common, and there was a good understanding between the two men. Glyn-Jones moved quickly, and on 1 June 1911 led a delegation that met Lloyd George and his senior civil servants and included the Society's president, secretary, council members and representatives from Scotland, Ireland, the Drug Companies' Association and the Chemists' Defence Association.

By all accounts Glyn-Jones handled the meeting very skilfully [23] and strongly advocated that any dispensing done under the new scheme should be 'under the strict control of a qualified chemist', and by a person or corporate body entitled to carry out the business of pharmacy. He also mentioned that pharmacists, like medical practitioners, would prefer control of their services to be in the hands of local health committees rather than friendly societies. In these points, the medical establishment supported the Society, with the president of the General Medical Council confirming its views in writing to the Chancellor on 12 July [24].

On 6 July 1911 over a thousand pharmacists met in London, the largest meeting of pharmacists ever held, under the Society's president and supported by the two pharmacist MPs. A resolution to parliament confirming the above points was enthusiastically supported, together with a request for payment on a scale, rather than a *per capita* system, and a request for pharmacists to be represented on local health committees, the Advisory Committee and the Insurance Commission. The committee stages of the bill that concerned pharmacy were reached early in August 1911 and the next reprint of the bill, incorporating agreed amendments, included the key paragraph [25]:

> The regulations shall prohibit arrangements for the supply of drugs and medicines being made with persons other than persons, firms or bodies corporate entitled to carry on the business of a chemist and druggist under the provisions of the Pharmacy and Poisons Act 1908, who undertake that all medicines supplied by them to insured persons shall be dispensed either by a registered pharmacist or by a person who, for three years immediately prior to the passing of this Act, has acted as a dispenser to a duly qualified medical practitioner or a public institution.

This last point was intended to avoid unemployment of doctors' dispensers as a result of the changes. In the event, few took up the opportunity.

Further negotiations

Glyn-Jones and the Society had won a substantial victory for pharmacy and escaped the drastic consequences of friendly society dispensing by unqualified persons. The bill completed its passage through the House of Commons on 6 December and received the royal assent on 16 December 1911, although it was not until 15 January 1913 that the medical and pharmaceutical benefits of the scheme came into effect. Negotiations between government and the BMA (then with a membership of over 25,000) were protracted. Lloyd George offered Dr Smith Whitaker, the medical secretary of the BMA, the appointment of deputy chairman of the Insurance Commissioners. He accepted and was appointed, to the dismay of the members. A protest meeting was called, at which there were angry speeches and cries of 'traitor' [26].

The dispute with the BMA continued, with demands for higher capitation fees and even, despite earlier attitudes, requests for doctors to be able to dispense for their own patients. Government did not accept the latter. The dispute was never formally concluded. The BMA held out, but had overplayed its hand [26] and by 11 January 1913 *The Pharmaceutical Journal* was reporting that 14,000 doctors had signed up for the scheme. Doctors who had been contracted to some friendly societies, often being paid as little as 4s a year per patient for consultation and medicines, realised that their income would be doubled by the scheme, without the expense of supplying drugs. Resistance by the BMA collapsed and the National Health Insurance Scheme commenced operation.

The scheme in practice

On Wednesday 15 January 1913 *The Pharmaceutical Journal* claimed 'the business of pharmacy entered a new era' [27]. This was a watershed for pharmacy in Britain. The Society had secured for pharmacists the exclusive right to dispense doctors' prescriptions for patients insured under the new scheme. There was nevertheless still nothing to prevent anyone, doctor or layman, from compounding and dispensing medicines provided payment was not by the National Insurance Fund and did not involve the sale of a poison. An exception to the rule for National Insurance dispensing by pharmacists was made for patients in rural areas where there was no pharmacy. In such areas, the doctor or his staff could dispense, an arrangement that still exists for National Health Service (NHS) patients today.

The new National Insurance Scheme applied only to those in employment. Dependants such as wives and children, who still paid privately or who were insured through friendly society or other schemes, could still have medicines supplied by the doctor. The Society hoped that the new arrangements would encourage doctors to cease dispensing altogether and write prescriptions for all their patients; a change that did slowly occur in some areas.

The impact on pharmacy

The impact on pharmacies was profound. On the first day many pharmacies received dozens of prescriptions where previously they had received few or none at all. Pharmaceutical wholesalers experienced an upsurge in demand for dispensing materials and some even ran out of dispensing equipment. Pharmacists had pressed for payment by item of service in accordance with a national scale and this arrangement became embodied in a regular publication, the Drug Tariff. Doctors initially issued prescriptions in duplicate, the top copy being stamped and priced by the pharmacist and submitted to the local insurance committee for payment.

Despite some initial problems the new scheme worked remarkably well. Almost 14 million people were covered initially, through 236 local insurance committees. Some administrative and accounting problems arose and some pharmacists were irritated by the need to submit prescriptions for payment to several different local insurance committees, as a result of working in a location where different administrative boundaries met.

By July 1914 the Drug Tariff was requiring insurance committees to avoid payment for proprietary products of undisclosed formula,

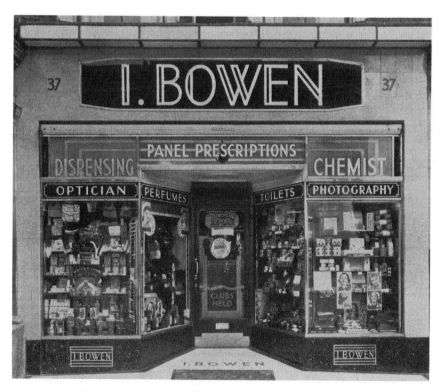

Figure 5.3 Pharmacy of I Bowen, offering National Insurance panel dispensing.

known as 'secret remedies'. Local formularies began to appear as an aid to the standardisation of common remedies, but it was not until 1929 that the National Formulary was introduced. The new arrangements soon settled down, and with the outbreak of war in 1914 the government had more pressing issues to attend to.

The National Health Service Act 1946

With only minor modifications the National Insurance Scheme served throughout the inter-war years. The earnings limit was successively raised, and additional categories of patient were admitted. For those not covered by the national scheme a wide variety of contributory insurance arrangements existed, often on a local basis but also through trade unions and friendly societies. There was a need to rationalise the whole process, and to have a single national system that applied to everyone. Even at the darkest point of the Second World War plans were being drawn up for such a system, a task that fell to William Beveridge.

The Beveridge Report was submitted to ministers of the wartime coalition government in 1942. A statement on the future social programme was made to the House of Commons in February 1943, accepting the report in principle, with an intention to institute a comprehensive medical service covering every man, woman and child in the country who wished to benefit from it. Discussions with concerned parties began and a White Paper was issued in 1944. At the general election of July 1945 the Labour Party was successful and Aneurin Bevan, the Minister of Health, became responsible for preparations for the new health service.

The National Health Service Bill

The National Health Service Bill was presented to parliament in March 1946 and the subsequent Act received the royal assent on 6 November 1946. There was a huge amount of organisational work to be done both before and after the passing of the Act. The service would be extended to cover medical, pharmaceutical, optical and dental benefits for the entire population. It would also integrate hospital services into the system; something that the 1911 Act had not attempted, with the exception of sanatoria for the treatment of tuberculosis. Not least, extensive consultations were necessary for the organisation of medical services and the remuneration of medical practitioners, pharmacists, opticians and dentists.

As in 1911, extended discussions took place between the government and the BMA. It was decided by government that the service would commence operation on the Appointed Day, which would be 5 July 1948. On that day the new scheme moved into action. As experience was gained, modifications were required, for example the NHS (Amendment) Act 1949 and the NHS Act 1951. Complex discussions about arrangements for the NHS followed, and there were numerous modifications and developments to the service over the years that followed [28].

As far as pharmacy was concerned, a well-tried system of working was already in existence under the 1911 Act, so that together with later modifications the introduction of the new scheme proceeded without undue difficulty. With the entry of millions of family dependants, previously excluded, into the scheme, dispensing activities expanded rapidly. The basic arrangements for the organisation of pharmaceutical services that had been established at the beginning of the 20th century remained largely unchanged at its end.

However, pharmacy had changed. During the 20th century pharmacy in Britain had developed from the situation where most prescriptions were dispensed by the doctors who wrote them, with pharmacists being largely dependent on counter trade, to a position where it was normal for medical prescriptions to be dispensed by duly qualified persons.

References

1. Hunt J A. William Allen – the First Member. *The Pharmaceutical Journal* 1994; 253: 941.
2. Holloway S W F. *Royal Pharmaceutical Society of Great Britain 1841 to 1991: A Political and Social History.* London: Pharmaceutical Press, 1991: 1.
3. Holloway S W F. *Royal Pharmaceutical Society of Great Britain 1841 to 1991: A Political and Social History.* London: Pharmaceutical Press, 1991: 147–184.
4. The National Insurance Bill [editorial]. *The Lancet* 1911; 1: 1362.
5. Holloway S W F. *Royal Pharmaceutical Society of Great Britain 1841 to 1991: A Political and Social History.* London: Pharmaceutical Press, 1991: 273–278.
6. Sir W S Glyn-Jones: His life and work. *The Pharmaceutical Journal* 1927; 65: 285–287.
7. The Anti-Cutting Record. *The Pharmaceutical Journal* 1895; 55: 404.
8. Hunt J A, Jones I F. Sir William Glyn-Jones – a pharmaceutical colossus. *The Pharmaceutical Journal* 1995; 255: 884–887.
9. The Chemists' Defence Association [annotations]. *The Pharmaceutical Journal* 1899; 63: 538.

10. Moreton Parry L. [Memorial tributes to William Glyn-Jones]. *The Pharmaceutical Journal* 1927; 65: 288.
11. Glyn-Jones W S. Drug Trade Appeal Fund [letter]. *The Pharmaceutical Journal* 1902; 69: 30.
12. Holloway S W F. *Royal Pharmaceutical Society of Great Britain 1841 to 1991: A Political and Social History.* London: Pharmaceutical Press, 1991: 274–305.
13. Report of the 67th Annual General Meeting of the Society. *The Pharmaceutical Journal* 1908; 80: 703.
14. Pharmacy in Parliament. *The Pharmaceutical Journal* 1909; 82: 553.
15. Little E M. *History of the BMA.* London: British Medical Association, 1932.
16. Grigg J. *Lloyd George – the People's Champion.* London: Methuen, 1978.
17. Hunt J A, Jones I F. David Lloyd George – his influence on pharmacy in Britain. *The Pharmaceutical Journal* 1994; 253: 912.
18. *Hansard.* Fifth Series. 1911; 25: 609.
19. Hunt J A, Jones I F. David Lloyd George – his influence on pharmacy in Britain. *The Pharmaceutical Journal* 1994; 253: 913.
20. The National Insurance Scheme [editorial]. *The Pharmaceutical Journal* 1911; 86: 617–618.
21. The National Insurance Scheme [editorial]. *The Lancet* 1911; 1: 1299.
22. The National Insurance Bill [editorial]. *The Lancet* 1911; 1: 1362–1363.
23. *Official Report of Deputations to the Chancellor of the Exchequer.* Deputation by the Pharmaceutical Societies of Great Britain and Ireland, Drug Companies Association etc. 1 June 1911, pp. 10–12. HMSO. Cd. 5869 October 1911. Public Record Office, Kew, Piece No. PIN3/4, p. 395.
24. Letter from the President of the General Medical Council to Lloyd George. *The Times*, 17 July 1911.
25. Reprint of Clauses 1–17 of the National Insurance Bill. HMSO. Cd. 5885. 1911, p. 25. Clause 14 (2) b) iii).
26. Vaughan P. *Doctors Commons – a Short History of the BMA.* London: Heinemann, 1959: 189–209.
27. National Insurance Dispensing [editorial]. *The Pharmaceutical Journal* 1913; 90: 90.
28. Ross J S. *The National Health Service in Great Britain.* Oxford: Oxford University Press, 1952.

Part Three

The practice of pharmacy

6

The development of pharmaceutical education

Melvin Earles

One of the important threads running throughout the history of pharmacy is the nature of the pharmacist's education and training. Early declarations about the roles of physicians and apothecaries invariably emphasised lengthy training, usually by means of an extended apprenticeship. Following the establishment of the Society of Apothecaries in 1617, entry was strictly regulated and subject to the passing of rigorous examinations, but the sale and supply of drugs and chemicals remained unregulated, and anyone was free to set themselves up in business in this way.

When the Pharmaceutical Society was founded in 1841 there was a developing tradition of academic pharmacy abroad. In France, six schools for the education of pharmacists were founded in 1803. There were schools of pharmacy in the German states, and in Bavaria study at a university became obligatory in 1808. A College of Pharmacy opened in Philadelphia in 1821 [1]. There was nothing comparable in Britain. Pharmaceutical subjects were taught in the Edinburgh Royal Dispensary, at Apothecaries' Hall in London and in the medical schools.

Pharmacy education in Britain, 1841 to 1887

There was no separate and distinct school of pharmacy, and training to practise as a chemist and druggist was by the traditional apprenticeship system. It was Jacob Bell's opinion that in Britain pharmacy had been 'degraded to the level of an ordinary trade divested of its scientific respectability'. The prime task of the new organisation was the advancement of chemistry and pharmacy and the promotion of a uniform system of education.

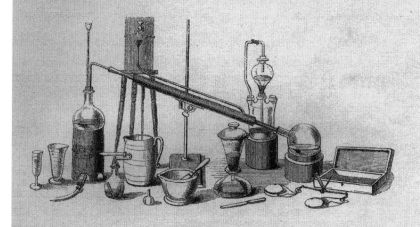

PRACTICAL PHARMACY:

THE ARRANGEMENTS, APPARATUS, AND MANIPULATIONS, OF THE PHARMACEUTICAL SHOP AND LABORATORY.

BY

FRANCIS MOHR, Ph. D.,

ASSESSOR PHARMACIÆ OF THE ROYAL PRUSSIAN COLLEGE OF MEDICINE, COBLENTZ;

AND

THEOPHILUS REDWOOD,

PROFESSOR OF CHEMISTRY AND PHARMACY TO THE PHARMACEUTICAL SOCIETY
OF GREAT BRITAIN.

ILLUSTRATED BY FOUR HUNDRED ENGRAVINGS ON WOOD.

LONDON:

TAYLOR, WALTON, AND MABERLY,

UPPER GOWER STREET, AND IVY LANE, PATERNOSTER ROW.

1849.

Figure 6.1 Title page of *Practical Pharmacy* by F Mohr and T Redwood, 1849.

The Society's school

As a result, one of the first tasks of the new Society was to establish its own school of pharmacy. It opened in Bloomsbury Square, London, in 1842. Bell announced that 'the foundation of education in our school is chemistry' [2]. This was a time when British chemists had created a popular interest in the subject and there was a growing appreciation of its contribution to the arts and manufacturing processes. Among the early members of the Pharmaceutical Society were several who had studied chemistry in Justus von Liebig's laboratory in Giessen. These men were aware of the importance of practical training in the science, and in 1844 a room in the School of Pharmacy was fitted out to teach practical chemistry, one of the first facilities of its kind in Britain.

Chemistry was taught in the school by George Fownes, who had studied with Liebig and whose *Manual of Chemistry* was then regarded as the most complete textbook in English. Medical botany was taught by Dr Anthony Todd Thomson and pharmacy by Theophilus Redwood. Redwood later became Professor of Chemistry and Pharmacy and was the author, with Francis Mohr, of *Practical Pharmacy* published in 1849. In 1844 Jonathan Pereira was appointed Professor of Materia Medica and taught at the school when he was compiling his encyclo-paedic *The Elements of Materia Medica and Therapeutics*. He was also the author of *Selecta e Praescriptis*, a small work for learning prescription Latin that was popular until overtaken by Joseph Ince's *Latin Grammar of Pharmacy*, first published in 1882.

The scheme for education began with a test in Latin before indenture. It was believed that this evidence of education would raise the standard of recruitment. The apprentice would attend a course of lectures in the applied sciences and sit the Minor examination, which would qualify him as an assistant to a chemist and druggist and entitle him to join the Pharmaceutical Society as an associate member. The more advanced Major examination would lead to the designation Pharmaceutical Chemist and qualify the candidate to become a full member of the Society.

Provincial schools

A plan for provincial schools was devised involving local member associations. Support was given in the form of a grant equivalent to a portion of the annual subscription for the area. Grants are recorded for members in Manchester, Norwich, Bath and Bristol. These schools bore

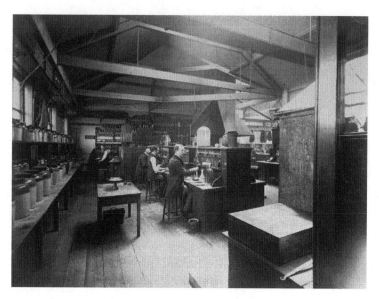

Figure 6.2 The 'major chemical laboratory', third floor, 17 Bloomsbury Square, c. 1883.

little resemblance to the London prototype. In most cases they involved lectures in a Mechanics Institute or medical school: for example in Manchester, lectures on chemistry and botany were held in the Pine Street medical school. In some cases there was also some form of rented property to act as a library and materia medica museum [3].

The provincial plan was not a success. At the time there were few local facilities for teaching science and in some parts of the country they were non-existent. When, for financial reasons, the Society withdrew the grant most of these local 'schools' closed down for lack of students. The reasons for this were two-fold: the long hours worked by apprentices, and the attitude of their masters, the majority of whom were opposed to interference by a London-based elite. To compensate, the London school was designated the 'national school', serving apprentices who lived in London and provincials who could afford a short sojourn in the capital. The school continues today as the School of Pharmacy, University of London, and throughout its long history its teachers and distinguished alumni have been a potent influence on the progress of pharmaceutical science and education. In the 1840s and for some years after, the school, beset with problems of student numbers and finance, was all there was to represent the Society's ambitions for pharmacy education [4].

Statutory qualification

In 1851 Jacob Bell, by then an MP, presented a bill to parliament that included a reference to an examination for qualification to practise as a chemist and druggist. This was lost at the committee stage following arguments based on free trade, and it did not appear in the 1852 Pharmacy Act [5]. Soon after this disappointment, government proposals concerning the sale of poisons indirectly threatened the Society's plans for education. Except for arsenic there were no restrictions on the sale of poisons, and a series of accidents and two notorious trials for murder involving strychnine excited considerable public concern. The government sought to restrict sales to a species of qualified person and proposed the granting of a licence by a Board of Examiners of which one was to be a member of the Pharmaceutical Society. The policy was vigorously opposed by Jacob Bell, with the country-wide support of chemists and druggists, who objected to having to apply for a licence to trade.

The Society was criticised for its successful opposition on a matter of public safety but Bell argued that the licence might come to be regarded as a licence to practise pharmacy and the public would make no distinction between a licensed chemist and a pharmaceutical chemist. If this were to happen there would be no incentive to take the Society's examinations [6].

Pharmacy education and the 1868 Act

The Pharmaceutical Society recognised the need for some form of regulation for the practice of pharmacy and the Council drew up a bill for a revised Pharmacy Act. Its object was to introduce the registration of qualified persons for the purpose of compounding the prescriptions of a medical practitioner. However, because most doctors did their own dispensing, many chemists and druggists rarely, if ever, saw a prescription.

Registration as a chemist and druggist was to be subject to the candidate passing the Minor examination. This was a concession to attract support for the bill. The Minor was originally designed for assistants and the Major, leading to the Pharmaceutical Chemist (PhC) qualification, was to be the qualification for conducting a pharmacy business. The upgrading of the Minor brought severe criticism from teachers at the School of Pharmacy. In putting forward this bill the Society hoped that a qualification based on pharmaceutical competence would ensure responsibility and indirectly solve the sale of poisons problem. There was opposition from the United Society of Chemists and Druggists, who claimed to represent the majority engaged in the trade. Founded shortly after the death of Jacob Bell in 1859, it united those who were critical of his regard for pharmacy as a profession. Their interest was in trade and they drew up an alternative bill relating qualification to the sale of poisons [7].

The two societies and government ministers were locked in debate for some time and the outcome was another disappointment for those with an interest in education. In 1868, parliament passed a new Pharmacy Act subtitled 'An Act to Regulate the Sale of Poisons'. It required that all persons, except those already engaged in business, be examined to test their practical knowledge and registered as chemists and druggists. The Pharmaceutical Society was to be the examining body.

There had been some discussion on this matter because the Society, having established a school, was regarded as an educating body and differed from other examining authorities such as the Royal Colleges and the Society of Apothecaries. To overcome this problem the Privy Council was given authority to see that the examinations were properly conducted. The examinations held in London and Edinburgh were oral tests. Questions were asked relating to items laid out on tables in the

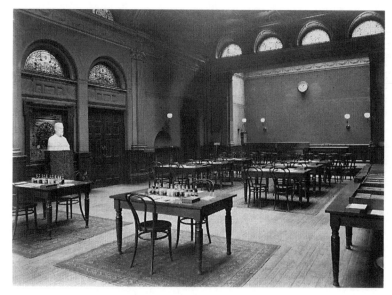

Figure 6.3 Examination hall, 17 Bloomsbury Square, c. 1883.

examination hall such as crude drugs, medicinal plants, chemical and pharmaceutical apparatus, pharmacopoeias and specimen prescriptions [8].

The Act fell short of the Pharmaceutical Society's ambition for a uniform system of education. There was a qualifying examination and this was generally acceptable. In the mid-19th century examinations were becoming commonplace and had reached into areas where appointments were hitherto matters of patronage, such as the Civil Service. They already complemented apprenticeships in a range of arts and crafts. The Society of Arts began its system of examinations in the 1850s and the Government Science and Art Department started a scheme of examinations in 1860. The latter were associated with classes in science, which was not the case for many pharmacy apprentices.

The candidate for the chemist and druggist examination had to prepare for it using whatever facilities were available to him (or her – the first woman to register as a chemist and druggist by examination was in 1869). For a second time membership groups were asked to organise some teaching for local apprentices. Of the 26 associations listed in 1869–70, only nine had succeeded in organising classes to cover all subjects, these having the advantage of improved local arrangements for teaching science that had developed since the founding of the Government Science and Art Department following the Great Exhibition of 1851.

The success of these local arrangements was variable. In Newcastle there were three failed attempts before reasonable success was achieved in 1886. Lectures were held every Friday from October to July in rooms rented by the North of England Pharmaceutical Association and courses in practical chemistry arranged in the Durham College of Science. There was a materia medica collection and a library purchased with a grant from the Pharmaceutical Society. The fee for the course was 5 guineas, with arrangements for students to pay for single subjects. Student numbers varied, causing severe financial problems. At one time of particular difficulty, N H Martin FLS, a leading figure in the Association, remarked 'registered chemists, as a body, do not believe in education and do not want it' [9].

Private schools

For apprentices unable to attend the School of Pharmacy in Bloomsbury or a provincial school there were the private schools. The first was the North London School of Chemistry, owned by J C Braithwaite, once an instructor at the School of Pharmacy. The South London School of Chemistry and Pharmacy opened in 1870, followed by the highly successful Westminster College of Pharmacy owned by G S V Wills PhC.

There were seven such schools in 1890 but only two were in the provinces, one in Liverpool and one in Manchester. A decade later there were 22 distributed around the country. Proprietary schools relied on student fees and their reputation, in what became a competitive situation, depended upon success in the qualifying examination. As a consequence, teaching was closely tailored to the requirements of the examination, a fault found in other areas of education in the 19th century.

A less respectable form of private enterprise was the 'crammer', a species of teacher engendered by the emphasis being placed on examination at the expense of education. These people moved into pharmacy after the 1868 Act and were roundly condemned at the British Pharmaceutical Conference in 1872 [10]. An example of the practice appeared in an advertisement announcing that 'the student's time will be principally employed in examination in which the questions are such that he may reasonably expect afterwards'.

There was no safeguard against superficial forms of training and failure rates in the examination were high. When this was investigated in 1881 it was found that the rates of failure in chemistry, botany and materia medica were twice those in the practical subjects of pharmacy, dispensing and prescription reading. The solution was to require a certificate of attendance at the recognised course of study and divide the examination into two parts, science and practice [11]. It was assumed this could be done by altering the bye-laws but the Privy Council informed the Society that the powers conferred by the 1868 Act referred to the conduct of the examination, not to the means of preparing for it!

Pharmacy education in Britain, 1887 to 1911

By this time there was sufficient evidence of advances in pharmacy and its constituent sciences to support the policy of a compulsory course of study, but there was persistent opposition. In 1887, a bill to amend the Pharmacy Act in favour of education and training was introduced into the House of Lords and favourably received. When it reached the Commons there were objections after it was pointed out that the membership of the Pharmaceutical Society was a fraction of the total number of practising chemists and druggists and was not therefore representative of the trade. When next the Society approached parliament, in 1890, it was not as a representative body but as an educating organisation, but the gambit failed when a Petition of Opposition was received [12].

D L S Cardwell, discussing general education, observed that 'the belief in individualism, the frequently expressed dislike of state interference, and central administration, were the three key factors responsible for many of the educational ills of the 19th century' [13]. There were, however, several other reasons for the failure to establish a uniform system of education for pharmacy in Britain at the time. Prominent among these was the conservative attitude of the very large majority of chemists and druggists on the register.

Expansion of the syllabus

At the turn of the century there had been major developments in the sciences related to pharmacy, including two relatively new disciplines, experimental pharmacology and bacteriology. Both of these were destined to enter the pharmacy syllabus. The growing reputation of pharmacy as an academic discipline was enhanced through a number of important initiatives: by the reports of the annual British Pharmaceutical Conference, which had been meeting since 1863, and by research papers from the School of Pharmacy. In 1901 three professors at the school became Recognised Teachers of the University of London and members of the Faculty of Science [14].

At the time a relationship was established with a university, pharmaceutical training was still locked into the 'examination enforces education' philosophy. It was not just the rank and file who were indifferent to a compulsory systematic scheme of education to complement the apprenticeship training. When the Society was endeavouring to persuade parliament to allow it to introduce a course of study Mr Wills, owner of the private Westminster school, said:

> In the name of reason, what can it matter to the examiners or to the public where or how a student obtained his knowledge? Is he qualified? That is the all important question.

The average candidate at this time supplemented home study with a voluntary attendance of about 3 months at a private school, or attended whatever courses the local technical institute could provide. The problems he or she faced are reflected in the examination results. In 1900 the failure rate in the Minor (or chemist and druggist) examination was reported by the London board of examiners to be 72% of candidates entered for the examination [15,16].

Legislation on education

Three Acts of Parliament helped to solve these problems. The Technical Instructions Act of 1889 was passed in response to a perceived weakness in technical instruction in Britain when compared with other trading nations [17]. Pharmacy courses started up in some of the institutions founded or upgraded as a result of the Act and developed into departments of pharmacy preparing students for the chemist and druggist and

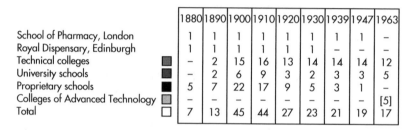

	1880	1890	1900	1910	1920	1930	1939	1947	1963
School of Pharmacy, London	1	1	1	1	1	1	1	1	–
Royal Dispensary, Edinburgh	1	1	1	1	1	1	–	–	–
Technical colleges	–	2	15	16	13	14	14	14	12
University schools	–	2	6	9	3	2	3	3	5
Proprietary schools	5	7	22	17	9	5	3	1	–
Colleges of Advanced Technology	–	–	–	–	–	–	–	–	[5]
Total	7	13	45	44	27	23	21	19	17

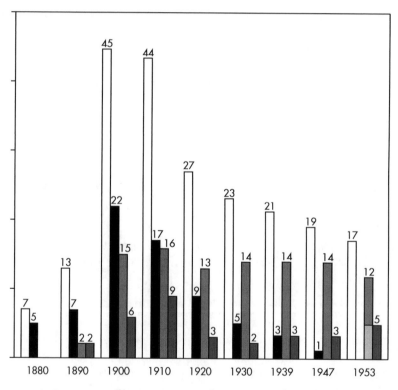

Figure 6.4 Institutions offering courses in pharmaceutical subjects in Great Britain, 1880–1963. Reproduced from [3], p. 81, by permission of the author.

PhC qualifications. The London polytechnics were one result of the Act. One of these was the South Western Polytechnic, which began a course of lectures in sciences related to pharmacy in 1896, and developed into a department of pharmacy that exists today as part of Kings College, University of London.

The second legislation to affect education was the Pharmacy Act of 1908. After long consideration this allowed the Pharmaceutical Society to make bye-laws to regulate courses of study and qualifying examinations. Shortly afterwards, Lloyd George's National Insurance Act of 1911 had an important impact on pharmacy education. The Act required that National Insurance dispensing must be carried out by contracted pharmacists. These decisions made it possible to introduce a compulsory course of study for a qualification officially related to dispensing of medical prescriptions as well as to the supply of scheduled poisons.

The examination that emerged was divided into two parts: Part I consisted of chemistry and botany, while Part II included materia medica, pharmacy and dispensing [18]. In addition to the prescribed course the candidate had to present evidence of having undertaken a period of apprenticeship or pupilage, as it was sometimes called. These regulations did not come into force until after the First World War, when the Society had its first opportunity to approve schools, a matter that was not referred to in the 1908 Act and was a sensitive issue with the private schools.

Pharmacy education in Britain, 1911 to 1946

Developments in pharmacy education were interrupted during the second decade of the 20th century by the First World War, but at the end of it large numbers of servicemen returned looking for training and employment. In 1919 the Pharmaceutical Society was asked by the Ministry of Labour to approve schools for training a large number of ex-servicemen in receipt of the government grant. A sufficient number of institutions were found for this purpose, but they were too numerous for the normal intake. It was decided that the number of schools approved for Parts I and II should be limited, but no restriction was placed on the number recognised for only Part I.

First degrees awarded

A very significant event in the history of pharmaceutical education in Britain occurred in 1924. The University of London, following representations by the Council of the Society, introduced a Bachelor of Pharmacy degree in the Faculty of Medicine. In the 19th century there had been several proposals for a degree in pharmacy but each was unrealistic at the time. In 1904 the University of Manchester introduced a BSc degree for pharmacy students, and in 1907 a degree in pharmacy was established in the University of Glasgow. Neither received recognition with regard to qualification [19]. The London degree was approved for registration as a Pharmaceutical Chemist, subject to a test in forensic pharmacy. The introduction of a degree was evidence, in contrast to the basic nature of the chemist and druggist course, that pharmacy as an academic discipline had advanced to university standard.

Students could read for the two-year internal BPharm degree at the School of Pharmacy or at the Chelsea Polytechnic, where there were Recognised Teachers. Within a short time provincial institutions were able to prepare students for the London External BPharm. Between the two world wars only a few students opted for the advanced pharmacy courses. In the Nottingham Department, from which 50–80 annually qualified with the chemist and druggist qualification, there were two BPharm and three PhC students in 1932; by 1939 there was little change, with four BPharm and two PhC students [20].

Pharmacy education in Britain, 1946 to 1986

In the years after the Second World War there were far-reaching changes in pharmacy education to meet the challenge of advances in pharmacotherapy and the demands of the NHS. It was also necessary to adapt to the 1944 Education Act, which had established a system of grants that encouraged school leavers to go straight into higher education. This meant that the apprenticeship or articled pupilage system would have to give way to a period of practical training following the qualifying examination. There was also a change in institutions teaching pharmacy. The private schools had served their purpose: some closed and others were taken over by local institutions. The last proprietary school was in Liverpool, taken over in 1949. Henceforth pharmacy would be taught in polytechnics, Colleges of Advanced Technology and university departments.

In 1946 the University of London announced the introduction of a three-year honours degree that would replace the two-year general degree. The post-war education policy of the Pharmaceutical Society, which was aimed at achieving degree standard for qualification, was based on the findings of a Committee of Enquiry set up after the constitutional changes of the 1933 Pharmacy Act [21–23]. The three-term chemist and druggist course was phased out and a single register of Pharmaceutical Chemists established. Those holding the chemist and druggist qualification were upgraded to PhC, and those who already held the PhC qualification were appointed Fellows of the Pharmaceutical Society of Great Britain (FPS).

In 1957 the entrance requirements for the PhC qualification were brought into line with the universities, and the course was extended to three years. This decision proved to be controversial. Some pharmacists thought it was unnecessary, others that it would deter candidates, laying the foundation for a future manpower problem.

Award of university status

With the PhC course matching the degree course in length it was only a matter of time before university status for pharmacy was introduced. The findings of a government review of higher education were published in 1963, and among its recommendations was the creation of new technological universities. A number of the institutions upgraded had departments of pharmacy [24]. With the polytechnics being able to award nationally approved degrees it was possible from 1967 for all persons seeking registration to practise pharmacy to be university graduates. The Pharmaceutical Society, having passed its school over to the University of London shortly after the war, now relinquished its role as an examining body, but retained powers to approve degree courses for pharmacy.

The curricula for the pharmacy degrees built up over the years were science-based. Under the headings of the four principal subjects pharmaceutics, pharmaceutical chemistry, pharmacognosy and pharmacology there were specific subjects such as pharmaceutical microbiology, medicinal chemistry, formulation, physical pharmacy, phytochemistry, radiopharmacy and others. These formed subjects for research, an activity that developed rapidly in the pharmacy schools as the institutions were upgraded to Colleges of Advanced Technology, polytechnics and then universities. Teaching in departments of pharmacy became research-informed, but with this came a problem experienced in other subjects – an academic career came to rely less on teaching and more on research output and research funding.

The problem with the established curricula was this: to what extent does a course based on scientific principles properly prepare an undergraduate to practise pharmacy? The question was not new or confined to Britain. The matter had been raised in the School of Pharmacy in the 1930s, when it was argued that perhaps there should be different courses for practice in retail, hospital and industry. In 1964 Sir Hugh Linstead, former secretary of the Pharmaceutical Society, observed: 'There is in most countries a certain tug-of-war between scientific and academic pharmacy on the one hand and the practitioners of pharmacy on the other.' This matter became acute with new and novel developments in the practice of the profession [25,26].

In 1957 C W Maplethorpe, chairman of the Pharmaceutical Society's education committee and a prime mover in the policy to advance pharmacy education, indicated the wider responsibilities that pharmacists were likely to meet. Writing in the *Future Pharmacist*, the journal of the British Pharmaceutical Students Association, founded to give students a voice in their affairs, he observed: '[the pharmacist] has a large contribution to make in deciding the form which treatment should take in particular cases and will be in a position to deal on equal terms with authorities in other fields including medicine.'

Taking up this theme again in 1966 he referred to the pharmacist acting as an adviser on drugs and medicines to the medical profession and protecting the public from dangers inherent in many new compounds [27]. Maplethorpe, by emphasising the necessity of pharmacists being trained to undertake a consultative role, was responding to the increase in the number and range of medicines, and to growing concern over their potential dangers, which had been highlighted by the thalidomide tragedy in 1961.

Emergence of clinical pharmacy

By the time qualification as a pharmacist was solely by means of a university degree, pharmacists in hospitals had already begun to leave the relative isolation of the dispensary and to work alongside medical staff in the practice of ward pharmacy. A new discipline, called clinical pharmacy, entered the curriculum, and this represented something of a revolution in British pharmacy. In the 18th and early 19th centuries the apothecaries had evolved into medical practitioners. In 1841, when the chemists and druggists founded their Society, the sensibilities of the medical profession demanded that the chemists avoided any undertaking that might be deemed an intrusion into medical practice.

Jacob Bell wished pharmacy to become a branch of medicine but one founded on the scientific principles of the calling [28,29]. When he wrote that the foundation of education in the school was chemistry, the word chemistry was printed in capital letters, suggesting that it was a political statement as well as one of intent. Medically related subjects, such as pharmacology, were later introduced into the pharmacy course, but for the first hundred years of the Society's history the term 'clinical' would have been avoided. Clinical pharmacy became a feature of a wider academic subject, 'pharmacy practice'. The first pharmacy practice research session was introduced into the British Pharmaceutical Conference in 1977.

Pharmacy education in Britain after 1986

In 1983 a committee was set up by the Nuffield Foundation to examine pharmacy (Chapter 7) [30]. It reported in 1986, and stated that the traditional division of pharmacy departments into four main subject areas with vested interests in staff, space and funding acted as a restraint on development. Recommendations included that subjects be grouped to demonstrate relevance to each other and to practice, and that teaching should concentrate on communication skills [31].

The conclusions of the Nuffield committee were not new to teaching staff who had already introduced elements of clinical and practice pharmacy into their courses. The report nevertheless sharpened the general response to the changing nature of practice. In the 10 years that followed, 16 university chairs in pharmacy practice were established and many teacher/practitioners recruited. To deal with the situation fully a longer course was necessary, but at the time of the Nuffield recommendations universities were involved in the reforms and rationalisations following the financial strictures imposed by Margaret Thatcher. As a result, academics had the procrustean task of fitting the new and enlarged practice subjects into a three-year course.

The four-year degree, 1997

A four-year course of study leading to the degree of Master of Pharmacy (MPharm) was introduced in 1997. The graduate who wishes to practise pharmacy is now required to undertake a postgraduate year of training under the supervision of a pharmacist and sit an examination conducted by the RPSGB before registration as a pharmaceutical chemist. The new course is by no means the end of the story. In 2003 a symposium on the development of a strategy for pharmaceutical education was organised by the RPSGB, the Academic Pharmacy Group and the Academy of Pharmaceutical Sciences. Among the matters discussed was 'professional training or science education?' This is a clear indication that Sir Hugh Linstead's scientist/practitioner contest is unresolved and remains a problem for the future, one in which increasing diversity in education is expected [32].

References

1. Sonnedecker G. *Kremers and Urdang's History of Pharmacy*, 4th edn. Philadelphia, PA: J B Lippincott, 1976.
2. The School of Pharmacy [report]. *The Pharmaceutical Journal* 1843; 2: 113–116.
3. Earles M P. The pharmacy schools of the nineteenth century. In: Poynter F N L, ed. *The Evolution of Pharmacy in Britain*. London: Pitman Medical, 1965: 81.
4. Wallis T E. *History of the School of Pharmacy*. London: Pharmaceutical Press, 1964.
5. Holloway S W F. *Royal Pharmaceutical Society of Great Britain 1841 to 1991: A Political and Social History*. London: Pharmaceutical Press, 1991: 179.
6. Earles M P. A history of the Society. *The Pharmaceutical Journal (Anniversary Supplement)*. 27 April 1991: S6–9.
7. Holloway S W F. *Royal Pharmaceutical Society of Great Britain 1841 to 1991: A Political and Social History*. London: Pharmaceutical Press, 1991: 208–215.
8. Trease G E. *Pharmacy in History*. London: Baillière, Tindall and Cox, 1964: 191.
9. Earles M P. Associations' Schools of Pharmacy. *The Pharmaceutical Journal* 1959; 183: 98–99.
10. Attfield J. *Yearbook of Pharmacy*. London: Pharmaceutical Society of Great Britain, 1872: 495.
11. Special committee to consider the relation to each other of pharmaceutical education and the pharmaceutical examinations [report]. *The Pharmaceutical Journal* 1881–2; 12: 148–149.
12. *Hansard's Parliamentary Debates*. 1887; 313: col. 463: 1888; 324: col. 697: 1891; 351: col. 15.
13. Cardwell D S L. *The Organisation of Science in England*. London: Heinemann, 1957.
14. Wallis T E. *History of the School of Pharmacy*. London: Pharmaceutical Press, 1964: 45.
15. Matthews L G. *History of Pharmacy in Britain*. Edinburgh: E & S Livingstone, 1962: 165.
16. Appointment of an assistant to the examiners [report]. *The Pharmaceutical Journal* 1900; 10: 366.
17. Argles M. *South Kensington to Robbins*. London: Longmans, 1964: 35.
18. Examination and Education Committee [report]. *The Pharmaceutical Journal* 1911; 86: 13.
19. Robinson B. *The History of Pharmaceutical Education in Manchester*. Manchester: University of Manchester, 1986: 114.

20. Trease G E. *Pharmacy in History*. London: Baillière, Tindall and Cox, 1964: 252.
21. *Report of the Committee of Enquiry Part II*. London: Pharmaceutical Society of Great Britain, 1941.
22. Pharmaceutical Society of Great Britain [report]. *The Pharmaceutical Journal* 1941; 147: 201–210.
23. Holloway S W F. *Royal Pharmaceutical Society of Great Britain 1841 to 1991: A Political and Social History*. London: Pharmaceutical Press, 1991: 411, 416.
24. *Higher Education* (The Robbins Report). London: HMSO, 1963–4.
25. Holloway S W F. *Royal Pharmaceutical Society of Great Britain 1841 to 1991: A Political and Social History*. London: Pharmaceutical Press, 1991: 407.
26. Wallis T E. *History of the School of Pharmacy*. London: Pharmaceutical Press, 1964: Foreword v.
27. Maplethorpe C W. Pharmaceutical education in 1966. *The Pharmaceutical Journal* 1966; 197: 491–503.
28. McMenemey W H. Education and the medical reform movement. In: Poynter F N L, ed. *The Evolution of Medical Education in Britain*. London: Pitman Medical, 1966: 137.
29. Bell J, Redwood T. *An Historical Sketch of the Progress of Pharmacy in Great Britain*. London: The Pharmaceutical Society of Great Britain, 1880: 118.
30. *Pharmacy: The Report of a Committee of Inquiry Appointed by the Nuffield Foundation*. London: Nuffield Foundation, 1986.
31. The Nuffield Report [current affairs]. *The Pharmaceutical Journal* 1986; 236: 348–369.
32. Is pharmacy education in crisis, or is it simply changing? *The Pharmaceutical Journal* 2003; 271: 790–791.

7

The development of community pharmacy

Peter G Homan

From earliest times the basis of pharmacy was the making and selling of medicines to the public. When man first started to trade in goods is lost in antiquity. Certainly medicine men in primitive tribes would have collected herbs and discovered or concocted medicinal remedies, the formula of which they would have kept secret, and used to barter. Egyptian medicine dates from around 2900 BC. Egyptian pharmacists were also priests, and practised their art in the temples.

It is impossible to give a date for the first community pharmacist. In Rome it is known that Archagathos the Greek opened a shop around 200 BC. This housed a pharmacy as well as a surgery and a hospital, a similar set-up to those found in Greece at that time. In medieval Europe it was the monasteries that carried out the dispensing of medicines. Later, private pharmacies were established and existed with public monastic pharmacies until the early 19th century. The first retail establishments appeared in Italy and France around the 11th century.

Early development of community pharmacy

The Arabs opened the earliest recorded pharmacy shops in public areas in the 8th century. With foreign trading in herbs and spices and Arab influences pharmacies started to appear in Europe around the 11th century. Soon after, Britain was importing the products that would lead to trading in pharmacy. In London, the first recorded shop dealing with the sale of medicines was opened by an apothecary in 1345 [1].

Italian and French pharmacists originated from pepperers and spicers who, in the 12th century, formed themselves into societies known as guilds. In Germany pharmacy was always controlled by the government of the time. Pharmacies in America were founded by immigrants during the late 17th century. Originally known as Apothecary

Shops (later to be called drug stores), the first to be opened is thought to have been in Boston in 1646 [2]. As well as the sale of drugs and proprietary medicines, the drug store would sell commodities 'such as paints, oils, varnishes, brushes, wallpaper and glass' [3].

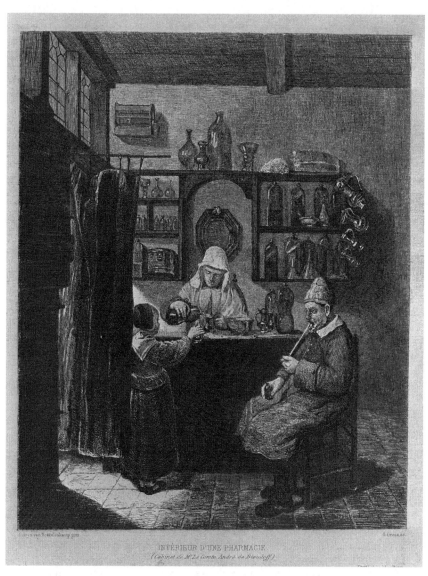

Figure 7.1 Interior of a 19th-century Dutch pharmacy showing a woman pharmacist at work. Engraving by Gustave-Marie Greux after Quiringh van Brekelenkam, 1875. Reproduced by permission of the Wellcome Library, London.

Developments in Britain

In 12th-century Britain there were two types of dealers in drugs: the pepperers were wholesalers, and the spicers were retailers. Spicers began to take on the dispensing and compounding of medicines, and by the end of the 13th century they were beginning to use the title 'apothecary'. In the 14th century the pepperers changed the name of their guild to the Grocers' Company and included the apothecaries as members. In 1617 the apothecaries formed their own guild, the Worshipful Society of Apothecaries.

Gradually the apothecaries became involved in the prescribing as well as the compounding of medicines. This put them into conflict with the College of Physicians and, at the same time, with chemists and druggists who were also dealing with drugs and dispensing medicines. In 1540 the College of Physicians had been empowered to 'search, view and see the apothecary wares, drugs and stuffs' in London. These powers were enhanced in 1618 when four members were authorised to survey and examine the stocks of 'apothecaries, druggists, distillers and sellers of waters and oils, and preparers of chemical medicines'.

The 1701 Rose Case (Chapter 4) led to the apothecaries being recognised as medico-pharmaceutical practitioners and, eventually, as general practitioners of medicine. Dispensing of medicines gradually became the work of the chemists and druggists.

Chemists and druggists

In Britain in the early 18th century druggists and chemists were mainly separate callings, which were gradually combined. Dual 'chemists and druggists' began to appear in the early 19th century. They were formed by the uniting of three factions: apothecaries who wished to continue as dispensers and suppliers of drugs; dispensary assistants who set themselves up as dispensing chemists; and druggists who were formerly members of the 'pepperers' section of the Grocers' Company.

As dealers in drugs and chemicals chemists and druggists set up shops to advise as well as sell to the general public. They did not feel 'governed' by the guild system that controlled the apothecaries but believed in a free trade to supply anybody with dispensed medicines and to sell them any of their trade goods. These goods of course included medicines and as chemists and druggists increased in numbers they became a major source of medical help to the general public, setting up shops on high streets throughout the nation.

By the early 19th century, chemists and druggists had diversified into many allied trades. In 1843 Jacob Bell wrote of 'three divisions', explaining that 'we have operative chemists, dispensing chemists, and manufacturing chemists, wholesale druggists, saline chemists, chemists and druggists who give their attention to particular classes of preparations; others who cultivate the sale of horse and cattle remedies; others who are between wholesale and retail and supply apothecaries with drugs. The nature of the retail trade also varies according to neighbourhood and the rank of the customers' [4].

Customers' orders and prescriptions would be assembled on the shop counter, which would serve jointly as a trading area and as a dispensary bench. In addition to dispensing and the sale of drugs and medicines, other goods and facilities were introduced including surgical instruments, toilet preparations, photographic equipment and chemicals, spectacles, dentistry and even minor surgery. Dentistry was widely practised until the Dental Act of 1921 restricted registration as a dentist to those who had undertaken approved courses of study or had worked as a dentist for seven years or more. The Chemists Dental Association was disbanded in 1949, only five members remaining at that date. A Society of Chemist Opticians was founded in 1905. Today the links are still to be seen in premises such as Boots Opticians.

Many well-known pharmaceutical companies had their foundations in chemist and druggist's shops. Manufacturers included Allen & Hanburys and Thomas Morson, wholesalers included John Bell and Croyden and Martindales. After the formation of the Pharmaceutical Society in 1841 examinations eventually led to two categories of person able to practise, pharmaceutical chemists, and chemists and druggists. In 1954 these categories were combined as pharmacists (Chapter 6).

Symbols of community pharmacy

The apothecary's 'shop' was more of a laboratory than a retail premises. It would have a dispensing and manufacturing department and a consultation and waiting area. The walls would be adorned with 'mystic' symbols of the apothecary's art such as stuffed crocodiles and narwhal horns (unicorn substitute). Delftware pill-tiles and drug jars bearing the arms of the Worshipful Society of Apothecaries might also be on view to show membership of that guild.

The chemist and druggist shops were much closer to shops as we know them today. The original windows consisted of hand-made glass panes measuring approximately 40 cm × 20 cm. Behind these would be shelves bearing storage bottles known as *carboys* (from the Persian word 'quarabah' meaning a large flagon, used for wine or rose water). These carboys would be used for storage and for preparing pharmaceuticals using the heat of the sun. As almost all pharmacies had them in their windows they became a readily recognisable symbol for a pharmacy.

Glass production improved with the manufacture of polished plate glass from 1773 and the advent of rolled glass in the second half of the 19th century. Shop windows could be made much larger, giving more display area. The true storage jars were moved to behind the counter and larger imitation storage jars known as *specie jars* were used for display. Carboys were developed into large elegant containers filled with coloured water. The storage containers that lined the shelves inside the shop were later deemed unsuitable for hygiene reasons, and their use was discontinued in the 1950s. Today, the 'green cross', introduced by the Pharmaceutical Society in 1984, has become the universal symbol for pharmacy in Great Britain.

Chemist multiples

The Apothecaries Act of 1815 specified that apothecaries had to be licensed by the Worshipful Society of Apothecaries of the city of London in order to practise. By this time most of the apothecaries had taken on the role of general medical practitioner. Clause 28 of the Act exempted chemists and druggists from the need to hold such a licence. As a result, the latter group increasingly took over the role of dispensing and selling poisons [5]. The clause stated that [6]:

> Nothing in this Act contained shall extend, or be construed to extend, to prejudice in any way to affect the Trade or Business of a Chemist and Druggist, in the buying, preparing, compounding, dispensing, and vending of Drugs, Medicines, and Medicinable (sic) Compounds, wholesale and retail; but all persons using or exercising the said trade or business, or who shall or may hereafter use or exercise the same, shall and may use, exercise and carry on the same trade or business in such manner, and as fully and amply to all intents and purposes, as the same trade or business was used, exercised, or carried on by chemists and druggists before the passing of this Act.

The Pharmacy Act of 1852 made it illegal for an unregistered person to practise as a chemist and druggist or as a pharmaceutical chemist. The Pharmaceutical Society was given more statutory power, and established a standard of qualification for pharmaceutical chemists. It separated pharmacists from other members of the medical profession.

The Pharmacy and Poisons Act of 1868 regulated the sale of poisons. It also stated that 'from and after 31 December 1868 it shall be unlawful for any person to sell or keep open shop for retailing, dispensing or compounding medicines, or to assume or use the titles 'chemist and druggist', or 'chemist', or 'druggist', or 'pharmaceutical chemist' in any part of Great Britain unless such person shall be registered under this Act'. It was assumed under the 1868 Act that retail trade in pharmacy, that is dispensing and the sale of poisons, would be conducted by individual proprietors. The Act, however, stated 'a person', but made no reference to a 'company'.

The Pharmaceutical Society v. the London and Provincial Supply Association

There was, at this time, a retail establishment in Tottenham Court Road, London called the London and Provincial Supply Association. The proprietor was an unqualified person, Mr Mackness, and the business had a drug department managed by a qualified person who in turn had two qualified people under him.

In 1878 the Pharmaceutical Society's solicitor wrote to the London and Provincial Supply Association indicating that the Society intended taking legal proceedings under the 1868 Act. The Society claimed that a Mr Mackness, an unqualified person, had illegally sold oxalic acid, although it was a qualified person who had made the actual sale. Mr Mackness pleaded guilty and paid a £5 fine to the Pharmaceutical Society rather than go to court. To end further violation of the law he converted the business to a limited liability company.

The Pharmaceutical Society decided to determine the legal position of this move and applied for a penalty under the 1868 Act against the London and Provincial Supply Association Ltd for unlawfully keeping open shop for the sale of poisons. The resulting judgement was that it was *not* unlawful for a qualified person to sell poisons on behalf of a company. Two years later, in 1880, the House of Lords ruled that the word 'person' under the 1868 Act did *not* include corporate bodies. This meant that companies could not only use restricted titles, but could sell poisons, provided that they were sold by a qualified person.

Jesse Boot

The first multiple shop company specialising in drugs was owned by Jesse Boot. Boot's father, John, had opened a herbal shop in Goose

Gate, Nottingham, 'The British and American Botanic Establishment'. John died in 1860 and Jesse, then aged only 10, helped his mother to run the shop. At the age of 21 he became a partner in the business, which became 'Mary and Jesse Boot Herbalist'.

Boot was a natural businessman. He decided that the best way to trade was to buy in bulk, sell cheaply and advertise heavily. His stock was increased to include household commodities such as soap and candles as well as proprietary medicines, all of which were sold at cut prices [7].

In 1877 Boot took over the business completely and continued his promotional advertising, culminating in a move to larger premises in Goose Gate in 1881. He had ten branches by 1883 and in that year employed his first pharmacist, Mr Cheers, who was quickly replaced by Edwin Waring. Waring built up the dispensing business at Boot's Goose Gate branch by undercutting the price of dispensed medicines. Also in 1883, Boot registered as a limited liability company, 'Boot and Company

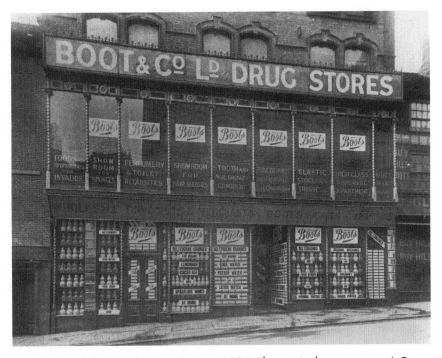

Figure 7.2 Boot's Goose Gate store, c. 1885. The original store was at 6 Goose Gate, but in 1881 Jesse acquired the site at 16–20 Goose Gate and completely redesigned the shop. The entire frontage was made from glass divided by iron columns and the space was used for eye-catching window displays. Reproduced by permission of Boots Group Archives.

Ltd'. He began to expand the business by purchasing more shops in Nottingham and, in 1884, in Sheffield. Soon Boot's shops were all over Britain, and by 1890 he had 110 branches. Boot continued to diversify, and he introduced lending libraries and even cafes into many of his branches [8].

The 1880s and 1890s saw rapid expansion of multiple pharmacies, particularly in the towns and cities. By 1890 there were three other firms with over ten branches: Taylors Drug Company (Leeds & Yorkshire), W T Warhurst (Liverpool) and Timothy White (Portsmouth). The 1890s saw the establishment of Day's Southern Drug Company in Southampton, Lewis & Burrows Drug Stores Ltd in London, and Mago Ltd in Birmingham. Other companies of note included Needhams Ltd (Yorkshire), the Sussex Drug Co. (Brighton), Hodders Ltd (Bristol), Wands (Leicester) and H B Pare (Manchester).

Opposition to the multiples

Company pharmacists were generally looked down upon by the proprietor pharmacists. Holloway quotes one who described 'registered chemists who, by their Judas-like treachery in selling their services to unqualified persons ... have degraded pharmacy, as carried on in joint stock drug stores, to the lowest depths of mere commercialism' [9]. However, there were redeeming features: the drug stores added dispensing and the sale of poisons, creating work for pharmacists; and pharmacists who could not afford their own premises could become managers and superintendents.

Competition amongst the multiples meant that working conditions were improved, as were the salary and status of pharmacists. Shorter working hours were offered, with no Sunday duties, and a half-day holiday each week. Qualified relief was provided to enable assistants to have a holiday. These were attractive conditions. By 1906, Boots had 329 branches and employed 434 qualified pharmacists.

Impact on proprietor chemists

The main problem for the proprietor pharmacists was that the multiples undercut them on price. One such was William Glyn-Jones (Chapter 5). Half of the trade in his shop in East London was the sale of proprietary medicines. Because he was having to cut prices to meet the competition, his profit was only about $7\frac{1}{2}\%$. He was, in some cases, paying the same price to buy the goods as the multiples were selling the goods. He believed that only 'resale price maintenance' (although this term was not in use at the time) would halt the march of the multiples and help the small man to survive. In 1896 he formed the Proprietary Articles Trade Association (PATA), to support those manufacturers who insisted that their proprietary medicines were sold at the full retail price.

Jesse Boot was worried that inability to cut prices would mean lost business. He was determined to smash the PATA. He and William Day (of Day's Southern Drug Company) decided to have a mammoth sale of PATA protected goods. They bought from every source, including community pharmacists. They stored the goods in a disused chapel in London, but there was a fire and the goods were destroyed. Some said this was divine intervention, but the publicity led to more small pharmacists realising the danger and joining the PATA. By 1898 membership was more than 3000.

The Drug Companies' Association

In 1899 the Pharmaceutical Society attempted to present a parliamentary bill to debar limited companies from dispensing or selling poisons. Boot and William Day responded by setting up the Drug Companies' Association. In the bill was a clause that particularly upset Jesse Boot. It

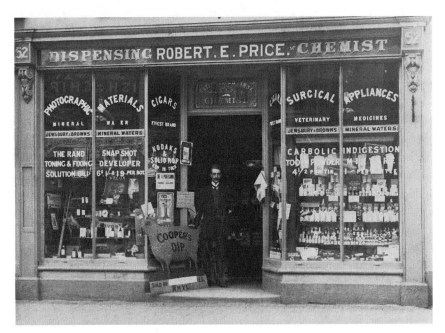

Figure 7.3 Shop front of Robert E Price, dispensing chemist, Rhyl, 1909.

was proposed that companies should be prevented from using the title of 'chemist and druggist'. Boot had spent a lot of money advertising Boots the Chemists. It was important that he kept the title as a trade name. The bill was put forward a number of times, and was actively opposed on each occasion by the Drug Companies' Association.

The government then put forward their own bill, which finally resulted in the 1908 Pharmacy Act. The new Act replaced the schedule of poisons from the 1868 Act; licensed listed sellers of poisons; extended the Pharmaceutical Society's powers of examination; and permitted limited companies to carry on the business of chemist and druggist.

Attached to the last point were strict conditions. The poisons department had to be under the control and management of a qualified superintendent or a qualified manager. The superintendent had to be a member of the board of directors. The Company could use some titles but not all. It could use any of four titles: 'chemist and druggist'; 'chemist'; 'dispensing chemist'; and 'dispensing druggist'. But the titles 'pharmacist', 'pharmaceutist' and 'pharmaceutical chemist' could only be used by a qualified person. Multiple chemists were here to stay.

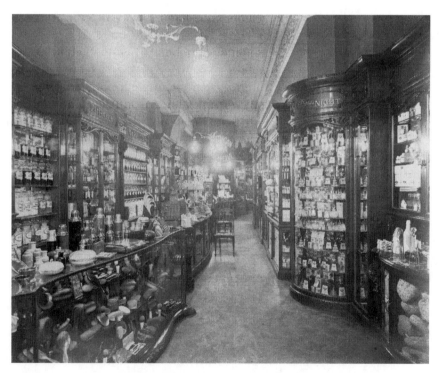

Figure 7.4 Interior of Heppell & Co. Chemists, Strand, London, 1912.

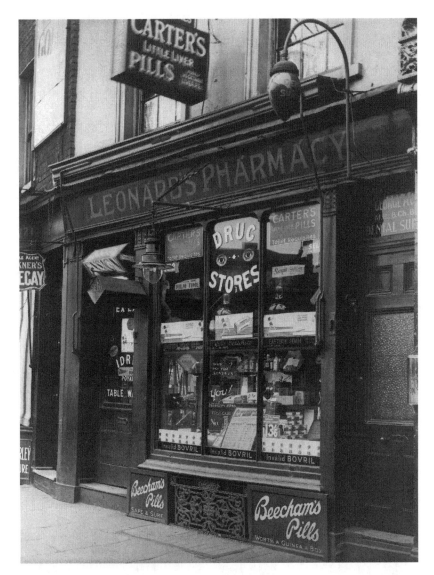

Figure 7.5 Leonard's pharmacy, London, c. 1930.

Self-service

Boot and his company found themselves opposing the Pharmaceutical Society at regular intervals throughout the 20th century. In 1952 Boots introduced a new trading method. Developed in the USA, it was named 'self-service'. Traditionally, all service in shops had been provided by asking an assistant for the goods required, and then paying that assistant.

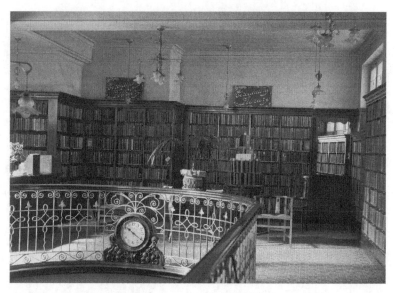

Figure 7.6 Boots Booklovers' Library, Southampton store, c. 1920s. Reproduced by permission of Boots Group Archives.

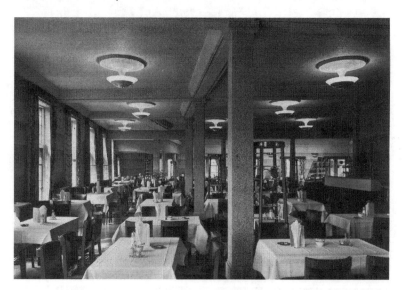

Figure 7.7 Boots café, Pelham Street, Nottingham, c. 1920s. Jesse Boot's wife, Florence, was responsible for introducing the libraries and cafés at the turn of the 19th century. They were designed to attract middle-class customers to the stores and Florence Boot chose the décor of each café herself. The book lending service was established in 1898; libraries were sited on the first floor or at the back of the branch to draw customers through as many departments as possible. Reproduced by permission of Boots Group Archives.

Now supermarket food shops had introduced a system whereby people selected their purchases and paid at a dedicated desk. Boots gave it a try.

The Pharmaceutical Society did not approve. It maintained that 'drugs and medicines are not ordinary commercial articles for which the limit of the market may safely be the desire and the capacity of the public to purchase them. It is not in the public interest that they should be subject to the ordinary conditions of trade and any and every method adopted to induce the public to buy them'.

The Society took High Court action in 1953 and lost. A Court of Appeal upheld the decision in favour of Boots. It should be noted that Boots only put remedies that were on general sale by other outlets on open display until late in 1980. Until that time all requests for medicines had to be made at the chemist counter. 'Self-service' later became known as 'self-selection'.

The Dickson Judgement

In 1955 the Council of the Pharmaceutical Society set up a committee to examine the general practice of pharmacy at that time, with particular reference to professional standards [10]. The committee submitted its

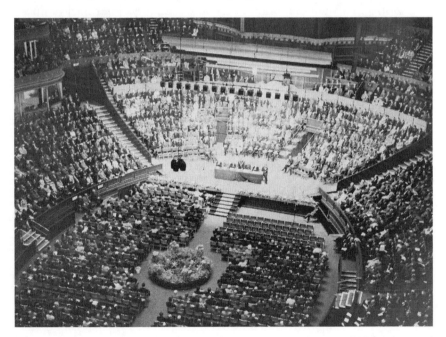

Figure 7.8 Special General Meeting of the Pharmaceutical Society, held at the Royal Albert Hall on 25 July 1965.

report in 1961, but the full report was only published in *The Pharmaceutical Journal* two years later, after the self-selection judgement [11].

Following publication of this report a motion was put before the Society's Annual General Meeting (AGM) in 1965, directing that new pharmacies must be situated in physically distinct premises and must confine their trading activity to the sale of pharmaceutical, professional and 'traditional' chemists' goods. The latter included toiletries, cosmetics and photographic items. There was such a large attendance at the AGM that no vote could be taken, and an adjourned AGM was arranged for 25 July 1965 to be held at the Royal Albert Hall.

Robert Campbell Miller Dickson, Retail Director of Boots, sought an injunction to stop the meeting on the grounds that the motion was outside the Pharmaceutical Society's powers and, being in restraint of trade, had no legal force. The injunction was refused on an undertaking that no attempt would be made to give the motion effect until after the judgement in the action to determine whether the object of the motion was within the power of the Pharmaceutical Society.

The AGM was held and the votes cast were 5026 for the motion and 1336 against. Over 6000 of the 29,000 registered pharmacists (20%) had attended and voted, and the Pharmaceutical Society had won a majority. At that time there were about 29,000 pharmacists on the register, about 75% of whom were in community pharmacy. Of 14,000 retail shops, 1100 were Boots. The hearing of Dickson versus the Pharmaceutical Society took place on 23 June 1966.

The High Court ruled that 'it is not within the powers of the Society to enforce the provisions of the motion on the ground that the said provisions are in restraint of trade'. The Court of Appeal confirmed this decision and in 1968 the House of Lords affirmed that 'it was not within the Society's main object of "maintaining the honour and safeguarding and promoting the professional interests of members".' It was a very expensive lesson for the Pharmaceutical Society to learn regarding its limitations.

Mergers of multiples

Of all companies The Boots Company had the greatest influence on the practice of community pharmacy in Britain. It grew as a result of both opening new branches and acquisitions. William Day, a co-founder with Boot of the Drug Companies Association, was forced to retire as a result of recurrent asthma, and Boot bought his 65 drug stores and two warehouses in 1901. Taylors Drug Stores, which from the start were one of

Boots greatest competitors, had opened stores in London in 1889, before Boot. Taylors merged with Timothy Whites to become Timothy Whites and Taylors, and this company, in turn, was taken over by Boots in 1968.

In 1989, Boots acquired Underwoods, which had a large number of pharmacy outlets in the London area, making Boots the largest retail chemist in Britain at the time. However, community pharmacies are a very dynamic part of the retail sector, and new entrants constantly appear. Lloyds Pharmacy now have the largest number of shops on the High Street. Its branches include many pharmacies that were originally part of old established companies such as Savory and Moore, Allens Chemist, Cross and Herbert, Kingswood GK, Lloyds Chemist, Hills Pharmacy and the wholesaler AAH.

In recent years supermarkets including Asda, Safeway, Tesco and Sainsbury have opened pharmacies in many of their stores. Superdrug, founded in 1964 as a drug store, was taken over in 1988 by Kingfisher Plc, who also owned Woolworths. Kingfisher sold Superdrug to Kruidvat in 2001. Since 2003 the company has been owned by A S Watson, part of Hutchison Whampoa. They have, since 1992, introduced pharmacies into many of their drug stores, and introduced pharmacy on the Internet.

Community practice

From the early days of chemists and druggists the selling of a range of commodities and services developed in pharmacies. Mainstays of the pharmacist included counter prescribing and the manufacture of his own medicines or *nostrums* as they were known. Pharmacists would have their own notebooks of preparations that would include medicines, cosmetics, toiletries and household accessories.

Until 1941, proprietary medicines were subject to tax under the Medicine Stamp Act, but this Act did not apply to articles of the pharmacist's own manufacture. A publication called the *Pharmaceutical Journal Formulary* ran from 1904 for many years, and included the formulas for a multitude of preparations that pharmacists could make themselves. It included many of the proprietary medicines available at the time. The *Chemist & Druggist* produced a similar publication called *Pharmaceutical Formulas*.

Dispensing prescriptions

At the beginning of the 20th century dispensing made up a small but important part of a pharmacist's income. Most dispensing was done by the doctors themselves. This was to change with the advent of the National Health Insurance Scheme. Both proprietor and company pharmacists were allowed to contract for the dispensing of National Insurance prescriptions, and the result was a three-fold increase in the numbers of prescriptions dispensed by pharmacists.

A further increase in the number of prescriptions dispensed occurred with the introduction of the NHS in 1948, resulting in community pharmacists becoming ever more dependent on the dispensing of prescriptions written by doctors for their livelihood. Today, over 70% of the income of a typical independent pharmacy comes from this source.

The Jenkin case, 1920

A major influence on pharmacy practice has been the powers of the Pharmaceutical Society. These powers have been tested in the courts and these cases are watersheds in pharmacy history. One such case was the Jenkin case in 1920.

In the aftermath of the First World War, the government was keen to reform industrial relations in Britain by setting up a number of schemes for negotiating wage rates and other working conditions. The Pharmaceutical Society promoted the setting up of a Joint Industrial Council for the whole of the pharmaceutical industry, including manufacturing, wholesaling and retailing. The Society's membership included both employers and employees, and it was well placed to preside over negotiations between them.

The Society's plans came up against some powerful opponents, notably Jesse Boot and pharmacists in Scotland. The latter obtained legal opinion on whether the Society had the powers under its Charter to become involved in negotiations about pay and conditions. The Society decided to test its powers in the courts. Arthur Henry Jenkin was a hospital pharmacist, and a member of the Society's Council. He took out an injunction to restrain the Council of the Society from undertaking a range of activities, including the regulation of pay and conditions of service, to function as an employers' association, and to provide legal and insurance services to members.

The injunction was granted. At a hearing on 19 October 1920, the Court decided that the Society did not have powers to regulate wages, hours of business, and the prices at which goods were sold, or to provide insurance or legal services. As a result of this decision, two months later a separate body, the Retail Pharmacists Union, was set up as a 'union of retail employer chemists for the protection of trade interests'. It was renamed the National Pharmaceutical Union in 1932, and the National Pharmaceutical Association (NPA) in 1977. The NPA was controlled by employers, and employees had little or no influence on its activities. At the same time Jesse Boot established a Managers' Representative Council to represent pharmacist-managers in his branches.

The Pharmacy and Poisons Act 1933

After the Jenkin Judgement the Society set about redefining its purpose. Indeed, it has been argued that the NPA is the true successor to the aims of the Society's founding fathers 'to protect the collective and individual interests and privileges of all its members, in the event of a hostile attack in parliament or otherwise'.

The 1933 Act clarified the relationship between the Privy Council, the Society's Council and its members. Registration as a pharmacist meant automatic membership of the Society. To enforce the Act the Society appointed pharmacists as inspectors who inspected conditions of storage of poisons and registers of sales.

The Society established the Statutory Committee, which had authority over pharmacists and over companies carrying on a business under the Pharmacy Acts. It first met in July 1934, the first pharmacist's name being removed from the register shortly after. Within a few years a Code of Ethics was produced and published. Today this is included in the Society's publication *Medicines, Ethics and Practice* [12].

The National Health Service Act 1948

The NHS initially gave free treatment and medicine to all. The numbers of prescriptions increased from 70 million in 1947 to 250 million in 1949 [13]. Sales of proprietary medicines were depressed and many of the popular brand names disappeared. However, with the introduction of charges for prescriptions and strong advertising by manufacturers of proprietary medicines, sales recovered and gradually increased.

In 1984 the government delivered a heavy blow to the NHS patient. After 1 April 1985 only certain medicines would be prescribable on the NHS. A multitude of medicines including cough remedies, digestives, laxatives and analgesics were no longer available on NHS prescription. Many were household names such as Benylin, Codis and Disprin. This was the Black List (which continues to be in force), and it lists medicines that cannot be prescribed on NHS prescriptions. It was bad news for patients and the manufacturers of medicines. However, the combination of the Black List and escalating prescription charges produced an increase in counter prescribing and over-the-counter medicine sales.

During the last two decades of the 20th century there was an increasing interest in complementary or alternative medicine. Homoeopathy, herbal medicine, aromatherapy, Bach Remedies and many more have added to the range of products sold and the scope of the expertise required by the pharmacist.

The Nuffield Report, 1986

The pharmacist in Britain had traditionally sold his wares and dispensed prescriptions. In the early days he had stood at his counter to serve his customers and prepare their prescriptions. The advent of the National Health Act had resulted in him moving into a dedicated area for the preparing of prescriptions – the dispensary – and this was where he spent his working day. In busy shops dispensing became so heavy that the pharmacist could spend very little time on the counter. Counter sales would be made 'under supervision' by sales assistants. In the 1980s the future role of the pharmacist as a healthcare professional came under discussion.

In October 1983 the Trustees of the Nuffield Foundation commissioned an inquiry into pharmacy. Its terms of reference were 'to consider the present and future structure of the practice of pharmacy in its several branches and its potential contribution to healthcare and to review the education and training of pharmacists accordingly'. In their report the Committee of Inquiry made a total of 96 recommendations, 26 of which related to community pharmacy [14].

To implement all of these recommendations for extended roles, the pharmacist would have had to leave his premises for periods of time in order to carry out such things as home visits. This brought in the question of supervision of the pharmacy. The Council of the RPSGB rejected any attempt to find alternative methods of supervision and issued a statement in 1989 stating 'every prescription for a medicine must be seen by a pharmacist, and a judgement made by him as to what action is necessary'.

An extended role

The pharmacist was tied to his pharmacy and unable to take up any extended role without the services of a second pharmacist. However, in

November 1990, a Joint Working Party of the Department of Health was set up to consider how the pharmacist's role might be extended.

Its report, *Pharmaceutical Care: the Future for Community Pharmacy*, was published in March 1992, and it made a total of 30 recommendations [15]. These included increasing the range of medicines available for sale by pharmacists, the maintenance of patient medication records by pharmacists, the extension of needle and syringe exchange schemes, participation in health promotion campaigns, and having separate areas for providing advice and counselling. The recommendations formed the basis for negotiations about the scope of community pharmacy over the years that followed. Many of these recommendations were adopted.

Community pharmacy present and future

The dispensing of prescriptions remains the pharmacist's speciality. He is now able to offer a collection and delivery service for the patient's convenience. Because of increased legislation on the manufacture and labelling of preparations the pharmacist's nostrums have virtually disappeared, but proprietary sales are high and the pharmacist's counter prescribing role is being aided by legislation to make many prescription items available over the counter.

Today, diagnostic services such as blood pressure monitoring and the sale of diagnostic tests for diabetes and pregnancy are commonplace. Large multiples are offering healthcare in the form of optometry, podiatry and dentistry. Community pharmacies have joined with doctors' surgeries in health centres where the patient can receive total healthcare. Pharmacies have gone on-line: medicines and prescriptions may now be obtained via the Internet.

Community pharmacy is continuously in a state of change. At this time there is discussion on repeat prescribing to allow pharmacists to renew patients' prescriptions without them needing to contact the surgery. Supplementary prescribing is being introduced to enable pharmacists to prescribe medicine for NHS patients. These activities have clear historical echoes in the role of the apothecary. Are pharmacists following the way of the apothecary towards the physician's role?

References

1. Grier J. *A History of Pharmacy*. London: Pharmaceutical Press, 1937: 38.
2. Cook E F, Martin E W (eds). *Remington's Practice of Pharmacy*, 10th edn. Eston, PA: Mack Publishing Company, 1948; 22.

3. Sonnedecker G. *Kremers and Urdang's History of Pharmacy*, 4th edn. Madison, Wisconsin: The American Institute of the History of Pharmacy, 1976: 155.

4. Bell J, Redwood T. *An Historical Sketch of the Progress of Pharmacy in Great Britain*. London: The Pharmaceutical Society of Great Britain, 1880: 119.

5. Matthews L G. *History of Pharmacy in Britain*. Edinburgh: E & S Livingstone, 1962: 115.

6. Apothecaries Act 1815, Clause XXVIII.

7. Chapman S. *Jesse Boot of Boots the Chemist: A Study in Business History*. London: Hodder and Stoughton, 1974.

8. Weir C. *Jesse Boot of Nottingham*. Nottingham: Boots Company plc, 1994; 46–47.

9. Holloway S W F. *Royal Pharmaceutical Society of Great Britain 1841 to 1991: A Political and Social History*. London: Pharmaceutical Press, 1991: 279.

10. Dale J R, Appelbe G E. *Pharmacy Law and Ethics*, 3rd edn. London: Pharmaceutical Press, 1983: 557.

11. Report of the Committee of Inquiry into the General Practice of Pharmacy. *The Pharmaceutical Journal* 1963; 190: 347–358.

12. *Medicines, Ethics and Practice. Number 26*. London: Royal Pharmaceutical Society of Great Britain, 2004.

13. Anderson S C. The historical context of pharmacy. In: Taylor K, Harding G, eds. *Pharmacy Practice*. London: Taylor and Francis, 2001: 3–30.

14. *Pharmacy: The Report of a Committee of Inquiry Appointed by the Nuffield Foundation*. London: Nuffield Foundation, 1986.

15. Department of Health and Royal Pharmaceutical Society of Great Britain. *Pharmaceutical Care: The Future for Community Pharmacy*. London: Royal Pharmaceutical Society of Great Britain, 1992.

8

The development of pharmacy in hospitals

Shirley Ellis

From earliest times the making and dispensing of medicines has not been limited to sale and supply to individuals. Medicinal preparations were used in a wide range of institutions where people were cared for collectively. Probably the first institutions where pharmacy was practised in Britain were the Roman military hospitals, or *valetudinaria* [1]. By medieval times a wide variety of institutions were in existence (Chapter 3). Pharmacy became an established activity in the early monasteries, which usually had their own hospital.

In this chapter the development of hospital pharmacy will be considered in four chronological periods. The first is the period before 1911, when the National Health Insurance Scheme was introduced. The second considers the first half of the 20th century, up to the formation of the NHS, in 1948; and the third takes the story up to publication of the Noel Hall Report in 1970. The final period reviews developments in the practice of hospital pharmacy from then up to the present day.

Hospital pharmacy before 1911

From the 6th century onwards monasteries were amongst the few places offering conditions favourable to the successful treatment of disease [2]. Each had its *infirmarian*, who was charged with finding 'whatever may be necessary in the way of medicines and comforts for the sick and keeping a good supply of ginger, cinnamon and peony ... so as to be able at once to minister some goodly mixture or cordial when it was required'. The dissolution of the monasteries by Henry VIII, between 1537 and 1547, also meant the loss of the hospitals, but the Mayor of London petitioned the king to restore those of St Bartholomew, St Thomas and Bedlam in London. These hospitals then employed an apothecary, in place of the *infirmarian*.

By the 18th century philanthropists were financing the building of hospitals [3]. One of the first departments to be established was the *elaboratory*, or apothecary's shop. The apothecary was expected to be resident in the hospital and his duties involved the administration of patient admissions and the assumption of responsibility for their care in the absence of the visiting medical staff and matron. This was in addition to the procurement and dispensing of medicines. Some participated in the committees that produced hospital pharmacopoeias for in-house use. Most hospitals required the apothecary to have served several years of apprenticeship under a member of the Society of Apothecaries. He was often helped in the preparation of medicines by the *elaboratarian*, who did the unskilled manual work; these staff later became known as dispensers.

Apothecary to pharmacist

In 1815 the Apothecaries Act effectively blocked the development of hospital pharmacy for some time, by setting up a series of lectures and examinations, leading to the Licentiate of the Society of Apothecaries. This was a much more medically orientated qualification. Most licensed apothecaries in hospitals became resident medical officers. This title was more consistent with their duties, although many continued to supervise the dispensing of medicines. Within a decade advertisements began to appear for 'apothecary's assistants in pharmacy departments', and later for 'pharmacists'.

After 1841 some of the larger hospitals required applicants to hold membership of the Pharmaceutical Society. The chief pharmacists at the three main London hospitals were described as 'men who stood for the highest standard of work, also for administration and practical economics in the running of their departments'. Training within the hospital service was uncommon, and at the beginning of the 20th century there were no apprentices in the big London hospitals. Most of the assistants were men who had just qualified [4].

Outside these hospitals over 60% of those working in hospital pharmacies were women. In 1908 Margaret Buchanan exhorted them to become registered pharmacists, and claimed that 'there have been not a few instances where women's business capacity and up-to-date knowledge of drugs and economical methods have led to practical appreciation on the part of management committees' [5]. Today, the percentage of pharmacists employed in hospital pharmacy who are women remains high, at 73.5% [6].

Professional associations

By the turn of the century there were enough pharmacists employed in London institutions to form a Poor Law Dispensers' Association. In 1909 this became the Public Pharmacist and Dispensers' Association. Membership consisted of registered pharmacists and holders of the assistant certificate of the Society of Apothecaries employed in hospitals and public dispensaries. Membership declined after the First World War, partly because membership was now restricted to registered pharmacists and partly through an inability to recruit members from amongst voluntary and teaching hospital staff. In 1923 a further merger took place, with pharmacist members of the Voluntary Hospital Officers' Association, creating the Guild of Public Pharmacists [7]. By 1921 most hospitals employed only pharmacists, although even 50 years later there was still no legal requirement to do so.

Hospital pharmacy, 1911 to 1948

At the beginning of the 20th century many hospital pharmacies were still undertaking the large-scale preparation of galenicals from crude drugs, an activity that had been going on for over 200 years. In addition, and in the interest of economy, many produced domestic products for the hospital such as soap solutions, denture powder and baking powder. Around 60% of medicines were still in liquid form, manufactured on the premises and supplied in large stock containers to the wards.

The 1911 National Insurance Act dramatically increased the number of prescriptions written in the community. This encouraged the development of pharmaceutical wholesaling, and the industrial-scale preparation of standard mixtures and galenicals. Hospital departments took advantage of this, buying in galenicals, and taking in-house manufacture into more specialised areas [8]. In 1938 the dispensary of one 200-bed provincial hospital was equipped with an autoclave, refrigerator, hot-air oven, two emulsifying and mixing machines and a still. It was making sterile glycerine, sterile sodium citrate for blood transfusions, zinc cream and paste, and dusting powders. Four varieties of cod liver oil emulsion with vitamin A concentrates and iron were prepared for distribution to surrounding health centres. They still prepared large quantities of soap solution. In addition, the pharmacist was responsible for the ordering and issuing of dressings, surgical sundries, glassware and instruments, and for arranging repairs to the latter, an activity carried on from the days of the apothecary.

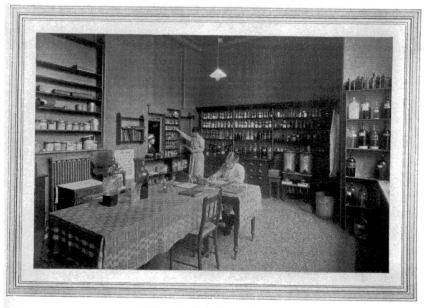

DISPENSARY, NEW HOSPITAL FOR WOMEN.

Figure 8.1 Dispensary of the New Hospital for Women, London, c. 1916. Reproduced by permission of the Wellcome Library, London.

A description of the new pharmaceutical department at Guy's Hospital, in 1940, reflects the pattern of dispensing at the time, with its central fixtures for stock mixtures in Winchester bottles and earthenware jars [9]. Another fixture holds metal containers for glycerine, liquid paraffin, malt extract, etc. Under the benches are drawers and cupboards for ointment containers, bottles, and all the normal requirements for dispensing. Cupboards on two walls above the benches accommodate the 'more out-of-the-way drugs, tablets and of course proprietaries'. In adjoining rooms the hospital prepared sterile intravenous solutions and injections, a large variety of tablets on a tabletting machine, and ointments using an end-runner mill.

The Pharmacy and Poisons Act 1933

The 1933 Pharmacy and Poisons Act reintroduced one of the apothecary's responsibilities that had been allowed to lapse: pharmacists were required to visit the wards. Their duties were primarily to inspect the storage of scheduled poisons, and to ensure that the appropriate signatures were obtained for their use. Many pharmacists took this opportunity to discuss other problems associated with medicines and their administration with nursing staff. This increased contact with ward staff led to requests for practical instruction in pharmacy and dispensing to nurses in training.

An inquiry into the hospital pharmacy service was carried out by the Pharmaceutical Society in 1939 [10]. It found that two-thirds of the 397 hospitals with more than 100 beds employed a full-time pharmacist, and that 50% of those with less than 100 beds used outside pharmacists to supervise dispensing. The number of patients treated, both as inpatients and outpatients, continued to increase, and other hospital departments, such as radiology, began to make demands upon the pharmacist's expertise and time. Some departments were involved in the recovery of silver from used X-rays, as a source of income, during the Second World War.

Therapeutic revolution

The therapeutic explosion of the post-war years changed the practice of hospital pharmacy; it was the start of a period in which innovations by hospital pharmacists led to the development of pharmaceutical equipment. Dispensing of tablets for individual inpatients gave way to the issue of ward stocks of commonly used drugs.

Nurses began to produce medicines lists, by which stock was selected from a cupboard, and administrations were made at the bedside. This became a common source of medication errors, and resulted ultimately in the development of the medicine trolley. All the medicines in use could be transported around the ward to each bedside, and selection could be made against the original prescription.

Bulk tablet production ceased in most hospitals in favour of direct purchase from the manufacturer, although some teaching hospitals still produce small quantities of special formulations. The preparation of infusions and sterile irrigations increased.

Aseptic dispensing

The arrival of multi-dose vials of penicillin powder, which had to be reconstituted before issue to the wards, brought not only a high daily workload but an appreciation of the dangers of bacterial contamination. Enclosed cabinets were designed, in which the vials could be manipulated through glove ports, thus protecting the product from contamination and the operators from developing allergies to penicillin.

They were cleaned with spirit before use each time. Over the next 60 years these aseptic cabinets increased in sophistication and efficiency, to meet the dual demands of mixing large-volume containers of nutrients for intravenous feeding, and the hazards to the operator of handling sterile radioactive and cytotoxic materials.

Hospital pharmacy, 1948 to 1970

The introduction of the NHS in 1948 was eagerly awaited by hospital pharmacists. They hoped that the setting up of a Pharmaceutical Whitley Council would result in a national pay structure that would recognise their worth, and end the influence of the poverty-stricken voluntary hospitals on remuneration. Unfortunately this was not the case: the salaries agreed were low and career prospects poor. However, the problems were recognised, and in 1953 a government subcommittee was set up under the chairmanship of Sir Hugh Linstead to 'review the arrangements for the provision of pharmaceutical services in hospitals and to advise on the most efficient and economical organisation of those services'.

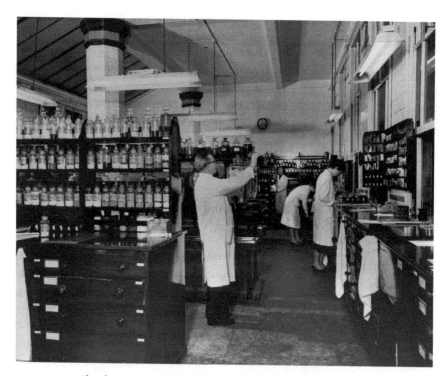

Figure 8.2   The dispensary, St Bartholomew's Hospital, 1959.

The Linstead Report

Linstead found that most pharmacies were efficient departments run on scientific and business principles despite poor facilities [11]. The range of activities observed was wide, and the report identified ten activities as the prime responsibility of pharmacy departments (Box 8.1). For the first time the pharmacist's responsibilities outside the pharmacy department were delineated. It opened the way for greater involvement on the wards, as well as reinforcing the investigative and development activities within the pharmacy itself. It also recognised the role played by teaching-hospital pharmacists in medical education, and recommended increased participation in medical decisions.

It was recognised that not all pharmacy departments were large enough to undertake all the functions, so a group pharmacy structure was established between adjacent hospitals. The group pharmacist had a professional managerial role over the whole group, although each pharmacist remained the employee of their Hospital Management Committee. Teaching hospitals retained their independence and medical school links under Boards of Governors. They were outside the Regional Hospital Board structure, but pharmacies linked to the same medical school often worked together on a voluntary basis.

Hospital pharmacy departments supported one another, each concentrating on the activities for which they were best equipped. Where hospitals were too small to have their own departments, pharmacists from another hospital within the group visited them to check ward

---

Box 8.1 Responsibilities of a pharmacy department (from the Linstead Report [11]).

The responsibilities of a pharmacy department include:

- providing, drugs, medicinal preparations, dressings, chemicals and pharmaceutical sundries, and ensuring the nature and quality thereof;
- ensuring their correct storage;
- dispensing prescriptions for in-patients and out-patients;
- preparing pharmaceuticals, including devising formulae for special needs;
- investigating pharmaceutical problems;
- assisting with the development of new treatments;
- promoting economy of use of medical supplies;
- assisting efficient prescribing through advice to prescribers;
- instructing users of medicines;
- training pharmacy students.

stocks and give advice. Staff shortages often made this arrangement unsatisfactory. The total pharmacy staff for England and Wales in 1955 was 1267 pharmacists and 858 technicians [12]. Group contracts for purchasing were set up in some areas to take advantage of bulk buying.

The Linstead Report recommended that some activities should cease; these included biochemical analysis, syringe sterilisation, and the purchase, storage and issue of surgical instruments and X-ray materials. The expansion of pathology services removed the need for the first, but the latter three persisted in many departments until Supplies and Central Sterile Supply Departments became fully operational in the 1960s. The supply of X-ray materials remained a bone of contention in some hospitals for many years. Pharmacists were happy to lose the procurement of films and developing fluids, but considered the new injectable diagnostic agents to be pharmaceuticals.

The Aitken Report

In 1958 the government initiated an inquiry into the control of dangerous drugs and poisons in hospitals. The subsequent Aitken Report [13] indicated that pharmacists were responsible for the safe and secure handling of medicines throughout the whole organisation, and not just within the pharmacy department. Thus when high levels of medication errors were detected on wards, pharmacists took the initiative. They set up multidisciplinary teams to examine drug administration and identify ways of reducing the risk [14]. Errors arose through illegible prescribing; inaccurate transcription of administration instructions by nurses onto medicine lists, which were then used for administration; failure to read labels or confusing labelling.

Within a decade systematised prescription sheets were introduced and, to avoid the need for nurse transcription of doses due while these were away from the ward for dispensing, ward pharmacists were introduced. Ward pharmacy duties included collecting details of new prescriptions for dispensing, and annotation of any prescriptions where the prescribed name differed from that on the stock container. Experiments were carried out using medicine trolleys with one drawer for each patient, and American systems in which unit-dose packs were preselected in the pharmacy and issued on a daily basis. Both systems transferred the responsibility for drug selection from the nurse to pharmacy staff. The reduction in medication errors observed was insufficient to justify the extra expense of unit doses in the UK at the time [15]. Education of prescribers was felt to be a more cost-effective approach, and many pharmacies introduced training sessions for junior doctors on appointment on the prescribing policies of the hospital.

Hospital pharmacy, 1970 to 1980

The activities being undertaken in hospital pharmacies in 1970 did not differ significantly from those proposed in the Linstead Report 15 years earlier, except in the emphasis on activities on the wards [16]. Bulk production of sterile infusions, irrigations, eye drops and single-dose injections was introduced, and the need to apply quality control to both purchased and internally manufactured products was stressed.

The hospital pharmacy service had by 1970 become a major contributor in the provision of pre-registration training for pharmacy graduates. Worries were still being expressed about the ability of pharmacists to fulfil their responsibilities in the face of chronic staff shortages. It was accepted that pharmacists had a responsibility to advise prescribers on the pharmacological value of the drugs available, and to ensure that prescribed drugs were of the nature and quality required. The Pharmaceutical Society recommended that if these responsibilities could not be met the pharmacist's workload should be reduced, not the standard of care. As a result many hospital pharmacies ceased dispensing for outpatients; patients were given prescriptions to be taken to a local pharmacy. This practice continues today as a means of relieving staff shortages in hospitals.

The practice of pre-packing standard quantities of analgesics and antibiotics labelled ready for dispensing by nurses to patients attending accident and emergency departments was also introduced to relieve pressure on pharmacy and nursing staff, especially outside normal hours. New labelling requirements set out in the Medicines (Labelling) Regulations of 1976 and the provision of child-resistant closures were applied here first. Hospitals were legally exempt from the requirements, but they were soon voluntarily applied to all outpatient dispensing in the interests of safety.

Hospital building programme

The 1970s was a decade of substantial hospital building in Britain, and the Department of Health developed a 'standard hospital plan', which was quick and economical to erect. The Best Buy Mark I contained only a small pharmacy, barely adequate for dispensing and ward supply. The Regional Pharmaceutical Officers Committee (RPhOs) contributed to the design of the Best Buy Mark II. This contained facilities for sterile production and tablet repackaging, as well as for extemporaneous non-sterile preparation. Four Best Buy hospitals were built in East Anglia alone. However, by the time the designs were perfected, outside influences and clinical progress rendered them inappropriate. During the 1980s the emphasis changed to a 'nucleus hospital plan', and although the RPhOs produced a blueprint for the pharmacy it reflected the requirements of the present service rather than anticipating future developments.

Medical gases

There was an extension of the pharmacist's responsibility for medical gases in 1972. Gases were always purchased as medicinal substances, but now pharmacists were asked to check new medical gas installations and piped gas systems, after shutdown for major repairs. One or more pharmacists in each district was specially trained for these duties and nominated as a 'suitably qualified person' to issue, with works staff, the authorisation to use the system when the work on it was completed and checked [17].

The Medicines Act 1968

Other legislation and external problems began to affect the hospital pharmacy service. In 1968 the Medicines Act introduced a licensing system for the production of pharmaceuticals, together with a code of practice, The Rules and Guidance for Good Pharmaceutical Manufacture and Distribution, usually known as 'The Orange Guide' [18]. Although Crown Immunity meant that the sanctions included in the Act could not be applied, health authorities were asked to comply with its recommendations as far as possible.

At the time of its introduction, many hospitals were manufacturing large quantities of intravenous fluids. However, in 1972, an incident involving the commercial supply of contaminated solutions resulted in further controls on hospital procedures, and many units found that the cost of introducing the new standards threw doubt on the economic case for continuing. Some hospitals switched their entire sterile production facilities to the production of bottled sterile water for operating theatres, along with bladder and wound irrigation solutions. Others ceased large-scale sterile production, sterile water being produced by central sterile supplies units. Some regions set up industrial-scale centralised sterile production facilities off-site, operated by hospital pharmacy staff. Some of these units pioneered the transition from glass to plastic containers.

By 1974 the practice of adding drugs to intravenous fluids was becoming widespread. A joint working party of the Standing Medical, Nursing and Midwifery, and Pharmaceutical Advisory Committees was asked to examine the risks, and to make recommendations on the responsibilities of the various professions [19]. It was agreed that admixture was a pharmaceutical operation and that ideally it should be carried out under the direct control of a pharmacist. Hospital pharmacists were asked to provide an individual dispensing service where possible, and where this was impracticable to advise on the policies, procedures and staff training for those involved. Thus the emphasis on sterile production changed in the early 1970s from bulk manufacture to complex aseptic dispensing, creating a need for technicians with new skills.

The Noel Hall Report

In 1970 a working party under Sir Noel Hall was set up to investigate the staffing situation and to make recommendations. The Noel Hall Report recommended restructuring the service on a larger scale to improve career opportunities, make better use of facilities and expertise, make greater use of support staff, and provide opportunities for further training and study for higher degrees [20]. The pharmaceutical industry supported the latter by awarding travelling scholarships and research awards through the Guild of Hospital Pharmacists [21].

Reorganisation along the lines proposed by Noel Hall began in 1971, with the appointment of regional and area pharmacists. However, the salaries were still too low to attract junior staff [22]. In 1974, reorganisation of the NHS structure reinforced the Noel Hall proposals by recommending a regional, area and district structure for the NHS as a whole. This enabled greater progress to be made [23].

Management structures

A number of senior management appointments were made: regional and area pharmacists became pharmaceutical officers, and a third tier, district pharmaceutical officers (DPhOs), were appointed. The higher levels were administrative posts based in the newly created offices with the rest of the management teams, but the DPhOs were frequently the chief pharmacists of the district general hospital, and remained based in their pharmacy departments. All officers were directly responsible to their employing health authority, giving an enhanced status to pharmacy.

The first newly created posts under the Noel Hall recommendations were those associated with the centralisation of technical services. They included regional specialists in quality assurance, drug information, radiopharmacy, and pharmaceutical research and development. Their role was to co-ordinate services across their region, ensure that the expertise and training of staff was adequate, set standards, and monitor their maintenance. Specialist advisory committees, with one representative from each region, were established to promote the sharing of good practice, and to promote the exchange of information between the Department of Health (DoH) and the hospital service. They met quarterly with the chief pharmacist and appropriate central technical staff at the DoH.

Hospital manufacturing

The 1975 circular HSC(IS)128 from the DoH applied the requirements of the Medicines Act to hospital manufacture and assembly [24]. The DoH set up a specialist production pharmacist advisory committee, to join those of RPhOs, quality assurance and drug information, to advise the DoH on the implications and implementation of the circular. Each region nominated the head of a production unit, although not all representatives had a regional responsibility.

Inspections were to take place in the same way as in the pharmaceutical industry. They would cover every aspect of the service – premises, procedures, materials, manufacturing methods and quality control. This required the separation of quality control and production activities within departments, including technical and support staff, and converted what had been largely a laboratory-based analytical quality control service into a much broader quality assurance activity. Inter-hospital, and eventually inter-regional sample testing (PITS) [25] was established to ensure consistency of laboratory standards throughout the service. It eventually involved over 40 laboratories.

Regional quality control pharmacists were given authority to inspect facilities, procedures and documentation in all hospital pharmacies within their region where manufacture or assembly was carried out. These internal NHS inspections supplemented those of the Medicines Inspectorate and by detecting problems early, helped to reduce the number of adverse reports, which could affect continuity of production. The increased demand for testing, and the sophistication and cost of the analytical equipment required, led eventually to the development of regional laboratories.

Through regional working parties of pharmacists involved in quality control and production, standard procedures and product specifications were drawn up. This assured purchasing pharmacists of the equivalence and quality of products, whichever hospital production unit made them. Product specifications are of particular value when requests from other hospitals reach a point where demand justifies a change from extemporaneous dispensing to a manufacturing process but is still insufficient to be attractive to the pharmaceutical industry.

Drug information services

In the 1970s the role of ward pharmacists extended to participation in ward rounds and direct contributions to patient care. The rapid growth in the number of pharmaceuticals entering the market made it impossible for individual clinicians or pharmacists to keep on top of the information required for their safe use. Drug information sections were established within hospital pharmacies to support ward pharmacists and to provide a query answering service for other staff. After the Noel Hall Report these units were supported by regional Drug Information Centres.

Regional drug information pharmacists recognised that the provision of unbiased information would require the critical assessment of a vast number of drug-related publications, and input from all those with appropriate expertise. They established a network to make best use of that expertise. Regular nationally circulated new-product evaluations and a computerised pharmaceutical information bank, *Pharmline*, were the result. To ensure that all material added to these databases was of consistent quality, standards were developed and training provided for all levels of drug information pharmacists, from ward-based to regional staff.

Specialist information centres on, for example, drugs in pregnancy, psychiatry or oncology, were established where there was a particular interest, and began to offer a service to their colleagues. Today, a national medicines information service serves the whole NHS from 270 departments and 15 regional centres [26].

Radiopharmacy

Radiopharmaceuticals are injectable solutions containing small amounts of radioactive material used in diagnosis. Traditionally doses had been prepared in physics laboratories within the radiotherapy department, but the development of scanners, generators of radioisotopes such as technetium^{99m} from molybdenum^{99m}, and the use of injectable short half-life products, necessitated the development of departments with aseptic dispensing facilities.

By 1980 there were 60 such departments. Regional centres provided for day-to-day needs in the local department, supplied material and provided advice to smaller district general hospital departments, provided training for pharmacists, and undertook research into new products and applications [27].

Hospital pharmacy, 1980 to 1990

Ward pharmacy changed gradually during the 1980s, from a stock control/supply function to a proactive service providing prescribing and administration advice to clinicians, nurses and patients, in addition to the drugs themselves. The Nuffield Report on Pharmacy in 1986 described hospital pharmacy as a 'clinical pharmacy service' [28]. It suggested that this implied 24-hour pharmacy cover. As a result most district general hospitals introduced an on-call system.

Some attempted residency schemes, but these proved inefficient of pharmacists' time except in the largest teaching hospitals. Later DoH Circulars supported the new clinical emphasis, seeing it as an improved use of pharmacy services, leading to better patient care and the cost-effective use of medicines. Particular emphasis was placed on the monitoring of drug therapy and the control of expenditure [29].

Clinical services

The development of clinical services was not uniform across the hospital service. Some pharmacists became specialists in a particular clinical field and provided an extended service to their wards or hospital. Many hospitals produced prescribing guidance and formularies. Teaching hospitals developed formulations and delivery systems to meet major clinical advances such as home dialysis, organ transplantation and chronic pain control. Greater use was made of technicians in order to free pharmacists' time, and an improvement in the career structure for technicians resulted.

By 1990, 97% of hospitals had a multidisciplinary Drug and Therapeutics Committee [30], which oversaw the content and implementation of the formulary and prescribing policies. Substitution of branded products by generic equivalents had been a long-standing practice within the hospital service. Monitoring prescribing to maximise this, and compliance with other hospital formulary recommendations, became an essential part of the ward pharmacist's duties.

The undergraduate pharmacy course did not fully meet the needs of the new clinical pharmacist and in-service clinical training programmes were set up in some hospitals. A masters course in clinical pharmacy was started in Manchester in 1978. Many other courses followed, and the content of the undergraduate course was adapted to meet the growing need. By 1990 almost all hospitals had pharmacists who monitored drug therapy, but a much smaller percentage were involved in medication history taking or patient counselling [31].

Standards of service

Clinical services were not the only service to develop unevenly, and following the Nuffield Report the RPhOs, with others, produced a set of *Standards for Pharmaceutical Services in Health Authorities in England* [32]. These set out the activities involved in the provision of a full service (Box 8.2), with criteria for measuring the level and quality of service provided in various sizes and types of hospital. These were commended to general managers at all levels of the NHS. In 1999, the NHS Quality Control Committee issued a guidance booklet on quality audits and their application to hospital pharmacy, and this has now been adopted as a key component of clinical governance.

In 1986, the Modern Materials Management Group (3M) reported on an *Investigation into the Provision of Pharmaceuticals to Health Authorities* [33]. This recommended that each Regional Health Authority (RHA) set up a 'short-line store' to handle low-volume/high-value lines. The report provided an impetus for the improvement and computerisation of regional contracting, drug purchase and stock control. It also signalled the devolution of responsibility for day-to-day work to technicians and clerical staff.

Loss of crown immunity

Further rationalisation of hospital manufacturing services occurred during the 1980s, when the DoH recommended that the economic viability of in-house manufacture should be assessed, and hospital production of commercially available products should cease. Although some regional centralisation occurred the full impact was not felt until

---

Box 8.2   Responsibilities of a hospital pharmaceutical service [33].

Activities undertaken in all pharmacies:

- establishing and maintaining safe systems of work for each section of the service;
- procuring pharmaceuticals, undertaking medicines utilisation review and maintaining stock control;
- distributing medicines;
- providing ward pharmacy, in-patient prescription monitoring, and clinical services where possible;
- manufacturing and assembling medicines;
- applying appropriate quality assurance for the level and type of activity undertaken;
- establishing and maintaining a local formulary and participating in the Drug and Therapeutics Committee;
- providing drug information services and monitoring the occurrence of adverse drug reactions.

Activities determined by clinical need or local circumstances:

- patient counselling and medication history services;
- therapeutic drug level monitoring services;
- intravenous additive and parenteral nutrition services;
- aseptic dispensing services;
- cytotoxic preparation and reconstitution services;
- radio-pharmaceutical services;
- participation in clinical trials.

1990, when the NHS lost its crown immunity, and production units required a licence from the Medicines Control Agency (MCA). The cost of upgrading smaller units to the required standard proved prohibitive in many cases, and technical services in these hospitals are now primarily concerned with aseptic preparation, non-sterile extemporaneous dispensing and repackaging.

Central intravenous additive services (CIVAS) are considered high risk, and are either controlled by the MCA, under special manufacturing licences, or by regional quality assurance pharmacists working to guidance issued as *Aseptic Dispensing for NHS Patients* [34], where production is on an individual patient basis. Such dispensing services are frequently operated and managed by suitably trained technicians, with pharmacists having overall responsibility.

Clinical trials impose a high workload on hospital pharmacies, especially in teaching hospitals. Pharmacists are usually involved at the start of each trial and play an active part in the Ethical Committee approval process. Their expertise became particularly important after medicines undergoing clinical trial no longer had to have a clinical trials certificate under the Medicines Act in 1981. The subsequent dispensing procedures and special patient counselling to maintain 'blind' studies involves all the pharmacy staff at ward level and in in-patient and out-patient dispensaries.

Hospital pharmacy since 1990

Since 1990 government pronouncements, economic pressure, changes in pharmaceutical education and pharmacists' preference have all moved hospital pharmacy into a more patient-orientated service. The more traditional duties of dispensing, ward supply and stock control and purchasing are largely carried out and managed by technicians, whose career structure has greatly improved. Hospital pharmacies in England and Wales are now staffed by 3837 pharmacists and 4023 technicians, with 39% of the latter in supervisory or managerial grades in 2001 [35].

Today pharmacists spend a greater part of their time outside the pharmacy department interacting with other health professionals, giving closer integration of pharmacy into the totality of patient care. At the same time senior staff are involved in many committees and working parties within the hospital where previously pharmaceutical expertise was only obtained on an *ad hoc* basis. Areas of involvement include clinical governance; risk management; clinical effectiveness audit; control of infection; health and safety and patient liaison.

The level of clinical pharmacy provision still varies between hospitals. The Audit Commission reported in 2001 that it represented less than 30% of the pharmacists' time in some hospitals but over 70% in others [36]. The components of the service also vary and can be divided between general services and those provided for specialised units (Box 8.3). An important role of hospital pharmacists remains the education of clinical and nursing staff about medicines and their uses.

In broad terms the duties and responsibilities of the 21st century hospital pharmacist and the earliest apothecaries do not differ significantly. It would appear to have gone full circle, from complete patient care through restriction to preparation and supply of medicines and back to a clinical role supported throughout by technical staff. However, the volume and potency of today's medicines, the risks attached to their use, and the confidence placed in the pharmacist by professional staff and patients suggest a parallel point on an ascending

---

Box 8.3 Components of a clinical pharmacy service.

Services common to all hospitals:

- prescription monitoring;
- providing prescribing advice to medical and nursing staff;
- detection and prevention of medication errors and detection and reporting of adverse drug reactions (CSM yellow card scheme);
- patient education and counselling;
- taking medication histories;
- establishing links with primary care on patient discharge;
- advising on pharmacokinetics and therapeutic drug level monitoring;
- clinical and professional audit.

Specialised services provided according to clinical need or local demand:

- anticoagulant services;
- pain management and palliative care;
- geriatric and paediatric services, including development of appropriate regimens;
- nutrition, selection, formulation, and preparation of nutrients;
- oncology, prescribing regimens and side-effect control;
- mental health, including monitoring and community support;
- renal services, development of treatment guidelines;
- HIV/AIDS services, including patient education and counselling.

---

spiral rather than a circle, with ample opportunities to continue the climb.

References

1. Whittet T D. The history of pharmacy in British hospitals. In: Poynter F N L, ed. *The Evolution of Pharmacy in Britain*. London: Pitman Medical, 1965: 17.
2. Poynter F N L. *The Evolution of Hospitals in Britain*. London: Pitman Medical, 1964.
3. Granshaw L. *The Hospital in History*. London: Routledge, 1989.
4. Taylor A L. Hospitals and pharmaceutical education. *Public Pharmacist* 1936; 1: 4.
5. Buchanan M. The present position of women in pharmacy. *The Pharmaceutical Journal* 1908; 80: 675–678.
6. *Summary of the 2002 Pharmacy Workforce Census*. London: Royal Pharmaceutical Society, 2003: 25.
7. Fish J W B. The Guild of Hospital Pharmacists 1923–1983. *The Pharmaceutical Journal* 1983; 231: 338.

8. Anderson S C. The historical context of pharmacy. In: Taylor K, Harding G, eds. *Pharmacy Practice*. London: Taylor and Francis, 2001: 17.

9. Moore J. Pharmaceutical department Guy's Hospital. *Public Pharmacist* 1940; 1: 4.

10. *Report of the Committee of Inquiry, Part II*. London: Pharmaceutical Society of Great Britain, 1941: 8.

11. *Report of the Sub-Committee on Hospital Pharmaceutical Services (Linstead Report)*. London: HMSO, 1955.

12. Steane M A S. *The Development of Hospital Pharmacy in England and Wales* (thesis). Bradford: University of Bradford, 1982.

13. *DHSS Report on the Control of Dangerous Drugs and Poisons in Hospitals (Aitken Report)*. London: HMSO, 1958: 18.

14. Crooks J, Calder G. Hospital pharmacists on the ward. *The Pharmaceutical Journal* 1966; 196: 242–244.

15. Ellis S. *Pharmaceutical Services and Patient Safety in Hospitals* (thesis). Bradford: University of Bradford, 1973.

16. Fitchett E. The pharmacist's role. *J Hosp Pharm* 1970; 28: 11–15.

17. *Piped Medical Gases, Medical Compressed Air and Medical Vacuum Installations, Permit to Work System*. HN (77) 45. London: DHSS, 1977.

18. Department of Health and Social Security. *Guide to Good Pharmaceutical Manufacturing Practice*, 1st edn. London: HMSO, 1971.

19. Breckenridge A. *The Report of a Working Party on the Addition of Drugs to Intravenous Fluids*. HC (76) 9. London: DHSS, 1976.

20. *Report of the Working Party on the Hospital Pharmaceutical Service (Noel Hall Report)*. London: HMSO, 1970.

21. Greenleaf J. The Guild of Hospital Pharmacists 1923–1983. *The Pharmaceutical Journal*, 1983; 231: 339.

22. Brookes W T. *History of the Guild 1983 to 1997*. London: Guild of Hospital Pharmacists, 1998.

23. *Management Arrangements for the Reorganised National Health Service*. London: HMSO, 1972.

24. *Application of the Medicines Act to Health Authorities*. HSC (IS) 128. London: Department of Health, 1975.

25. Beaumont I M. Quality assurance. In: Stephens M, ed. *Hospital Pharmacy*. London: Pharmaceutical Press, 2003: 83–86.

26. Golightly P. Medicines information. In: Stephens M, ed. *Hospital Pharmacy*. London: Pharmaceutical Press, 2003: 91–120.

27. McCarthy T, Steane M A. Specialised but not isolated. *The Pharmaceutical Journal* 1980; 224: 597–598.

28. *Pharmacy: The Report of a Committee of Inquiry Appointed by the Nuffield Foundation*. London: Nuffield Foundation, 1986.

29. Department of Health. *The Way Forward for Hospital Pharmaceutical Services*. HC(88)54. London: DoH, 1988.

30. Fitzpatrick R. Strategic medicines management. In: Stephens M, ed. *Hospital Pharmacy*. London: Pharmaceutical Press, 2003: 157–160.

31. Child D, Cooke J. Clinical pharmacy services. In: Stephens M, ed. *Hospital Pharmacy*. London: Pharmaceutical Press, 2003: 124–146.

32. Watling J J (ed.). *Standards for Pharmaceutical Services in Health Authorities in England*, 2nd edn. London: Regional Pharmaceutical Officers Committee, 1989.

33. MMM Consultancy Group Ltd. *Investigation into the Provision of Pharmaceuticals to Health Authorities*. London: MMM Consulting, 1986.

34. Department of Health. *Aseptic Dispensing for NHS Patients*. EL(97)52. London: DoH, 1997.

35. NHS Pharmacy Education and Development Committee. *Hospital Pharmacy Staffing Surveys*, 2001 and 2002.

36. Audit Commission. *A Spoonful of Sugar – Medicines Management in NHS Hospitals*. London: Audit Commission, 2001.

9

The development of the pharmaceutical industry

Judy Slinn

Today, the pharmaceutical industry is dominated by large multinational corporations, which are characterised by a 'combination of research prowess and marketing power' [1]. It also encompasses a wide variety of small and medium-sized enterprises, some of which have found specialised niche activities for themselves, many of which remain national in the scope of their operations. This configuration is the result of almost two centuries of development and while, as we shall see, the most rapid growth of the industry has taken place since 1945, the significant shift from the making of medicines on a domestic basis to the industrial manufacture, first of the ingredients and some medicines, then of the drugs themselves, is a phenomenon of the 19th and early 20th centuries.

That change was driven by a combination of economic, social and political factors, including urban growth and prosperity, the incidence

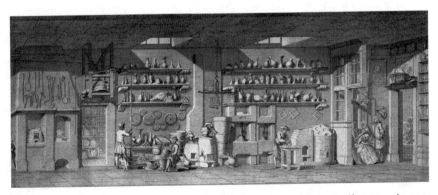

Figure 9.1 Production before the Industrial Revolution: Ambrose Godfrey Hanckwitz's laboratory in Maiden Lane, London, was constructed for scientific experimentation but was subsequently used for pharmaceutical processes, as depicted in this 1706 engraving by George Vertue.

of disease, the development of scientific, medical and technological knowledge and its diffusion, the growth and structure of national healthcare systems and of consumer demand and consumerism, each closely related to the others and of varying significance at different times. This chapter explores these changes in four broad chronologically divided periods. The first describes the origins of the industry in the 19th century; the second takes us from around 1890 to the outbreak of the Second World War; the third from 1939 up to the 1970s; and the fourth through the last two decades of the 20th century. The chapter begins, however, with a discussion of the nature of the pharmaceutical business today.

The business of making medicines

The business of the pharmaceutical industry may be described as the manufacture and processing of raw materials into medicines that prevent, treat or cure disease and illness, and the distribution, marketing and sale of those medicines in a finished form [2]. The variety of forms includes tablets, capsules, powders, ointments and syrups, as well as drugs, vaccines and sera in forms that can be injected into the body. For some of the many individual companies constituting the industry, the business also includes the search for and discovery of new compounds through extensive research and development (R&D); these have to be formulated and tested extensively to establish their safety and medicinal efficacy to the satisfaction of the regulatory authorities before they can be marketed.

Some of the industry's products are prescription-only medicines (those not advertised to the public are known as ethical medicines). The most profitable of these are usually the most recent discoveries, protected by patent and – after the patent expires – by brand name. Other products are generic medicines, that is, not protected by patent or brand name (although manufacturers may try to differentiate them by trade marks and their own name), while others are sold as proprietary or over-the-counter products. The market remains heterogeneous by virtue of the 40 or so therapeutic subgroups into which its products divide.

At the end of the 20th century, worldwide sales by the pharmaceutical industry were valued at approximately US$350 billion, and were expected to rise to a figure of US$500 billion within 5 years. Some 80% of those sales were made in ten countries, more than half of them in the two largest markets in the world, the USA and Japan [3]. The industry making those sales was dominated by a relatively small number of large multinational corporations, mainly based in the USA and Europe, whose names and businesses are increasingly global in their scale and scope.

The extent of globalisation, however, should not be exaggerated. As a study sponsored by the United Nations Industrial Development Organisation (UNIDO) in the early 1990s showed, 'the bulk of the world's pharmaceuticals are manufactured in a very few industrialised countries. The pattern of drug consumption is much the same: over three-quarters of all medicines are sold in industrialised countries, with the remainder being purchased by households in developing countries' [1].

These factors are necessarily reflected in this account of the growth of the industry, with its focus on developments in Europe (particularly in Britain, France, Germany and Switzerland) and the USA.

Origins in the 19th century

The isolation and identification of the alkaloids (see Chapter 10) in the early years of the 19th century was a significant factor in the development by a number of retail pharmacies of separate manufacturing establishments. Most medicines then offered by medical practitioners and pharmacies, for which there was an increasing demand in the countries experiencing the first industrial revolution [4], were based on plant extracts, mineral salts and inorganic chemicals [5]. The extraction and

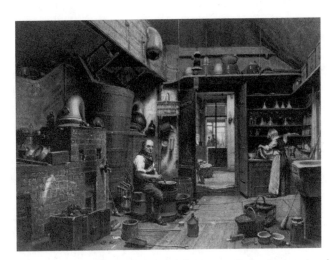

Figure 9.2 Laboratory of John Bell & Co.'s pharmacy, Oxford Street, London, 1842. The laboratory man is John Simmonds, who had worked there since its opening in 1798. Mezzotint by J G Murray after a watercolour by W H Hunt.

purification processes necessary, as well as some of the finishing formulation, outgrew the back rooms of the retail premises and could be carried out more efficiently and safely on a larger scale on an industrial basis.

Origins in Great Britain

For example, in Britain in 1806 the partnership of William Allen and Luke Howard, owners of a century-old pharmacy at Plough Court in the City of London, was amicably dissolved. While Allen retained the retail business, known later as Allen & Hanburys, Howard developed a manufacturing business based on mercurial preparations, chemicals used in medicines and a specialisation in quinine (Chapter 10). It was not until 1874 that Allen & Hanburys took the further step of establishing its own separate manufacturing plant at Bethnal Green [6].

Similarly, in the second half of the century Thomas Morson, who had a thriving wholesale and retail pharmacy business in London, established a separate factory to manufacture alkaloids [7]. At a time when family-owned businesses dominated most industries, such a separation might sometimes take place for family reasons, but was underpinned by a perception of the opportunities offered in an expanding market. Arthur Cox had established himself as a 'chemist and druggist' – the usual nomenclature in Britain at that time – in Brighton in 1839. For some years Cox worked on developing a technique for coating pills to disguise the unpleasant taste of the contents while ensuring the contents would be ingested. In 1854 a patent for his coating, a tasteless non-metallic film that gave his pills an 'elegant pearl-like appearance', gave him a 14-year monopoly to establish the brand. In 1871 he separated the business of manufacturing, which he continued to own and run, moving it into new premises, while he handed the retail shop to his son of his first marriage. The manufacturing business was to provide for the family of Cox's second marriage [8].

However, it was not only the retail pharmacists who expanded into manufacture. Several businesses were established during the 19th century as 'manufacturing chemists', founded by young men who had qualified, by apprenticeship, as pharmacists but had no direct connection with retailing. Examples of such businesses include that which became known as May & Baker, which began to manufacture in Battersea in 1834; and that known as Whiffens, similarly located in Battersea, which grew from the mid-1850s when Thomas Whiffen joined a small business making fine chemicals there [9].

Origins in the USA

In the early years of the 19th century, many of the retail pharmacies supplied a growing export trade to British colonies across the world, including the former colony in North America. The war of 1812, however, disrupted the trade and as a result, between 1818 and 1822, six fine chemical manufacturers established businesses in and around Philadelphia to supply the rapidly growing populations of the American east coast [10]. Most of these, including for example Smith Kline & French, survived to become well-known multinational pharmaceutical corporations in the 20th century. At that time, however, their product portfolios were very similar to those of their former suppliers in Britain, reflecting also the medical and scientific knowledge of the time. They included alkaloids such as morphine and quinine as well as acids, essential oils, plant extracts and mercury.

By mid-century more manufacturers had established themselves elsewhere in the USA. In 1858 Squibb opened a laboratory in New York to supply medicines to the US army, specialising in the production of high purity ether and chloroform for use as anaesthetics. Demand for the industry's products rose during the American civil war in the 1860s. In the expansionary period that followed, new businesses were established across the country, including Parke Davis in Detroit in 1866, Eli Lilly in Indianapolis in 1876, Upjohn in Michigan in 1885, and Abbott and G D Searle, both in Chicago in 1888 [11].

Origins in Germany

In Germany, too, the first pharmaceutical manufacturers show a similar pattern of development, as retail pharmacists branched out into separate manufacturing establishments. E Merck, originating as a pharmacy in 1668, started to produce alkaloids on an industrial scale in 1827, at a factory in Darmstadt. Over the next few decades it became the largest German supplier of fine chemicals. Elsewhere in Germany, Riedel's 'Schweizerapotheke' became well known for its alkaloids [12]. Ernst Schering founded his pharmacy in Berlin in 1851 and some four years later started manufacturing products for sale to other pharmacies [13]. C F Boehringer was involved in establishing a pharmacy in Stuttgart in 1817 and some ten years later added a manufacturing plant to the business. It was the next generation of the Boehringer family who integrated and developed a quinine business acquired by the founder and then moved all production to a new, larger factory at Mannheim [14].

Pharmacy, however, was not the only mainspring of pharmaceutical manufacturing in Germany. The production of dyestuffs, derived from coal tar distillates, was a branch of the chemical industry in which Germany came to excel in the second half of the 19th century, creating a position as a world leader that continued virtually unchallenged until the Second World War. It was in the major firms of the German organic chemical industry that, in the last two decades of the 19th century, new chemical compounds for medicinal use were discovered and developed. The first dyestuffs company to prepare pharmaceuticals was Hoechst, based in Frankfurt, which in 1888 introduced two analgesics – firstly antipyrin (phenazone), followed soon after by amidopyrine (brand name Pyramidon).

In the same year Bayer, founded in 1861, introduced a competitive product, acetophenetidin (phenacetin), followed quickly by two sedatives, sulphonmethane (sulphonal) and sulphonethylmethane (trional). At that time both Hoechst and Bayer were large companies, larger than any elsewhere in Europe or in America. In the 1880s Hoechst employed 2000 men in all [12]. Bayer employed about 1000 men, and 27 chemists in its research department, according to one of May & Baker's partners, Thomas Tyrer, who negotiated an agency agreement with Bayer for May & Baker to sell phenacetin and sulphonal in Britain. In contrast, May & Baker at that time employed probably not much over 100 men and had no research department [15].

Dyestuffs and mass production

In Britain, France and the USA attempts to develop a successful dyestuffs industry to challenge the German dominance had largely failed. That is not to say that there were not small dyestuffs companies and in France in the late 19th century, for example, Usines de Rhône had a small dyestuffs business and started making pharmaceuticals. In Switzerland, four firms developed in the second half of the century, all based in Basle, which manufactured dyestuffs, albeit using intermediates imported from Germany. The most significant of these were CIBA, the product of an 1884 merger of smaller businesses, Geigy, which had grown out of a dry saltery business established in 1758, and Sandoz, formed in 1876. In the 1880s CIBA and Geigy also began to manufacture pharmaceuticals and in 1896 Hoffman-La Roche was established as a pharmaceutical manufacturer.

By the 1890s, pharmaceutical products discovered as a result of scientific research in organic chemistry were beginning to move to centre

stage in the industry. By then too there had been technological developments, which played a significant role in a move towards mass production. For centuries pills, like those made by Cox's, had been largely
hand-made, but a method of mass production for sugar-coated pills
developed in France was further refined in the USA in the 1860s by
William Warner, one of the Philadelphia manufacturers [16]. In the
1870s Parke Davis developed the gelatine capsule, which was not only
easier for patients to swallow but also permitted a greater precision of
dose. Machinery to compress powders into tablets was developed in
Europe and in the USA in the 1860s.

The firm that became best known for its use of this machinery was
that of Burroughs Wellcome, established in London by two young
American pharmacists in 1880. Not only was it the first business in the
British industry to use the 'detailing concept' for its marketing, but it
also embarked on litigation in 1903, to defend the firm's trademark,
Tabloid, registered in 1884. The case attracted press attention, gener-
ating a good deal of useful publicity, while the success of the action fixed
the link between *Tabloid* and Wellcome inextricably in the public mind
[17]. Burroughs Wellcome came to occupy a central position in the
British industry in the early 20th century.

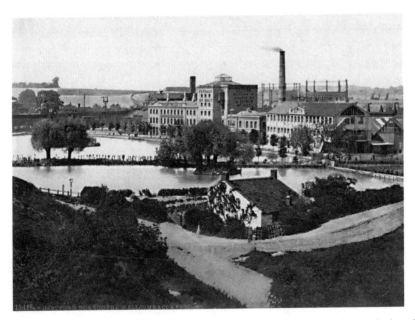

Figure 9.3 Burroughs Wellcome's factory at Dartford, Kent, c. 1896. Reproduced
by permission of GlaxoSmithKline.

Developments from 1890 to 1939

The origins and development of the pharmaceutical industry through the 19th century came from these two separate and distinctive directions. Over the next half century, these more or less integrated, so that we can speak more accurately of one pharmaceutical industry, rather than of pharmacy on the one hand and organic chemistry on the other. One historian of medicine has suggested that 'the study of materia medica developed during the 19th century into laboratory-based pharmacology. Meanwhile drugs research and manufacturing became inseparably linked' [18]. It was a process which was not perhaps quite as complete as that quotation might suggest by the end of the 19th century, but it was certainly well under way.

Research-led expansion before 1914

It has been argued that, in the USA, the 1890s were watershed years, for two reasons. The first was that some companies began to use scientifically and medically trained people in a systematic fashion; they were able to do so because medical schools started to include scientific medicine, particularly bacteriology, in their curriculum. The second was that the decade was characterised by significant growth in the industry, as there were new opportunities for the exploitation of national markets. Companies such as Parke Davis, Upjohn and Lilly grew rapidly, while Smith Kline & French became the largest of the Philadelphia manufacturers [19]. All of them enlarged not only their manufacturing operations but also their sales forces to reach the fast-growing urban populations across the USA, as the economy expanded.

The opportunities offered in the American market did not go unnoticed in Europe, and the German pharmaceutical companies were not slow in starting to make their presence felt there. Schering had developed a large international trade in which exports to the USA played an important part. Hoechst had a growing portfolio of bacteriological products including diphtheria serum introduced in the 1890s, while after the turn of the century it developed cocaine substitutes such as procaine hydrochloride (Novocain), and in 1910–11 arsphenamine (Salvarsan), the first of the organo-arsenic compounds to offer an effective treatment for syphilis. Bayer's development of aspirin, launched in 1898, led to successful sales worldwide, enhancing its position as the largest German chemical company.

In the first decade of the 20th century Bayer introduced a number of sedatives, including the barbiturate barbitone (Veronal), which it

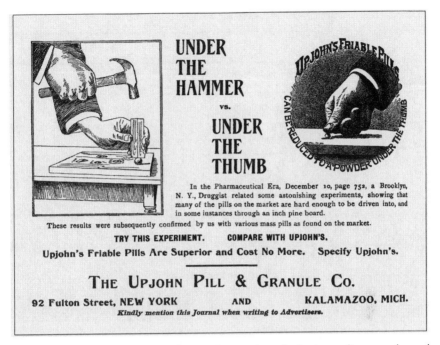

Figure 9.4 Advertising assumed a significant role in the business climate at the end of the 19th century. This advertisement was placed in the *American Druggist and Pharmaceutical Record* in 1897 and is reproduced with permission of the American Institute of the History of Pharmacy from its Kremers Reference Files.

licensed from Merck, who discovered it in 1904. Merck itself established a sales office in New York in 1891, under the direction of young George Merck, whose father ran the German factory. By 1897 sales in the USA topped US$1 million. George Merck became a US citizen in 1902 and shortly afterwards began manufacturing at Rahway in New Jersey and in St Louis [20]. By 1913 Merck employed 2000 people in its US operations.

Growth also took place elsewhere in the world. In Scandinavia the Swedish firm, Astra, was established in 1913. Developments in Norway in the late 19th century involving 'substantial population growth, considerable health problems and rapidly developing healthcare services' brought a virtual explosion in the market for medicines. To satisfy this demand, several pharmaceutical businesses were established, including that of Nyegaard & Co, which moved rapidly from agency to wholesaler to, in 1911, manufacturer; its most significant product then was a tablet of aspirin (acetylsalicylic acid), known by the brand name Globoid [21].

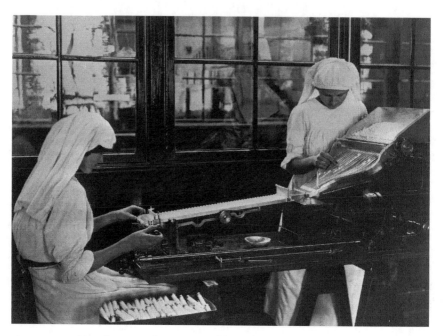

Figure 9.5 Manufacture of aspirin tablets at Wuppertal Elberfeld, c. 1910. Reproduced by permission of Bayer AG.

Developments in Great Britain

In Britain, Allen & Hanburys enjoyed a 'period of spectacular growth' between 1893 and 1918, although it included the development of related but non-pharmaceutical businesses, such as milk products and surgical instruments. The company's turnover doubled between 1911 and 1918, approaching £800,000 in the latter year. Over a similar period, 1911 to 1917, May & Baker more than tripled its turnover. Meanwhile the growth of the business of Burroughs Wellcome led to the establishment in 1894 of Physiological Research Laboratories and in 1896 of Chemical Research Laboratories. It was scientifically qualified staff from these laboratories who, over the next two decades, were instrumental in establishing research and development at Boots, British Drug Houses and Glaxo, thus stimulating further industry expansion.

There were, too, new factories established by Hoechst and Bayer, as well as by the US company, Parke Davis. In 1891 Parke Davis opened its first sales office in London. Eight years later the company bought land at Hounslow, where it built warehouses and then, in 1907, a factory [22]. Other American companies contented themselves for the time being with the use of agents to market and distribute their products in Britain and in the countries of the British empire: Smith Kline & French, for example, had a longstanding relationship with A J White and its subsidiary, Menley and James.

Impact of the First World War

This rapidly growing internationalism in the industry was inevitably disrupted during the First World War. In Britain, German products could no longer be imported, German patents and trademarks were suspended and the subsidiaries of German companies were closed down. British companies were encouraged by the government to start the manufacture of organic chemicals to replace the previously imported German drugs such as Salvarsan. Through its connection with the French company, Poulenc Frères, May & Baker had access to the French-developed arsenicals and was licensed, alongside Burroughs Wellcome, to manufacture them. This led directly to a close relationship with the newly established Medical Research Committee, later Council (MRC), which was responsible for testing the arsenicals, as well as to expansion of the

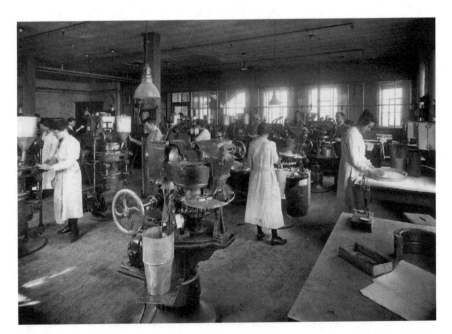

Figure 9.6 Tablet production at Boots' Island Street works, probably 1910s. Reproduced by permission of Boots Group Archives.

business in the shape of a new manufacturing plant and the growth of the company's scientific research. A number of companies, including Boots, began to manufacture aspirin and other synthetic drugs previously imported from Germany [23].

In the USA, after its entry into the war in 1917, the patents for German products were abrogated to US manufacturers, enabling companies like Abbott to add barbiturates and anaesthetics to their product portfolio and expand their operations [24]. The ties between Merck's subsidiary in the USA and its parent company in Germany were severed during the war, a break that became permanent, each thereafter pursuing its own path. Merck Inc. became and stayed an American company, merging in 1927 with the Philadelphia company, Powers-Weightman-Rosengarten (itself the product of an earlier 1904 merger). Similarly in 1929 Sharp and Dohme, manufacturing chemists, merged with the Mulford company, which had specialised in biological products and vaccines.

The inter-war years, 1918 to 1939

The inter-war years have been characterised as the age of vitamins, insulin, hormones and the sulpha-drugs [25], all of which provided stimuli to the growth of the industry even during the world economic depression. Insulin, discovered and developed in Canada (see Chapter 10), represented prestige and growth not only for Lilly, which was closely involved in the project, but also to the companies chosen as licensees to produce it [26]. New hormonal preparations emerged from research by a number of companies, among them the German company Schering (now merged with Kahlbaum and part of a larger combination, Kokswerke & Chemische Fabriken) and the US company Parke Davis, which continued to grow its business with the introduction to the market of thyroxine and other hormonal products.

More than three decades of work on accessory food factors – known as vitamins from 1912 – bore fruit in the early 1920s and, by the end of that decade, had brought a new company into the British industry. The Glaxo Department of the Nathan trading company (it became Glaxo Laboratories in 1935) started to manufacture vitamins to enhance the baby food it manufactured from dried milk [27]. Some pharmaceutical companies were attracted to the business of synthesising and manufacturing vitamins, including the Swiss company Hoffman-La Roche and American companies such as Abbott Laboratories. In the USA, the value of the wholesale vitamin market grew from less than

US$5 million in 1925 to just under US$100 million in 1939, to represent more than 10% of the market [25].

Sulpha-drugs were discovered in Germany (see Chapter 10) in the early 1930s. Further development took place in France, at Rhone-Poulenc, the company created by merger in the late 1920s when it also acquired May & Baker in order to access the British empire markets. The development of the sulphonamide, sulphapyridine (M&B 693), gave an impetus to May & Baker's growth in the late 1930s. The link between successful performance, growth and innovation, so well exemplified by the German companies, led an increasing number of companies in Europe and the USA to start to invest in R&D. In the USA, companies began to build up their own research and development departments, as much as the circumstances of the depression allowed, as well as to initiate and foster links with academic and scientific institutions whose research might feed into the discovery and development of new products [28].

In the late 1930s, two US companies followed in the footsteps of Parke Davis in establishing themselves as manufacturers in Britain. Abbott Laboratories set up a small factory in Perivale, west London, in 1937, principally to manufacture thiopentone sodium (Pentothal), its new anaesthetic whose fast action and quick recovery time made it an ideal drug to use on the battlefield. In 1939, Lilly started manufacture at the new factory it had built at Basingstoke [29].

Early mergers and amalgamations

Although amalgamation and growth had led to the emergence of large chemical companies in the USA, and in Britain to the creation of Imperial Chemical Industries (ICI), in part as a response to events in Germany, companies like Du Pont in the USA and ICI in the UK did not enter the pharmaceutical industry at this time. By contrast, in Germany there had been several movements towards the creation of larger units in the chemical industry; these culminated in the creation in 1925 of IG Farben, which, through Bayer and Hoechst, came to occupy an important place in the pharmaceutical industry. Merck, Boehringer and Knoll were also amalgamated into a larger unit.

These combines were larger than any other pharmaceutical corporation in the world at that time and, not surprisingly, the innovatory advantage in organic chemicals remained with Germany. This was clearly reflected in the distribution of world pharmaceutical exports in 1938. Of the four major drug-exporting countries, German exports represented 39% of the total, the USA 13%, the UK 12% and Switzerland 7% [30]. It was then hardly surprising that at the outbreak of war in 1939 Britain found, as in 1914, its supplies of some major medicines (not least the anti-malarial drugs) abruptly cut off.

Developments from 1939 to 1980

That shortage of drugs in Britain brought ICI into pharmaceuticals at last, but there were few other initiatives in the industry. Six years of war in Europe, however, diverted all corporate resources and attention to meeting the wartime need for drugs as specified in a national formulary. Government controls of industry took state involvement in industry in most countries, certainly in Britain and in Germany, to unprecedented levels. The pharmaceutical industry's capacity and operations expanded, if not always in the directions they had previously planned.

The development of penicillin during the Second World War (Chapter 10), with its much publicised and apparently almost magical conquest of infection not only eclipsed the discovery of the sulpha-drugs, generally taken as the starting point of the therapeutic revolution, but also had far-reaching effects on the post-war growth and structure of the industry internationally. In the development process itself, under-taken in the USA, Pfizer, hitherto a fine chemical manufacturer, played a significant role in making possible the large-scale manufacture of penicillin using deep fermentation technology. This was shared with other US companies and, after the war, a number of European companies bought licences to use it. Penicillin pointed the way to the discovery of streptomycin, followed by the development of other antibiotics launched in the 1950s.

Expansion in the 1950s

In the post-war years a combination of factors drove the industry through a period of exponential growth. A world market estimated to be worth US$600 million before the war reached US$4000 million by the mid-1950s, and US$7000 million by the end of the 1950s [25]. Other sources suggest even faster growth: Green states that 'between 1939 and 1959 sales of pharmaceuticals increased from US$300 million to US$2.3 billion' [31]. In the USA where the growth was fastest, another measure of it is the increase in the number of salesmen, from a pre-war 2000 to 15,000 in 1959. The indirect nature of the transaction by which patients accessed medicine, through prescription by doctors, led to similar growth of sales forces in Europe. This was part of the transformation of the major companies into 'vertically-integrated research- and information-intensive 'specialty' manufacturers ... whose products were protected by patents, promoted by brand names, and usually purchased only with a doctor's prescription' [32].

While the therapeutic revolution with its new and much more effective drugs represents one force driving the growth, the expansion of the market owed much to the rising expectations of good health among consumers and the start of the long post-war boom which lasted until the 1970s and brought increasing affluence to developed countries. Post-war reconstruction in Europe meant this development lagged behind that in the USA, but by the 1950s the countries of Europe and elsewhere were catching up. In Japan, post-war reconstruction included the development of a pharmaceutical industry, which began R&D (particularly on antibiotics) in the 1950s and which bore fruit several decades later.

The inauguration of the NHS in Britain in 1948, with healthcare accessible to all and free at the point of delivery (including free medicines until 1952, when prescription charges were introduced) increased the market for pharmaceuticals. Social insurance in France and other European countries played a part in rising demand and nationally many of the companies of the pre-war industry began the process of transformation that was already well advanced in the US companies. National differences in innovation, however, remained [33]. The failure of France and Japan to join the innovation competition has been attributed in part to the price regulatory schemes in operation as well as the structure of healthcare delivery [34].

In Germany, IG Farben was demolished and Bayer, Hoechst and BASF emerged as individual companies, as did Merck and Schering. In 1955 the national distribution of world pharmaceutical exports reflected the predominance of the USA with its 34% share, while the UK had 16%, Germany 10% and Switzerland 14%. By 1963 a levelling out process was taking place, with the US share at 25% and that of Germany at 15%; by 1975 Germany's share was 16%, the USA and the UK had a 12% share each and Switzerland stayed at 14% [30]. These national shares then remained much the same for the rest of the century.

The globalisation of pharmaceutical manufacturing

To the major corporations, however, nationality became an increasingly peripheral concern in these years. Most of the US corporations established manufacturing subsidiaries, some of which also carried out

R&D in Europe, principally in the UK, in the early 1950s. Some, such as Pfizer, established themselves from scratch, while others like Merck and Smith, Kline & French bought old British companies – Morsons and Menley & James respectively – as a base for development. The UK was attractive to them as a European base 'because of its outstanding academic system and expertise in disciplines related to medicinal research, the much lower salaries of highly trained researchers, and the common language and heritage' [35].

Other British companies drew together to defend themselves against possible US takeover, as did Glaxo and Allen & Hanburys, who merged in 1957. In the 1960s, Glaxo went on to acquire a number of other smaller British companies to grow its operations but, ironically, when a takeover bid came, it was not from a US company but from Beechams, a company that had transformed itself by the establishment of R&D and discovery of the semi-synthetic penicillins from a proprietary pill maker into a pharmaceutical company. The bid was resisted and failed [36].

By the early 1970s, when that took place, not only was the therapeutic revolution over, but increasing regulation to ensure product safety, introduced in most countries in the wake of the thalidomide tragedy in 1961, was making the time between the discovery of a new compound and its launch on the market much lengthier, eating into patent life. The R&D process itself was also becoming much more expensive. These factors, *inter alia*, played a part in the changes in the industry over the last two decades of the 20th century.

Developments from 1980 to 2000

Scientific research, particularly in molecular biology, led to discoveries in the 1970s such as that of the technique of recombinant DNA (popularly known as gene splicing), which formed the basis of what became known as the biotechnology industry [37]. This new industry developed rapidly in the USA in that decade, mostly in small firms, often spin-offs from universities. In the 1980s government initiatives and finance, particularly in Britain and Germany, stimulated biotechnology development in Europe.

The response of the pharmaceutical industry was varied. Some companies rapidly internalised biotechnology knowledge and processes; some invested in biotechnology companies (the Swiss company Roche made a large investment in the first US biotech company Genentech). Almost all of them developed a complex network of agreements whereby the pharmaceutical companies provided finance, development expertise and marketing services in exchange for licences to new products [38]. As the pharmaceutical industry's own rate of innovation slowed down, biotechnology appeared to offer the best prospect of new products.

Another significant feature of the early 1980s was the spiralling costs of healthcare in the developed countries. Demographic changes showed a higher proportion of older people in these countries, many of them troubled with chronic diseases requiring extensive and expensive medication. Governments looked for ways of containing their drugs bills. In some countries there was nothing new about this. In the UK a price regulation scheme had been in operation since the 1950s, but a list of products not to be prescribed (referred to as 'the black list' in GP surgeries and pharmacies), was finally introduced in the 1980s [39]. This had long been opposed by the industry's powerful trade association, the Association of the British Pharmaceutical Industry (ABPI). Government pressures were also brought to bear on doctors to prescribe economically and, where possible, generically. As the cost of discovering and developing new products continued to rise, so too did marketing costs, as the companies sought maximum penetration of world markets for new drugs to maximise profits.

Mergers and acquisitions in the 1980s and 1990s

In the mid-1980s a period of intense restructuring in the industry began, as companies searched for cost reductions and critical mass through mergers and acquisitions. Some of this activity was national in its scope; examples include the acquisition in the USA of Searle by Monsanto in 1985 and the merger of Bristol-Myers and Squibb in 1989; and in Switzerland the merger of CIBA-Geigy (which had merged in the 1970s) with Sandoz to produce Novartis. However much of it was transnational; SmithKline Beckman merged with Beecham in 1989; the Swedish company, Astra, merged with Zeneca (ICI pharmaceuticals, demerged from its parent); and the Swedish company Pharmacia merged with the American company Upjohn. This process continued through the 1990s, with Glaxo's acquisition of Wellcome in 1995, followed by the merger of SmithKline Beecham and Glaxo Wellcome in 2000, the same year as Pfizer's merger with Warner Lambert and further acquisition of Pharmacia-Upjohn.

German companies had held back from this process until Hoechst and Rhône-Poulenc pooled their pharmaceutical interests in a new Franco-German company, Aventis. As old names disappeared and new ones appeared it is impossible as yet to be sure how much growth this consolidation has generated or, indeed, whether the restructuring is yet complete. The creation of a successful industry manufacturing generics in India in recent decades and the possibility of such growth in other Asian countries experiencing rapid industrialisation (for example China) adds a new dimension to an already complex industry profile.

Challenges and opportunities

As this brief overview has shown, patterns of growth in the pharmaceutical industry were, until the last two decades of the 20th century, predominantly national, although the national players were sustained and stimulated from the beginning by international trade. In the last half century the use of patents and brand names has been a force encouraging international development and globalisation. Common features in the growth and development of the industry can be distinguished and national differences accounted for by the different times at which industrialisation and urbanisation took place.

However, there have been other influential factors, including the structures of healthcare systems, medical practices and the diffusion of scientific and technological knowledge. The ability of many of the industry's companies to collaborate within a framework of competition has been a noticeable feature of its development, and has secured the transfer of technology across national boundaries. A symbiotic relationship with the chemical industry has characterised the industry since the late 18th century, while in the 20th century fluid boundaries with first the food and later the biotechnology industry has led to considerable expansion.

While the impact of thalidomide, the adverse effects of some of the anti-inflammatory drugs and, most recently, of some of the anti-depressants may have diminished the high expectations of the industry prevailing in the middle of the 20th century, there are no obvious signs of falling consumption. There are, however, a number of challenging issues surrounding the industry in an age of consumerism. These include the cost and type of marketing, the industry's involvement in safety regulatory procedures and its accountability; resolution of some, or all of these issues will be required if the industry is to continue to grow.

References

1.   Ballance R, Pogany J, Forstner H. *The World's Pharmaceutical Industries.* Aldershot: Edward Elgar, 1992: 4.

2. Reekie W D. *The Economics of the Pharmaceutical Industry*. London: Macmillan, 1975.

3. IMS Health (2000). Global pharmaceutical market growth accelerates to 11% in 1999. http://www.ims-global.com/insight/report/market_growth/products0600.htm (accessed 14 January 2005).

4. McCraw T K, (ed.). *Creating Modern Capitalism*. Cambridge, MA: Harvard University Press, 1997.

5. Matthews L G. *History of Pharmacy in Britain*. Edinburgh: E & S Livingstone, 1962.

6. Tweedale G. *At the Sign of the Plough: 275 Years of Allen & Hanburys and the British Pharmaceutical Industry 1715–1990*. London: John Murray, 1990.

7. Liebenau J, Morson, T. In: Jeremy D, ed. *Dictionary of Business Biography*, Vol. 4. London: Butterworths, 1985: 346–347.

8. Slinn J. *Pills and Pharmaceuticals. A H Cox & Co Ltd. 1839–1989*. Barnstaple: A H Cox & Co Ltd, 1989.

9. Liebenau J, Whiffen, T. In: Jeremy D, ed. *Dictionary of Business Biography*, Vol. 4. London: Butterworths, 1985: 763–765.

10. Liebenau J. *Medical Science and Medical Industry: The Formation of the American Pharmaceutical Industry*. London: Macmillan, 1987.

11. Achilladelis B. *Innovation in the pharmaceutical industry*. In: Landau R, Achilladelis B, Scriabine A, eds. *Pharmaceutical Innovation Revolutionizing Human Health*. Philadelphia: Chemical Heritage Press, 1999: 49.

12. Haber F L. *The Chemical Industry During the Nineteenth Century*. Oxford: Clarendon Press, 1958: 46, 48, 133, 136.

13. Kobrak C. *National Cultures and International Competition: The Experience of Schering AG, 1851–1950*. Cambridge: Cambridge University Press, 2002.

14. Fischer E P. *Selling Science: The History of Boehringer Mannheim*. Mannheim: Boehringer Corporation, 1992.

15. Slinn J. *A History of May & Baker 1834–1984*. Cambridge: Hobsons, 1984: 44–47.

16. Porter R. *The Greatest Benefit to Mankind. A Medical History of Humanity from Antiquity to the Present*. London: Harper Collins, 1997.

17. MacDonald G. *In Pursuit of Excellence*. London: Wellcome Foundation, 1980.

18. Porter R. *The Greatest Benefit to Mankind. A Medical History of Humanity from Antiquity to the Present*. London: Harper Collins, 1997: 448.

19. Liebenau J. *Medical Science and Medical Industry: The Formation of the American Pharmaceutical Industry*. London: Macmillan, 1987: 30.

20. Galambos L, Sturchio J. *Values and Visions: A Merck Centenary*. New Jersey: Merck & Co, 1991.

21. Amdam R P, Sogner K S. *Wealth of Contrasts: Nyegaard & Co 1874–1985*. Norway: Ad Notam Gyldendal, 1994.

22. Deeson T. *Parke-Davis in Britain: The First Hundred Years*. Eastleigh: Parke-Davis & Co, 1995.

23. Slinn J. Research and development in the UK pharmaceutical industry from the nineteenth century to the 1960s. In: Porter R, Tiech M, eds. *Drugs and Narcotics in History*. Cambridge: Cambridge University Press, 1995.

24. Slinn J. *Abbott Laboratories in the UK*. Cambridge: Granta Editions, 1999.
25. Goodman J. Pharmaceutical industry. In: Cooter R, Pickstone J, eds. *Medicine in the Twentieth Century*. Amsterdam: Harwood, 2000: 141–154.
26. Bliss M. *The Discovery of Insulin*. London: Faber and Faber, 1988.
27. Davenport-Hines R P T, Slinn J. *Glaxo: A History to 1962*. Cambridge: Cambridge University Press, 1992: Chapter 4.
28. Swann J P. *Academic Scientists and the Pharmaceutical Industry*. Baltimore: John Hopkins University Press, 1988.
29. Kahn E J. *All in a Century: The First 100 Years of Eli Lilly & Co.* Indianapolis: Eli Lilly & Co, 1976.
30. Broadberry S. The performance of manufacturing. In: Floud R, Johnson P, eds. *The Cambridge Economic History of Modern Britain. Structural Change and Growth, 1939–2000*, Vol. 3. Cambridge: Cambridge University Press, 2004: 76.
31. Green J A. Attention to 'details': Etiquette and the pharmaceutical salesmen in postwar America. *Social Studies of Science* 2004; 34(2): 271–292.
32. United Nations. *Transnational Corporations and the Pharmaceutical Industry*. New York: United Nations, 1979: 2.
33. Hancher L. *Regulating for Competition*. Oxford: Clarendon Press, 1990.
34. Howells J, Neary I. *Intervention and Technological Innovation*. Basingstoke: Macmillan, 1998.
35. Achilladelis B. *Innovation in the pharmaceutical industry*. In: Landau R, Achilladelis B, Scriabine A, eds. *Pharmaceutical Innovation Revolutionizing Human Health*. Philadelphia: Chemical Heritage Press, 1999: 99.
36. Jones E. *The Business of Medicine*. London: Profile Books, 2002.
37. Galambos L, Sturchio J. Pharmaceutical firms and the transition to biotechnology: a study in strategic innovation. *Business History Review* 1998; 72(2): 250–278.
38. Gambardella A. *Science and Innovation*. Cambridge: Cambridge University Press, 1995.
39. Slinn J. Regulating the cost and consumption of prescription pharmaceuticals in the UK 1948–1967. *Business History* 2005; 47 (forthcoming).

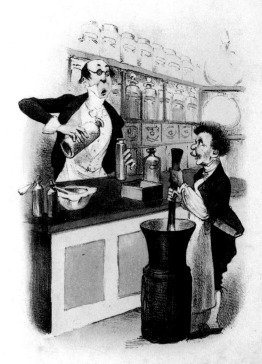

Plate 13 'Notions of the Agreeable no. 21', cartoon published by W Spooner, Strand, London, c. 1830–40. Such sketches give an idea of how pharmacies were equipped before the invention of photography, as well as of contemporary social attitudes.

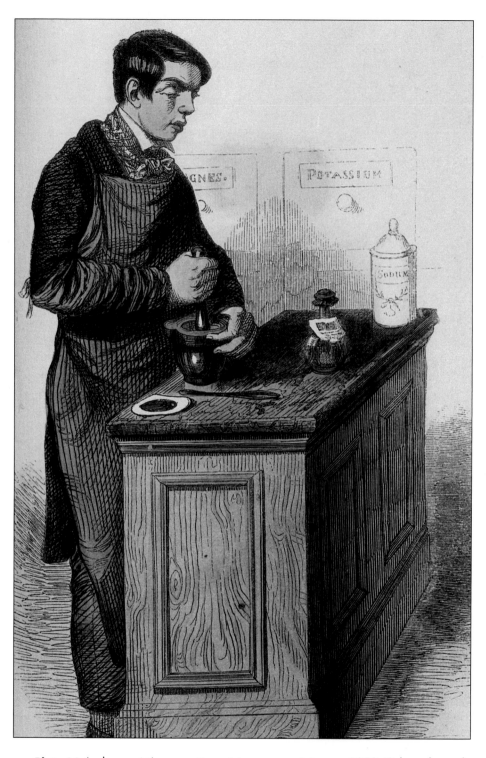

Plate 14 A pharmacist's apprentice mixing a prescription, c. 1850. Coloured wood engraving by J I Grandville, thought to be after J-I-I G Slypulkowski. Reproduced by permission of the Wellcome Library, London.

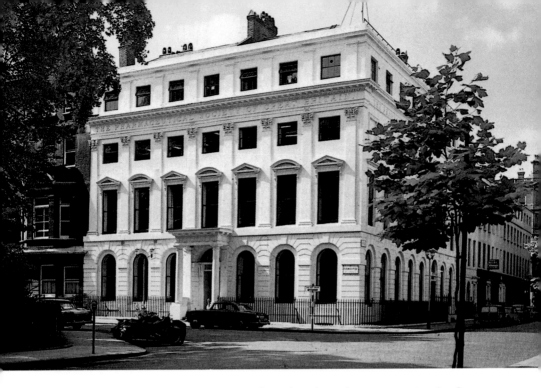

Plate 15 The Pharmaceutical Society was based at Bloomsbury Square, London from the end of 1841 until the early 1970s, when its 17th-century building, which had subsequently been remodelled by John Nash, was scheduled for demolition to make way for a new British Library.

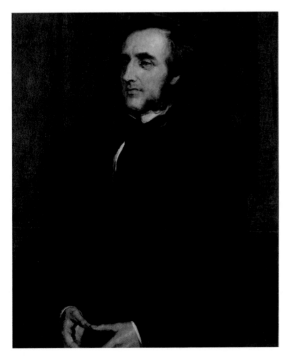

Plate 16 Jacob Bell portrayed by his friend, Sir Edwin Landseer, a few days before his death in 1859.

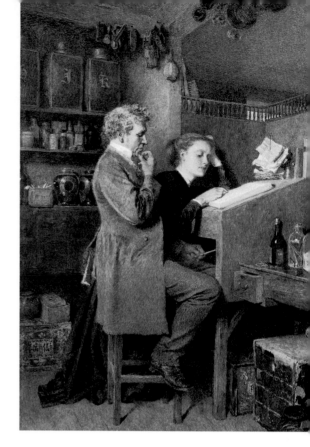

Plate 17 Something wrong somewhere. Painting by Charles Green, 1890. Reproduced by permission of the Victoria & Albert Museum.

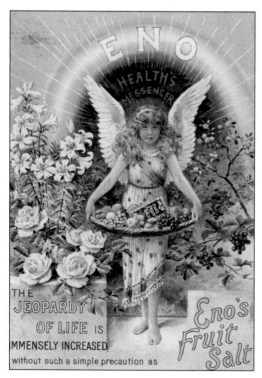

Plate 18 Advertisement for Eno's Fruit Salt dating from the 1890s. Reproduced by permission of GlaxoSmithKline and by courtesy of The History of Advertising Trust Archive. 'Eno's' and 'Eno's Fruit Salts' are registered trademarks of the GlaxoSmithKline group of companies.

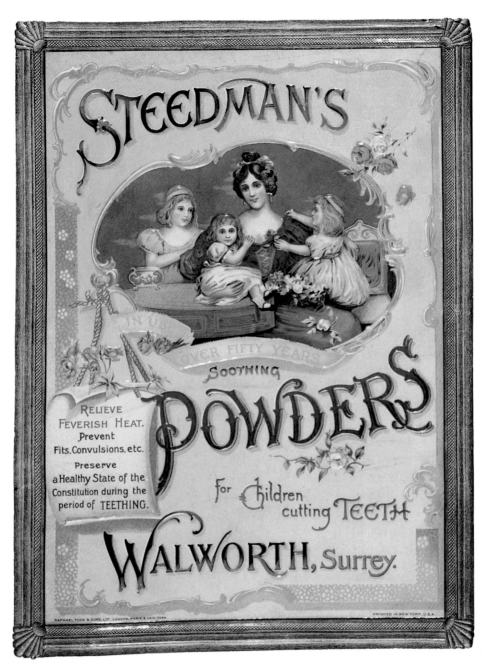

Plate 19 Between 1850 and 1900 a six-fold growth in annual sales of proprietary medicines stimulated competition and expenditure on promotion, as in the Eno's example (Plate 18) and this advertisement for Steedman's powders.

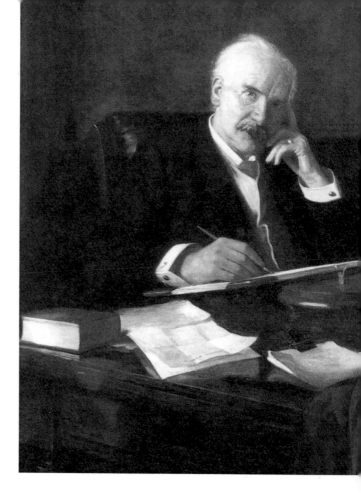

Plate 20 Sir Jesse Boot, Lord Trent of Nottingham. Painting by N Denholm Davis, 1909. Reproduced by permission of Boots Group Archives.

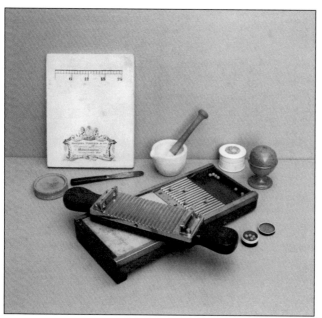

Plate 21 The practice of hand making batches of pills as and when required continued well into the 20th century. The equipment shown here comprises a mahogany and marble pill machine with brass cutters, graduated pill tile dating from about 1830, mortar with long-handled pestle, boxwood pill rounder, boxwood pill silverer, short spatula, porcelain pot for varnishing pills and cardboard flanged pill box.

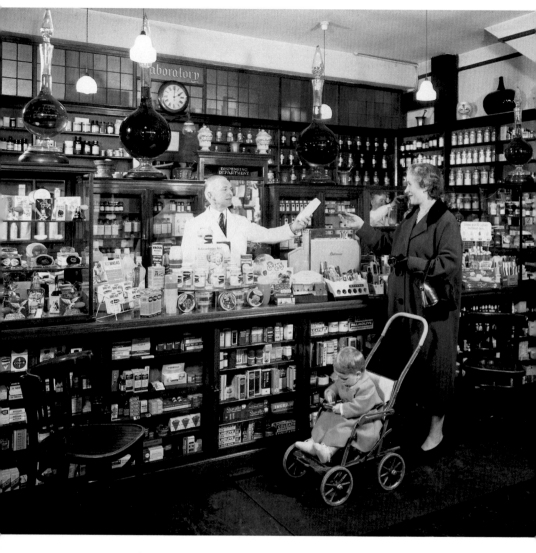

Plate 22 Interior of R J Mellowes' pharmacy, Enfield, Middlesex, 1959.

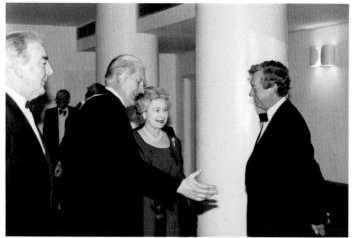

Plate 23 Visit by Her Majesty Queen Elizabeth II to the Royal Pharmaceutical Society's headquarters at 1 Lambeth High Street on the 150th anniversary of the granting of its Royal Charter on 18 February 1993.

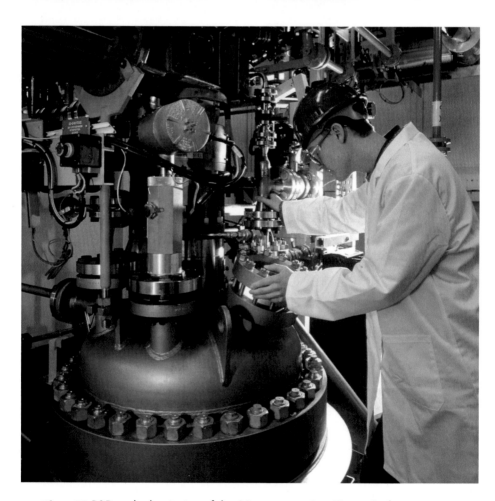

Plate 24 R&D at the beginning of the 21st century: AstraZeneca's chemistry laboratory at Charnwood, Leicestershire. Photograph reproduced by permission of AstraZeneca PLC.

Part Four

The products of pharmacy

10

From alkaloids to gene therapy: a brief history of drug discovery in the 20th century

Viviane Quirke

The 20th century saw a vast increase in the number of therapeutic innovations. These peaked in the 1940s, 1950s and 1960s, in a cluster often referred to as the 'therapeutic revolution', which included technological devices as well as drugs [1]. This chapter focuses on the history of drug discovery, because drugs themselves have played a central role in the history of pharmacy, and because they occupy a special place in the therapeutic arsenal available to the medical profession and to patients.

Four main periods of development are distinguished: firstly, the period up to the start of the First World War; secondly, between 1914 and the start of the Second World War; thirdly, during the war itself; and finally in the last 50 years. The chapter begins with an account of the changing nature of drug discovery in the 20th century, and of some of the factors that produced these changes.

The changing nature of drug discovery

The history of drug discovery in the 20th century is one of major shifts. There was the almost total replacement of galenicals by the products of the global pharmaceutical industry, which transformed the practice of pharmacy. From the making of medicines, the pharmacist became involved in the supply of pharmaceutical products, and then mainly in the provision of information about them.

At the beginning of the 20th century there was still room for the individual inventor in pharmaceutical development, but today the physician or pharmacist working in a backroom office has largely been replaced by the research team, working in an industrial laboratory, usually in collaboration with scientists in universities, hospitals and independent institutes [2]. The laboratory itself changed, from a small-scale, mostly analytical laboratory, to a large-scale research and development (R&D) laboratory, often built on greenfield sites separate from the factories manufacturing the drugs.

At the same time, the methods and instrumentation used in drug R&D altered beyond recognition. To the chemical methods and instrumentation for the production of alkaloids and subsequently, of synthetic organic chemicals, and to the bacteriological methods for the manufacture of vaccines, were added, to name but a few: pharmacological methods for the detection and measurement of drugs in isolated tissues or whole animals and for an understanding of drug action; biochemical methods for toxicity and distribution studies and for the testing of compounds in biochemical systems; physical methods and instrumentation for structure-activity studies and drug design. In the last quarter of the 20th century, computers, molecular biology and biotechnology also played a significant role in pharmaceutical R&D [3].

Thus, to borrow an expression from the physical sciences, the 20th century saw a shift 'from Little Pharma to Big Pharma'. At the same time, there was a change in the geographical centre of drug discovery,

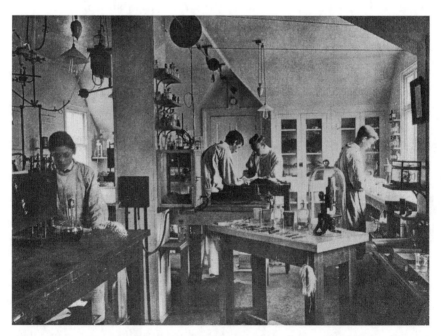

Figure 10.1 Experimental pharmacology laboratory of the Wellcome Physiological Research Laboratories, Brockwell Hall, 1909. Reproduced by permission of the Wellcome Library, London.

first from Germany to the USA, and then to a more balanced situation between western countries. More recently, the rise of a generic pharmaceuticals industry in developing countries such as India, has begun to alter this balance, although it is debatable whether its activities would qualify as 'therapeutic innovation'.

Successive waves in the predominant approaches to therapy took place, with immunotherapy gradually being superseded by chemotherapy, and replacement therapy blossoming as a complementary approach in the period between the two world wars [4]. As effective remedies for infectious diseases were discovered, the emphasis on infectious diseases was replaced by a newer focus on chronic disorders. These are now increasingly perceived as 'genetic' diseases, have already had a considerable impact on the practice of pharmacy, and promise to transform it even further in the decades to come. However, whether gene

---

Box 10.1 Chronology of principal therapeutic discoveries, 1900 to 1945.

1903 Barbitone (Veronal). Developed by E Fischer and J von Mering in Germany: hypnotic.
1910 Arsphenamine (Salvarsan). Paul Ehrlich and Hoechst, Germany: anti-syphilitic.
1919 Thyroxine. Isolated by E C Kendall, Mayo Clinic, USA: active principle of thyroid gland.
1922 Insulin. Isolated by Banting, Best, MacLeod, and Collip at Toronto University, the Connaught Laboratories, and Eli Lilly: pancreatic hormone.
1928 Alexander Fleming observes the antibacterial action of the mould *Penicillium notatum* (Inoculation Department, St Mary's Hospital, London).
1930s Synthetic vitamins. Vitamins A, B, C and D isolated.
1932 *Prontosil rubrum*. Action discovered by Gerhard Domagk at Bayer, Germany: antibacterial.
1935 Ernest Fourneau's team at the Pasteur Institute in Paris identify *p*-amino-benzenesulphonamide (sulfanilamide) as the active principle in *Prontosil*.
1938 Howard Florey's team at Oxford takes up the study of penicillin and develop the first broad-spectrum antibiotic.
1940 Fildes and Woods, working at the Middlesex Hospital, London, unravel the mechanism of action of sulfanilamide, and refer to it as 'competitive antagonism'.
1944 Streptomycin. Action discovered by Selman Waksman, Rutgers University, USA and Merck: anti-tubercular antibiotic.

Main sources: Various chronologies in Weatherall M. *In Search of a Cure: a History of Pharmaceutical Discovery*. Oxford: OUP, 1990, and Bartlett S. *Medicines Research in Britain* on www.abpi.org.uk (accessed 30 March 2005).

therapy will replace chemotherapy as the main angle of attack against chronic diseases at the beginning of the 21st century remains to be seen.

The factors that produced these shifts were complex. As well as advances in science, technology and medicine, there were important social, economic and political factors. Among these, the roles of two world wars, the growth of national health systems, the rise in public expectations of health services and drug safety regulation stand out. However, the drugs themselves also contributed to these shifts, by providing a stimulus for subsequent scientific and technical improvements, by capturing the public's imagination with tales of 'miracle cures', and by posing a challenge to health departments and regulatory authorities.

This chapter focuses on just a few of these discoveries. They were often associated with important events, and had a crucial impact not only on modern medicine and pharmacy, but also on therapeutic innovation in the 20th century. The major drugs discussed in the first half of the 20th century are summarised in Box 10.1.

Drug discovery before 1914: from alkaloids to Salvarsan

Medicinal plants have always played a special part in the treatment of disease. However, it was not until the beginning of the 19th century that the first active principal was successfully extracted from a plant. This was the narcotic principle of opium, which was alkaline and formed salts with acids, and was later named morphia, then morphine [5]. There followed the isolation and identification of many other plant alkaloids, including emetine from the ipecacuanha root for the treatment of dysentery and quinine from cinchona bark for the treatment of malaria.

Quinine

The prevalence of malaria in various parts of Europe in the early part of the 19th century provided a stimulus for the large-scale processing of cinchona bark and other plant alkaloids, often by pharmaceutical manufacturing businesses, such as Merck in Darmstadt. They not only built factories to carry out the manufacture of the drugs, but also developed the chemical expertise required for selecting plant material of suitable quality for their production.

The demand for quinine was high, and supplies of cinchona were hard to come by. Attempts were therefore made to synthesise it chemically. It was one such unsuccessful attempt, by the young English chemist William Henry Perkin at the Royal College of Chemistry in London (later to become Imperial College), which led to the synthesis of the first artificial dye, mauveine or aniline purple, from benzene, a by-product of the coal tar industry. In fact, quinine was not synthesised until 1944. However, the synthetic route to quinine never became a viable alternative to the production of analogues by then being developed for the war effort.

The synthetic dyestuffs industry that emerged out of the discovery of mauvine soon diversified into pharmaceuticals. It became an enterprise of considerable size in Germany, where it benefited from a number of favourable conditions such as German unification, the annexation of Alsace-Lorraine and a new patent law. This created the basis for the expansion of a powerful German pharmaceutical industry that would dominate the sector until the 1920s [6].

Synthetic chemicals

Meanwhile, the discovery of synthetic chemicals with anaesthetic properties, such as chloroform, which was given to Queen Victoria during childbirth, stimulated the interest of medical practitioners in such chemicals, and led to a search for other novel compounds with specific pharmacological activities. Among them were hypnotics such as Veronal (the barbiturate barbitone), antipyretics and analgesics.

The most significant of these, aspirin, had been synthesised by Charles Gerhardt in 1853, but lay forgotten on the chemists' shelves for almost a half-century. Although the fundamental mechanism of action of aspirin was discovered by John Vane in 1971, novel properties of this amazing compound are still being found today [7].

Vaccines and sera

In parallel with these efforts at curing illness, a new approach aimed at preventing infectious diseases, which had been shown to be caused by germs, became established in the last decades of the 19th century. This approach was called 'vaccination' (from Latin *vacca*, meaning cow, as in cowpox), by analogy with variolation (from Latin *variola*, meaning smallpox), which had long been practised in countries such as India and China to protect people against smallpox.

At the end of the 18th century, Edward Jenner in England, followed at the end of the 19th century by Louis Pasteur in France and Robert Koch in Germany, built not only upon this ancient tradition, but also (in the case of Pasteur and Koch) upon new knowledge about the bacterial causes of infectious diseases.

Pasteur showed that it was possible to protect birds from fowl cholera, and sheep from anthrax, by inoculating them with attenuated strains of the causative bacteria. He then developed a vaccine against rabies, caused by a virus, which was effective even after the patient had been infected. His demonstration on a young boy from Alsace who had been bitten by a rabid dog, and was saved by his new vaccine, caused a sensation [8]. He was able to obtain enough funds from an international public subscription to create the Pasteur Institute in Paris, founded in 1888. Its purpose was four-fold; to produce the rabies vaccine, to distribute it from a dispensary, to carry out research into infectious diseases and to teach microbiology.

The Pasteur Institute provided an inspiration for other medical research institutions elsewhere [9]. Robert Koch's Institute for Infectious Diseases was founded in 1891 in Berlin; the British Institute for Preventive Medicine (later renamed the Lister Institute, after the surgeon Joseph Lister, best known for promoting the use of antiseptics in surgery) was created in London in 1893 [10].

The discovery of diphtheria antitoxin by Emil von Behring and Shibasabuto Kitasato at the Koch Institute in 1891 stimulated pharmaceutical firms in countries such as Britain, France and the USA, as well as Germany, into producing vaccines and antitoxins [11]. Before long, many of these firms, such as Parke-Davis of Detroit, would become involved in the production of other biologicals, including organ and glandular extracts.

Chemotherapy

It was in Germany that the chemical capabilities of the dyestuffs industry were combined with the bacteriological and immunological expertise of the medical research institutes to produce a development that would have a profound and long-term impact on drug discovery in the 20th century. Indeed, chemotherapy emerged at the Institute for Experimental Therapy in Frankfurt-am-Main, created with the support of the Prussian

State as well as the local chemical industry for one of Koch's former research assistants, Paul Ehrlich [12].

Ehrlich developed the theory of chemotherapy, based on his concept of chemoreceptors, groupings of atoms by which chemical substances could attach themselves to the bacterial cell, in the same way as microscope stains attached themselves selectively to certain tissues, and antitoxins to bacterial toxins [13]. He put it into practice with Salvarsan, also known as compound 606 or arsphenamine. This was a 'magic bullet' capable of attacking the microorganisms responsible for syphilis without killing its human host.

Thanks to Ehrlich's extensive network of international contacts, Salvarsan became widely known. Further arsenicals followed, beginning with Neo-Salvarsan, which, being more stable and easier to use, had marked advantages over its predecessor. Although these drugs were eventually superseded by penicillin, Ehrlich's work provided a model for the search for chemotherapeutic agents throughout the interwar period and beyond.

Drug discovery from 1914 to 1939: from Salvarsan to the sulphonamides

Shortly after the launch of Salvarsan, the First World War broke out, and this was to reveal the extent of the German monopoly on synthetic drugs. The conflict interrupted supplies of Salvarsan and other German imported drugs, on which many countries had become reliant, even those that also had a strong chemical industry, like Switzerland [14]. However, at the same time, it offered a justification for the abolition of German patent rights in countries at war with Germany. It therefore led to a certain amount of technological transfer, and created the impetus for the production of synthetic chemicals by pharmaceutical companies, such as Boots and Burroughs Wellcome, which built up the necessary expertise, often in collaboration with academic departments [15].

However, until the experiments with *Prontosil Rubrum* by Gerhard Domagk in 1932 led to the discovery of sulfanilamide in 1935, chemotherapy failed to fulfil its early promise. Moreover, it was not until Raymond Ahlquist proposed his dual-receptor theory for adrenergic nerves in 1948 that the receptor concept provided a fruitful basis for therapeutic innovation [16].

For this reason, the period that followed the First World War is often considered as a low point in the history of drug discovery. Chemotherapy sank into the doldrums, competing at first unsuccessfully with immunotherapy, at a time when anti-sera proliferated, often with little effect, against a number of infectious diseases, for example strepto-coccal or pneumococcal infections. Nevertheless, the interwar years also saw important achievements in the budding field of replacement therapy, against deficiency diseases caused by a lack of vitamins or hor-mones in the body. Interestingly, in this area the most significant devel-opments occurred mainly in Britain and North America.

Vitamins

The word vitamin was coined by a Polish chemist, Casimir Funk, when he was a guest worker at the Lister Institute in 1912. The Institute later became involved in a research project, sponsored jointly by the newly formed Medical Research Committee (which became the Medical Research Council), to study rickets in post-war, famine-stricken Vienna. This led to the identification of the anti-rachitic factor, vitamin D. Other vitamins followed, and by the 1930s most of them had been isolated, their structures worked out, and their chemical synthesis realised. This was the stimulus for some companies, such as Glaxo, previously milk product and baby food manufacturers, to enter the pharmaceutical sector [17].

Hormones

There were a number of important milestones in the field of hormones during this period. These included the isolation of the active principle of the thyroid gland by E C Kendall at the Mayo Clinic in Rochester, Minnesota, in 1919; the extraction of the pancreatic hormone insulin, by F Banting, J J R Macleod, C Best and J B Collip in 1922 at the University of Toronto; and the characterisation of steroid hormones by various researchers in the 1920s and 1930s.

However, the discovery of insulin was perhaps the most significant from the point of view of the history of therapeutic innovation [18]. The lack of insulin had been shown to cause diabetes mellitus. It provided an early example of a fatal disease that could be controlled by a drug, although requiring skilful management on the part of the physician and the patient. It played an important part in the development of biological standardisation [19] and of academic-industrial relations [20]. Further-more, in certain countries with a limited chemical industry (for example Denmark) it played a key role in the growth of an indigenous pharma-ceutical industry [21].

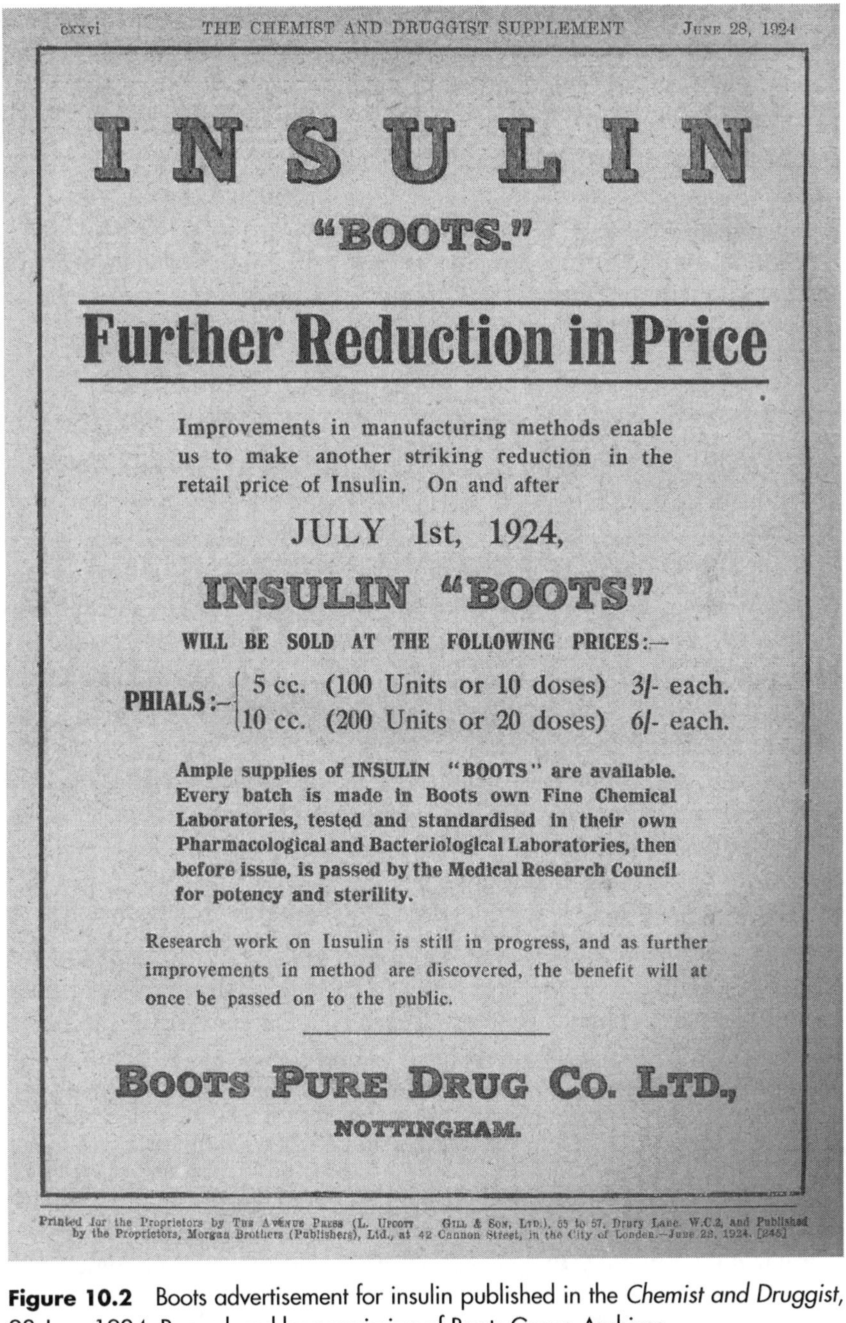

cxxvi THE CHEMIST AND DRUGGIST SUPPLEMENT JUNE 28, 1924

INSULIN

"BOOTS."

Further Reduction in Price

Improvements in manufacturing methods enable us to make another striking reduction in the retail price of Insulin. On and after

JULY 1st, 1924,

INSULIN "BOOTS"

WILL BE SOLD AT THE FOLLOWING PRICES:—

PHIALS:— 5 cc. (100 Units or 10 doses) 3/- each.
10 cc. (200 Units or 20 doses) 6/- each.

Ample supplies of INSULIN "BOOTS" are available. Every batch is made in Boots own Fine Chemical Laboratories, tested and standardised in their own Pharmacological and Bacteriological Laboratories, then before issue, is passed by the Medical Research Council for potency and sterility.

Research work on Insulin is still in progress, and as further improvements in method are discovered, the benefit will at once be passed on to the public.

BOOTS PURE DRUG CO. LTD.,
NOTTINGHAM.

Printed for the Proprietors by THE AVENUE PRESS (L. UPCOTT GILL & SON, LTD.), 55 to 57, Drury Lane, W.C.2, and Published by the Proprietors, Morgan Brothers (Publishers), Ltd., at 42 Cannon Street, in the City of London.—June 28, 1924. [245]

Figure 10.2 Boots advertisement for insulin published in the *Chemist and Druggist*, 28 June 1924. Reproduced by permission of Boots Group Archives.

Such is the significance of insulin that it continued to be a focal point for scientific research and therapeutic innovation for much of the 20th century: from the determination of its primary structure by Fred Sanger using sequencing methods in 1955, and the elucidation of its complete 3D structure by Dorothy Hodgkin using X-ray crystallography in 1969, to the development of Humulin, the first biotechnology drug, by Eli Lilly using recombinant DNA techniques in 1982 [22]. The arrival of human insulin has greatly reduced the dependence on pig and beef insulins. Today, insulin remains a privileged target for novel therapeutic approaches, such as cloning.

Antibacterials

Meanwhile, the search for chemical agents to treat bacterial infections continued, especially in the Bayer laboratories, now part of the chemical group IG Farben, where it was modelled on Ehrlich's research programme. In 1932, the director of research in experimental pathology there, Gerhard Domagk, carried out experiments on mice infected with streptococci using a red dye, named *Prontosil rubrum*. He found that the animals treated with the compound survived, while the controls died. Later, thanks to *Prontosil*, Domagk succeeded in curing his own daughter from a streptococcal infection. By 1935, clinical trials were under way, and the results of Domagk's experiments and early clinical tests were published [23].

The study of Prontosil was taken up by numerous centres in Germany and abroad, including the Therapeutic Chemistry Department of the Pasteur Institute in Paris. There, Ernest Fourneau's team was unhindered by a tradition in synthetic dye chemistry, unlike their German counterparts. They showed that, contrary to the popular belief that the power of dyes to destroy bacteria came from their ability to colour their vital elements, Prontosil was broken down in the body, and that its active principle was the colourless compound p-aminobenzene-sulphonamide (sulfanilamide).

Because this compound had been known for a long time, it could not be patented, and this dashed Bayer's hopes of being able to corner the market for sulpha-drugs. It enabled other manufacturers to develop similar compounds. Other drugs, all based on the sulfanilamide molecule, soon followed. Sulfanilamide (Septoplix) was launched in 1933 by Rhône-Poulenc, which had a long-standing collaborative arrangement with Fourneau. Sulphapyridine (M&B 693), which became famous for saving Winston Churchill's life when he suffered from pneumonia during the Second World War, was developed in 1937 by the British subsidiary of Rhône-Poulenc, May & Baker [24].

By effectively breaking the German monopoly on synthetic drugs, the discovery of the antibacterial action of sulfanilamide spurred some chemical companies into embarking on pharmaceutical research [25]. It led Imperial Chemical Industries (ICI), who would become important players in the history of therapeutic innovation during and after the Second World War, to develop sulphadimidine (Sulphamezathine), for a time the most widely used sulpha-drug in Britain [26].

Drug discovery from 1939 to 1945: synthetic anti-malarials, compound E and penicillin

At the start of the Second World War, the production of sulpha-drugs was well under way outside Germany. Nevertheless, as had been the case in the First World War, supplies of other German synthetic drugs, including pamaquine (Plasmaquin) and mepaquine (Atebrin), were once again interrupted. When the conflict extended from Europe to the Far East, this not only exposed the troops to malaria, but also cut off the route to Java, the main source of quinine. This might have created major difficulties for the Allied war effort, but it had been foreseen, and projects to synthesise novel anti-malarials began before the Japanese attack on Pearl Harbor in December 1941. These culminated in the development of proguanil (Paludrine) by ICI in 1945, and Chloroquine by Winthrop in 1946.

Soon after Dunkirk in May 1940, Anglo-American discussions started with a view to setting up lend-lease agreements, by which the USA would provide Britain with material support. As a result of these discussions, co-operative research programmes were initiated in order to pool British and American scientific knowledge and technical expertise. The best known of these are the radar and atom bomb projects, but there were also collaborative schemes to develop pharmaceutical products. Following a rumour that adrenal cortical extracts were being administered to German aircraft pilots to improve their ability to fly at high altitudes, this work included compound E (later known as cortisone), as well as synthetic anti-malarials [27].

By 1942, the programme to produce penicillin in large quantities for the treatment of war wounds, and to find a synthetic route to its manufacture, dominated the Allies' co-operative ventures in pharmaceuticals. Such was the importance of penicillin that after the war it would serve as a blueprint for other collaborative schemes, and would become a reference point for many biomedical research projects, not only in Britain and America, but in other countries also [28]. For this reason, the story of penicillin deserves to be told here in some detail.

Penicillin

The ability of the mould *Penicillium notatum* to inhibit bacterial growth had been known for a long time. An early study of the 'struggle for life' between bacteria and *Penicillium* had been made in 1876 by the physicist John Tyndall in his laboratory at the Royal Institution in London [29]. However, it was Alexander Fleming's chance observation of the mould's activity against staphylococci in 1928, and his subsequent study of the antibacterial substance it secreted, which he named 'penicillin', that provided the basis for the development of the drug by Howard Florey's team at the Sir William Dunn School of Pathology in Oxford 10 years later.

The declaration of war in 1939 did not curtail Florey's plans. On the contrary, it gave special urgency to the project to study microorganisms with known antibacterial activity. This now focussed on penicillin. Florey devised a series of experiments that helped to establish penicillin as a new kind of chemotherapeutic agent, less toxic than the sulphonamides, by then the medical profession's favourite means of treating bacterial infections, and active against staphylococci, against which most of the sulpha-drugs had no effect [30].

The team's preliminary results were published in *The Lancet* in 1940. Early clinical tests were carried out using the limited quantities made in the School of Pathology by Norman Heatley in 1941. Before the report was published, Florey and Heatley flew to the USA, with the MRC's and the British government's blessings, in the hope of getting the large-scale manufacture of penicillin started there.

The outcome of this visit, and of the combined British and American efforts that followed, was the mass production of the drug using deep fermentation rather than surface culture methods. These were developed by the North Regional Research Laboratory at Peoria, Illinois, and perfected by different American companies under the aegis of the Office for Scientific Research and Development (OSRD) [31]. Penicillin therefore became available in large enough quantities for the D-day landings. Supplies for the wider public were available sooner in some countries than in others, depending on how quickly firms either took up American licences or developed deep fermentation themselves.

The impact of penicillin on therapeutic innovation in the second half of the 20th century was immense. The penicillin industry that emerged from the war included newcomers to the pharmaceutical sector from the fermentation industries, whose expertise would later contribute to the growth of the new biotechnology in the 1970s [32]. It also included countries such as Japan [33]. Although deep fermentation was never completely superseded, the search for a synthetic route eventually led to the first semi-synthetic penicillin, ampicillin. This was active against Gram-negative bacteria (left untouched by penicillin), and was aptly named Penbritin by Beechams in 1959 [34].

The antibiotic era

Penicillin was hailed as the culmination of the chemotherapeutic approach in medicine [35]. Several pharmaceutical firms that had hitherto steered away from chemotherapy, such as the manufacturers of galenicals, Allen & Hanbury's, now adopted this approach in their search for novel remedies [36]. The search for further sources of antibiotics continued. This led to the development of methods for the mass screening of microorganisms, and to the discovery of numerous other antibacterial substances [37].

So began what has been described as 'the antibiotic era' [38]. Penicillin was followed by streptomycin, the first effective chemotherapeutic treatment of tuberculosis, one of the great killers of the late 19th and early 20th centuries [39]. The large-scale streptomycin trials devised by Austin Bradford Hill under the auspices of the Medical Research Council became the model of the modern randomised clinical trial, with important consequences for drug discovery in the second half of the 20th century.

The new era heralded by penicillin and its successors appeared to spell the end of infectious diseases. Together with the great vaccination campaigns of the post-war years, it helps to explain the new optimism and faith in modern medicine that reigned in this period, before bacterial resistance became a serious problem. It opened up a window of opportunity for some companies, such as ICI, to embark on ambitious programmes to tackle chronic as well as acute diseases [40]. At the same time, it put pressure on the newly established health services, as it led to an increase in public expectations and a spiralling rise in national drugs bills, the legacy of which continues to be felt today.

International dimensions

The American pharmaceutical sector, and to a lesser degree its British counterpart, had emerged victorious from the war. By contrast, like

Germany itself, the German pharmaceutical industry had been beaten. The links between German industry and Hitler's brutal racial policies led to the dismantling of the almighty IG Farben [41]. German scientists, especially biologists tainted by their association with eugenics, were for a time excluded from the international scientific community. This, compounded by the effects of emigration of Jewish scientists in the 1930s, led to delays in the development of a German school of molecular biology, and to a need on the part of researchers and companies alike to 'catch up' with developments abroad [42].

However, what of countries, like France, which had experienced defeat and occupation? In an interesting twist to the story, it seems that isolation from the main thrust of Allied research programmes could be favourable to pharmaceutical discovery. A particularly striking example of this can be found in the history of the first psychotropic drug (i.e. a drug affecting mood): chlorpromazine, discovered by Rhône-Poulenc (see below).

Unaware in 1944 that an American team at Iowa State College had succeeded in synthesising phenothiazine amines, but had found these compounds useless as anti-malarials, the French team pressed on with their research and found that, although ineffective against malaria, they had anti-histaminic properties. This led them not only to develop promethazine (Phenergan), for the treatment of allergies, but also to synthesise compound RP 3276, which was to form the core of the chlorpromazine molecule (Largactil). As the Director of Pharmaceutical Research at Rhône-Poulenc, Pierre Viaud, conjectured later: if in 1944 the French had known of the Americans' work, they would probably have abandoned their own.

Drug discovery from 1945 to 1995: from cortisone to gene therapy

The period following the Second World War saw an explosion in the numbers of new drugs being developed and marketed. Some of them had their origins in wartime projects. However, many others were the product of increased investments in pharmaceutical and biomedical research in the aftermath of war, and of the mass market for drugs created by the new national health services.

The magnitude of this increase has been vast, and this section can do little more than touch on a number of the most significant developments. These have extended across all pharmacological groups, from antibiotics to drugs for cancer, heart disease and mental illness. The main subject areas discussed here are corticosteroids, chlorpromazine, receptor-blockers, anti-cancer drugs, immunosuppressive agents and antiviral drugs. Those covered are summarised in Box 10.2.

Corticosteroids

Cortisone had been synthesised from bile acids by Merck during the war using a method devised by Kendall. However, it was the dramatic demonstration of the efficacy of the drug against rheumatoid arthritis made by Philip Hench, a colleague of Kendall, at the Seventh International Congress of Rheumatology in New York in 1949, that caused the 'outpouring of steroidal investigations' that gave us many of the drugs we know today [43].

By the mid-1950s, the serious side-effects brought on by the high dosage levels required to treat rheumatoid arthritis led to the development of cortisone analogues with reduced toxicity and enhanced physiological activity. Thus, as the role of cortisone in the treatment of rheumatoid arthritis started to wane, the central role that corticosteroids came to play in modern therapeutics began to emerge [44]. Like cortisone, these appeared to be a 'panacea' against a number of diseases of unknown causes, but which share the common feature of excessive inflammation, such as allergy, acute infections and autoimmune disorders. Since the 1990s, there has been 'somewhat of a rehabilitation of corticosteroids in rheumatoid arthritis' [45].

By providing a treatment for such a wide range of diseases, corticosteroids transformed the outlook of several medical specialties, including ophthalmology, gastroenterology, respiratory medicine, dermatology and nephrology, as well as rheumatology. Moreover, because it was soon realised that treatment with cortisone had to be sustained over a long period of time, raising issues of appropriate dosage and long-term patient care, rheumatoid arthritis became the prototype of a chronic illness [46]. Hence, corticosteroids provided pharmaceutical companies with a privileged angle of attack in the search for drugs against chronic diseases.

Thus, the discovery of cortisone had a great impact, not only on medicine, but also on the pharmaceutical industry. In some firms, shortages of bile acids or of dollars with which to import intermediates from the USA led to the development of non-steroidal anti-inflammatory drugs (NSAIDs), such as Boots' ibuprofen (Nurofen). In others, they prompted a search for alternative sources of raw material and for new means of producing corticosteroids.

Box 10.2 Chronology of selected therapeutic discoveries, 1945 to 1995.

1949 Compound E (cortisone). Shown to be active in rheumatoid arthritis by P Hench of Mayo Clinic, USA, using sample prepared by Merck.
1952 Salk developed polio vaccine in USA.
       Chlorpromazine (Largactil). Rhône-Poulenc: psychotropic drug.
1953 Mercaptopurine (Puri-Nethol). Burroughs Wellcome: anti-leukaemic.
1957 Halothane (Fluothane). ICI Pharmaceuticals: non-flammable anaesthetic.
1959 Ampicillin (Penbritin). Beechams: semi-synthetic penicillin.
1960 Chlordiazepoxide (Librium). Roche: anxiolytic and tranquilliser.
1962 Diazepam (Valium). Roche: anxiolytic and tranquilliser.
       Norethisterone (Anovlar). Schering: oral contraceptive.
       Azathioprine (Imuran). Wellcome: immunosuppressive and anti-arthritic.
1964 Ibuprofen (Brufen). Boots: NSAID for arthritis and inflammation.
1965 Propranolol (Inderal). ICI Pharmaceuticals: beta-blocker.
1966 Allopurinol (Zyloric). Wellcome: for the treatment of gout and arthritis.
1969 Salbutamol (Ventolin). A&H/Glaxo: β_2-stimulant for the treatment of asthma.
1970 Levodopa for Parkinson's disease.
1971 Mechanism of action of aspirin discovered by John Vane.
1973 Tamoxifen (Nalvadex). ICI Pharmaceuticals: for breast cancer.
1976 Atenolol (Tenormin). ICI Pharmaceuticals: β_1-blocker for the treatment of hypertension.
       Cyclosporine (Sandimmun). Sandoz: for transplantation.
       Cimetidine (Tagamet). SK&F: H_2-antagonist for the treatment of peptic ulcers.
1981 Captopril (Capoten). Bristol-Myers Squibb: ACE inhibitor for hypertension.
1982 Human insulin (Humulin). Eli Lilly: first pharmaceutical product of recombinant DNA.
1985 Aciclovir (Zovirax). Wellcome: antiviral against herpes simplex.
       Human growth hormone. Genentec/Eli Lilly: for dwarfism.
1986 Orthoclone. Ortho: for transplantation. First licensed human monoclonal antibody.
1987 Zidovudine (AZT, Retrovir). Wellcome: AIDS treatment.
1989 Simvastatin (Zocor). Merck Sharp & Dohme: for lowering blood lipids.
1990 First gene therapy experiment in a person with adenosine deaminase deficiency.
1992 Paclitaxel (Taxol). Bristol-Myers Squibb: for breast and ovarian cancer and leukaemia.
1995 Interferon beta-1b. Schering Health Care/Biogen: treatment for multiple sclerosis.

Main sources: Various chronologies in Weatherall M. *In Search of a Cure: a History of Pharmaceutical Discovery.* Oxford: OUP, 1990, and Bartlett S. *Medicines Research in Britain* on www.abpi.org.uk (accessed 30 March 2005).

This resulted in the development of biosynthetic methods from plant materials by Upjohn, Schering and Syntex almost simultaneously, using microorganisms as reagents in a process that would not only 'revolutionise the steroid industry' [47], but pave the way for the new biotechnology of the 1970s. Durey Peterson, who developed biosynthetic methods for the production of cortisone at Upjohn, has described how these methods 'spurred similar investigations of other substances using microbiological conversions', including antibiotics [48].

Chlorpromazine

Like cortisone, the psychotropic chlorpromazine (Largactil) had a momentous effect on therapeutic innovation in the second half of the 20th century. This drug, which calmed disturbed patients until then locked up in mental hospitals, led to a new, open-door policy in the treatment of the mentally ill. Thanks to the efforts of the French psychiatrists Jean Delay and Pierre Deniker, and to a well orchestrated marketing campaign on the part of Rhône-Poulenc, the use of chlorpromazine spread rapidly to Britain, the USA, and further afield [49].

Chlorpromazine transformed the practice of psychiatry, by emphasising the chemical aspects of mental disorders, and created a new discipline: psychopharmacology [50]. It stimulated a search for other psychotropic drugs, such as the benzodiazepines used as sedatives and hypnotics, and led to what David Healy has described as 'the anti-depressant era' [51]. However, the proliferation of such drugs on the market, the commercial interests tied to their sale, and their administration by a sometimes over-enthusiastic medical profession to an ever-widening patient base, including children, have also raised doubts about their use and abuse.

Receptor-blockers and stimulants

Although the first psychotropic drugs were developed without any clear understanding of their mechanism of action, the receptors for many of the neurotransmitters present in the brain were later identified. Other areas of research that were to benefit from the study of receptors were cardiovascular, respiratory and gastric medicine. This happened after the beta-blockers had begun what has been called the 'age of the receptor' [52].

The first clinically useful beta-blockers were synthesised at ICI's new pharmaceutical laboratories at Alderley Park, in Cheshire, where the British physiologist James Black arrived in 1958 [53]. There he was responsible for the project to find remedies against coronary artery disease, within a wider programme to develop cardiovascular drugs. Applying Ahlquist's theory of alpha- and beta-adrenoreceptors, which was then just beginning to gain acceptance, Black reasoned that, instead of trying to *increase* the supply of oxygen for the heart, as was being done at the time with nitrites, it might be possible to *reduce* the demand of oxygen, by blocking the beta-adrenoreceptors in the heart [54].

By 1960, Black and his team had developed pronethalol, which was launched under the brand name Alderlin in 1963. However, because it had been found to cause tumours in mice, it was withdrawn from the market, and replaced by propranolol (Inderal) in 1965. Following extensive trials, propranolol became the favourite treatment for cardiac arrhythmia, as well as for angina. After it had been found to reduce blood pressure, it was also used to treat hypertension [55].

The success of propranolol, and the size of the market it targeted, led to an active search by companies in Britain and elsewhere for new beta-blockers with different properties, for the treatment of different conditions. Although in hypertension the beta-blockers have to some extent been superseded by other drugs, such as the ACE inhibitors, they are still among the most widely used heart drugs today [56]. Moreover, by giving substance to the receptor concept, they prompted a search for further receptor-blockers and stimulants, for use in gastric and respiratory medicine.

An important breakthrough was the development by David Jack's team at Allen & Hanbury's (which later became part of Glaxo, now GlaxoSmithKline), of the bronchodilator salbutamol (Ventolin) for the treatment of asthma [57]. In gastroenterology, it was the development by Black (from 1964 at Smith Kline & French) of the histamine H_2 antagonist cimetidine (Tagamet) for the treatment of peptic ulcers [58].

For his contribution to medicine, James Black received the Nobel Prize for Physiology and Medicine in 1988, jointly with the American biochemists George Hitchings and Gertrude Elion. This was the first time the Nobel Prize had been awarded to scientists working in the pharmaceutical industry. The next section looks at Hitchings and Elion's contribution, which was made in the American laboratories of Burroughs Wellcome.

Anti-cancer agents

Thanks to the vast sums of money from public and private sources invested in cancer research, this most dreaded disease provided an important focus for pharmaceutical and biomedical investigations in the 20th century. However, progress in cancer therapy usually resulted from the convergence of many different areas of therapeutic research, not all of which were originally concerned with cancer.

During the Second World War, renewed fears about chemical gas attacks led researchers at Yale University, under contract with the US Office of Scientific Research and Development (OSRD), to make a pharmacological study of nitrogen mustards. These exhibited anti-tumour properties, which were studied on both sides of the Atlantic once the American workers had shared their results with their British colleagues. The outcome of this research was the use of nitrogen mustards as the first anti-cancer chemotherapeutic agents. A search for other compounds exhibiting a similar alkylating action (i.e. combining chemically with cellular constituents) began, and thereafter chemotherapy became closely associated with the fight against cancer.

Other therapeutic innovations were also tried against cancer, including steroid hormones and antibiotics. Following the discovery in the early 1950s of natural sources of steroids in plants such as the Mexican wild yam, and of therapeutic properties in *Rauwolfia serpentina* (Indian snakeroot: for hypertension), and more pertinently here *Catharanthus rosea* (Madagascar periwinkle: for leukaemias and lymphomas), there was renewed interest in plants as a potential source of anti-cancer drugs. They became the object of a vast screening effort led by the National Cancer Institute, in collaboration with the US Department of Agriculture, one product of which was Taxol [59].

Anti-metabolites

A different angle of attack was the search for anti-metabolites. This was to prove fruitful not only against cancer, but against other diseases as well, in particular disorders of the immune system and viral infections. Like the search for alkylating agents, it can be traced to a discovery made during the Second World War, but this time in Britain.

In 1940, Paul Fildes and Donald Woods at the Middlesex Hospital in London worked out the mechanism of action of sulfanilamide. They found that sulfanilamide competed with *p*-aminobenzoic acid (PABA), a substance chemically related to sulfanilamide, and a component of folic acid indispensable to the microbes poisoned by the drug. They named this action 'competitive antagonism' and argued that the presence of PABA prevented the microbes from developing, allowing them to be overcome by the body's natural defences. Before long these ideas would guide the search not only for antibacterials, but also for anti-cancer agents.

In 1942, George Hitchings was appointed to the American laboratories of Burroughs Wellcome. The programme on which he worked was based on his knowledge of folic acid, of its role in the synthesis of nucleic acids, and therefore also in growth [60]. In 1944, he was joined by Gertrude Elion, who was to be his close collaborator for the rest of his career [61]. Although the team's strategy was primarily led by their ideas about drug action and the anti-metabolites they made [62], a major impetus for their research was cancer, and Burroughs Wellcome had an arrangement with the Sloan-Kettering Institute (later the Memorial Sloan-Kettering Cancer Center) in New York to screen their compounds. By the late 1940s, Hitchings and Elion had identified two promising groups: purine analogues and 2,4-diaminopyrimidines.

Purine analogues

Elion's work focused on the purines, which would prove to be the most fruitful part of the programme. It was she who synthesised 6-mercaptopurine in 1951. Almost at once, it became involved in a 'myriad biochemical studies'. Mercaptopurine, or 6-MP as it was usually shortened to, was tested in leukaemia patients at the Sloan-Kettering Institute, and was approved by the Food and Drug Administration (FDA) in 1953 (marketed under the brand name Puri-Nethol).

Eventually mercaptopurine was used in combination with other drugs and radiation treatment, and made childhood leukaemia one of the more curable forms of cancers. It is often considered as a landmark discovery in the history of the pharmaceutical industry, for it was one of the first clinically useful chemical derivatives of a component of DNA. It gave substance to the idea of antimetabolites, and led to a prolonged search for the 'magic bullet' against cancer [63].

Mercaptopurine was important also in that it gave the Burroughs Wellcome team the confidence to pursue the nucleic acid anti-metabolite route. It was followed by several 'spin-offs'. Further studies of mercaptopurine showed it to exert its action by suppressing the body's immune response. In 1957 azathioprine (Imuran), a longer-acting derivative of mercaptopurine, was used as an immunosuppressive in transplant patients and to treat autoimmune diseases (mainly arthritis). Further studies of mercaptopurine also showed that it is broken down in the body by xanthine oxidase, the same enzyme that converts purines into uric acid, the build-up of which causes gout.

In the 1960s the purine analogue allopurinol (Zyloric) was developed for its treatment, and was approved in 1966 by the FDA. The group later applied their knowledge of nucleic acid metabolism to the problem of viruses, and developed aciclovir (Zovirax), launched in 1985, and to this day one of the most successful antiviral drugs.

Beyond the 20th century

By 1975, the pace of innovation had begun to slacken, not only at Burroughs Wellcome, but elsewhere. Many have explained this by the drastic tightening of safety regulations that occurred in the wake of the thalidomide tragedy of 1961. Another explanation has been that the easiest drugs were discovered first, often by accident, and that the purposeful search for novel remedies, based on an understanding of the underlying mechanisms of disease, takes much longer.

As the numbers of blockbuster drugs, which have helped to keep pharmaceutical companies in profit in the face of growing competition and rising costs, have begun to dwindle, firms have turned to mergers and acquisitions as a means of achieving economies of scale and scope. However, whether such mergers are conducive to innovation has been the subject of controversy.

Meanwhile, the new biotechnology has benefited from this dearth of new drugs, tapping into public anxieties about the end of the 'age of optimism'. In the 1970s biotechnology became an important focal point for national scientific and industrial policies, with the USA leading the way. However, the extent to which it has fulfilled its early promise in the field of human healthcare is questionable. There have been some successes, as with human insulin, interferon and human growth hormone, but the true benefits of these, often expensive, new drugs compared with their predecessors are unclear.

Nevertheless, there is no doubt that biotechnology has transformed therapeutic innovation at the end of the 20th century. It has brought back the inventor, in the person of the scientist-entrepreneur heading start-up companies. It has pushed Big Pharma into strategic alliances with start-ups and academia, and has led to the growth of what has been termed the 'bioscience industry'. At the beginning of the 21st century it continues to promise us new and better medicines, targeting the individual patient rather than the disease, and new and better therapies, such as therapeutic cloning and gene therapy.

References

1. Le Fanu J. *The Rise and Fall of Modern Medicine*. London: Abacus, 2000.
2. Sneader W. *Drug Prototypes and their Exploitation*. Chichester: John Wiley & Sons, 1994: 10.
3. Clark C R, Moos W H. *Drug Discovery Technologies*. New York: John Wiley & Sons, 1990.
4. Weatherall M. *In Search of a Cure: A History of Pharmaceutical Discovery*. Oxford: Oxford University Press, 1990.
5. Sneader W. *Drug Discovery: The Evolution of Modern Medicines*. Chichester: John Wiley & Sons, 1985: 2, 6–7.
6. Beer J J. *The Emergence of the German Dye Industry*. Urbana, IL: University of Illinois Press, 1959.
7. Rinsema T J. One hundred years of aspirin. *Medical History* 1999; 43: 502–506.
8. Geison G E. *The Private Science of Louis Pasteur*. Princeton, NJ: Princeton University Press, 1995.
9. Bynum W J. *Science and the Practice of Medicine in the Nineteenth Century*. Cambridge: Cambridge University Press, 1994: 152–157.
10. Chick H, Hume M, Macfarlane M. *War on Disease: A History of the Lister Institute*. London: Deutsch, 1971.
11. Liebenau J. Ethical business: the formation of the pharmaceutical industry in Britain, Germany and the US before 1914. In: Davenport-Hines R T P, Jones G, eds. *The End of Insularity: Essays in Comparative Business History*. London: Cass, 1988: 117–129.
12. Liebenau J. Paul Ehrlich as a commercial scientist and research administrator. *Medical History* 1990; 34: 65–78.
13. Parascandola J. The theoretical basis of Paul Ehrlich's chemotherapy. *Journal of the History of Medicine* 1981; 36: 19–43.
14. Riedl R A. A brief history of the pharmaceutical industry in Basel. In: Liebenau J, Higby G J, Stroud E C, eds. *Pill Peddlers: Essays on the History of the Pharmaceutical Industry*. Madison, WI: American Institute of the History of Pharmacy, 1990: 49–72.
15. Slinn J. Research and development in the UK pharmaceutical industry from the nineteenth century to the 1960s. In: Teich M, Porter R, eds. *Drugs and Narcotics in History*. Cambridge: Cambridge University Press, 1996: 168–186.
16. Black J W. Ahlquist and the development of beta-adrenoceptor antagonists. In: Hoffbrand B I, Shanks R G, Brick I, eds. *Ten Years of Propranolol: A Symposium on the History and Future of Beta-blockade*. Amsterdam: University of Amsterdam, 26–28 September 1975.
17. Davenport-Hines R, Slinn J. *Glaxo: A History to 1962*. Cambridge: Cambridge University Press, 1992.
18. Bliss M. *The Discovery of Insulin*. Toronto: McClelland & Stewart, 1982.
19. Sinding C. Making the unit of insulin: standards, clinical work, and industry, 1920–1925. *Bulletin of the History of Medicine* 2002; 76: 231–270.
20. Liebenau J. The MRC and the pharmaceutical industry: the model of insulin. In: Austoker J, Bryder L, eds. *Historical Perspectives on the Role of the Medical Research Council*. Oxford: Oxford University Press, 1989: 163–180.

21. Kragh H. The take-off phase of Danish chemical industry, ca. 1910–1940. In: Travis A S, Schröter H G, Homburg E, Morris P J T, eds. *Determinants in the Evolution of the European Chemical Industry, 1900–1939: New Technologies, Political Frameworks, Markets and Companies*. Dordrecht: Kluwer Academic, 1998: 321–339.

22. Homan J D H, Tepstra J. Insulin. In: Parnham M J, Bruinvels J, eds. *Discoveries in Pharmacology, Vol. 2: Haemodynamics, Hormones and Inflammation.* Amsterdam: Elsevier, 1984: 431–460.

23. Lesch J E. Chemistry and biomedicine in an industrial setting: the invention of the sulfa-drugs. In: Mauskopf S H, ed. *Chemical Sciences in the Modern World*. Philadelphia, PA: University of Pennsylvania Press, 1993: 158–215.

24. Slinn J. *A History of May & Baker, 1834–1984*. Cambridge: Hobsons Limited, 1984: 124–125.

25. Kennedy C. *ICI: The Company that Changed our Lives*. London: Hutchinson Limited, 1986: Chapter 8.

26. Reader W J. *Imperial Chemical Industries: A History. Volume 2: The First Quarter-Century, 1926–1952*. London: Oxford University Press, 1975: 458.

27. Rasmussen N. Steroids in arms: science, government, industry and the hormones of the adrenal cortex in the United States, 1930–1950. *Medical History* 2002; 46: 299–324.

28. Quirke V. Experiments in collaboration: the changing relationship between scientists and pharmaceutical companies in Britain and France, 1935–1965. D Phil thesis, Oxford University, 2000.

29. Crellin J K. Antibiosis in the nineteenth century. In: Parascandola J, ed. *The History of Antibiotics: A Symposium*. Madison, WI: American Institute of the History of Pharmacy, 1980: Chapter 6, pp. 5–13.

30. Quirke V. Howard Florey – medicine maker. *Chemistry in Britain* 1998; 34: 35–38.

31. Hobby G. *Penicillin: Meeting the Challenge*. Yale: Yale University Press, 1985.

32. Bud R. *The Uses of Life: A History of Biotechnology*. Cambridge: Cambridge University Press, 1993.

33. Yasigawa Y. Early history of antibiotics in Japan. In: Parascandola J, ed. *The History of Antibiotics: A Symposium*. Madison, WI: American Institute of the History of Pharmacy, 1980: Chapter 6, pp. 69–90.

34. Lazell H G. *From Pills to Penicillin: The Beechams Story*. London: Heinemann, 1975.

35. Goldsmith M. *The Road to Penicillin: A History of Chemotherapy*. London: Lindsay Drummond, 1946.

36. Tweedale G. *At the Sign of the Plough: 275 Years of Allen & Hanburys and the British Pharmaceutical Industry 1715–1990*. London: John Murray, 1990.

37. Tansey E M, Reynolds L A, (eds.). *Wellcome Witnesses to Twentieth Century Medicine. Volume 6, Post Penicillin Antibiotics: from Acceptance to Resistance?* London: Wellcome Trust, 2000: 59.

38. Moberg C L, Cohn Z. *Launching the Antibiotic Era: Personal Accounts of the Discovery and Use of the First Antibiotics*. New York: Rockefeller University Press, 1990.

39. Waksman S A. *The Conquest of Tuberculosis*. London: Cambridge University Press, 1964.

40. Quirke V. From evidence to market: Alfred Spinks' 1953 survey of new fields for pharmacological research, and the origins of ICI's cardiovascular research programme. In: Berridge V, Loughlin K, eds. *Medicine, the Market and the Mass Media: Producing Health in the Twentieth Century*. London: Routledge, in press.

41. Hayes P. *Industry and Ideology: IG Farben in the Nazi Era*. Cambridge: Cambridge University Press, 1987.

42. Deichmann U. Emigration, isolation and the slow start of molecular biology in Germany. In: de Chadarevian S, Strasser B, eds. Molecular Biology in Post-War Europe. Special issue of *Studies in History and Philosophy of Biology and Biomedical Sciences*, 2002; 30: 449–471.

43. Johns W F. *Steroids*. London: Butterworths, 1973: Preface.

44. Slater L B. Industry and academy: the synthesis of steroids. *Historical Studies in the Physical and Biological Sciences* 2000; 30: 443–479.

45. Karsh J, Heteny G. A historical review of rheumatoid arthritis treatment: 1948–1952. *Seminars in Rheumarism and Arthritis* 1997; 27: 57–65.

46. Harpuder K. Basic medical principles in the treatment of the chronically ill patient. *Journal of Chronic Diseases* 1956; 4: 170–176.

47. Szpilfogel S A. Adrenal cortical steroids and their synthetic analogues. In: Parnham M J, Bruinvels J, eds. *Discoveries in Pharmacology. Volume 2: Haemo-dynamics, Hormones and Inflammation*. Amsterdam: Elsevier, 1984: 253–284.

48. Peterson D H. Autobiography. *Steroids* 1985; 45: 1–17.

49. Swazey J. *Chlorpromazine in Psychiatry: A Study of Therapeutic Innovation*. Cambridge, MA: MIT Press, 1974.

50. Tansey E M. 'They used to call it psychiatry': aspects of the development and impact of psychopharmacology. In: Gijswijt-Hofstra M, Porter R, eds. *Cultures of Psychiatry and Mental Health Care in Postwar Britain and the Netherlands*. Amsterdam: Rodopi, 1998: 79–101.

51. Healy D. *The Antidepressant Era*. Cambridge, MA: Harvard University Press, 1997.

52. Cuthbert A W. Men, molecules and machines. *Trends in Pharmacological Sciences* 1979; 3: 1–3.

53. Quirke V, Black, James Whyte. *Encyclopaedia of Life Sciences, Vol. 3*. London: Nature Publications Group, 2002: 300–301.

54. Gerskowitch V P, Hull R A D, Shankley N P. The 'pharmacological tool-maker's rational approach to drug design: an appreciation of Sir James Black. *Trends Pharmacol Sci* 1988; 9: 435–437.

55. Shanks R. The discovery of beta adrenoceptor blocking drugs. In: Parnham M J, Bruinvels J, eds. *Discoveries in Pharmacology. Volume 2: Haemodynamics, Hormones and Inflammation*. Amsterdam: Elsevier, 1984: 38–72.

56. Opie L H, Yusuf S. Beta-blocking agents. In: Opie L H, Gersh B J, eds. *Drugs for the Heart*, 5th edn. Philadelphia, PA: W B Saunders Co., 2001: 11–12.

57. Jones E. *The Business of Medicine*. London: Profile Books, 2001: 329–332.

58. Ennis M, Lorenz W. Histamine receptor antagonists. In: Parnham M J, Bruinvels J, eds. *Discoveries in Pharmacology. Volume 2: Haemodynamics, Hormones and Inflammation*. Amsterdam: Elsevier, 1984: 623–645.

59. Goodman J, Walsh V. *The Story of Taxol: Nature and Politics in the Pursuit of an Anti-cancer Drug*. Cambridge: Cambridge University Press, 2001: Chapter 1.

60. George K H. George H Hitchings, 1905– : American pharmacologist. In: McMurray E J, Kosel J K, Valada R M, eds. *Notable Twentieth Century Scientists, Volume 2*. Reading: Gale Group, 1996: 933–934.

61. Marshall L. Gertrude Bell Elion, 1918– : American biochemist. In: McMurray E J, Kosel J K, Valada R M, eds. *Notable Twentieth Century Scientists, Volume 1*. Reading: Gale Group, 1996: 583–584.

62. Hitchings G. Chemotherapy and comparative biochemistry. G H A Clowes Memorial Lecture. *Cancer Research* 1969; 29: 1895–1903.

63. Giner-Sorolla A. The excitement of a suspense story, the beauty of a poem: the work of Hitchings and Elion. *Trends in Pharmacological Sciences* 1988; 9: 437–438.

11

From electuaries to enteric coating: a brief history of dosage forms

William A Jackson

Primitive man almost certainly took the leaves, stems, roots, barks and berries of single herbs (herb simples) internally for the relief of various symptoms. Roots and barks might be chewed; leaves would be applied externally, along with animal fats, to help heal wounds and abrasions. Herbs were also probably used for inhalation, with patients placing them on the fire and inhaling the vapours produced. Later, combinations of herbs would be used, and they would have been incorporated into materials such as fats, oils and honey.

In time these raw materials were increasingly processed in some way before being taken. They might be boiled to extract the goodness. They might be dissolved in a solvent, ground up, or diluted with something else. Something sweet might be added to improve the taste, something aromatic to improve its smell, or a dye to improve its colour. The result was the final dosage form in which the medicine was taken by mouth, applied to the skin, or inserted into a bodily orifice. This chapter describes some of the many dosage forms that have been employed both internally and externally, to cure or alleviate the physical ills of mankind.

Greek and Roman medicines

Humoral medicine, based on the four humours (Chapter 2), formed the basis of orthodox treatment until the 19th century [1]. During the classical period a number of dosage forms were used, including ointments, oils, powders, pills, pessaries, gargles and eye lotions. Enemas, also known as clysters or glysters, were liquids that were injected into the rectum using a horn as a funnel, or an animal bladder attached to a greased tube that was inserted into the anus. Hot fomentations, such as a sponge soaked in hot water, bran boiled in diluted vinegar and sewn into a bladder, or toasted millet in a woollen bag, were applied to relieve pain.

Cerates were external applications, usually made from oil, wax and powders, and were stiffer than poultices, which were similar dressings used to retain heat in a specific area [2]. Minerals as well as herbs and animal derivatives were used therapeutically, and a greasy clay rich in minerals, found on islands such as Lemnos, was formed into discs that were stamped to show their place of origin. These were known as terra sigillata, or sealed earth [3].

Perhaps the most important medicines from this period were the medicinal treacles or theriacs, originally taken to treat venomous bites or stings, but later becoming known as universal antidotes. They normally had a large number of ingredients, sometimes more than 70, and were made using honey [4]. Their use persisted into the 19th century.

Scribonius Largus, the Roman physician who came to Britain as a medical officer with the legions of Augustus, used preparations that included chemical as well as animal and herbal constituents. These remedies were probably used by important citizens in the larger cities and towns as well as by the army. However, most ordinary people would be treated with largely herbal remedies.

Arab medicines

Two of the books written by Avicenna (Chapter 2) contained instructions on preparing medicines, along with many formulae and a section on poisons. Avicenna is thought to have been responsible for introducing the practice of gilding and silvering pills [5]. The Arabs used sugar obtained from sugar cane, originally cultivated in India, and later in Persia, Cyprus, Sicily and Spain [6]. They introduced a number of sweet preparations including syrups, conserves, confections, electuaries and juleps.

Syrups were made by boiling a liquor with sugar. Conserves were prepared by mixing flowers, herbs, roots, peels or fruits with sugar to preserve them. Confections were made by mixing the dried and powdered ingredients with syrup or honey to the consistency of a thin electuary. Electuaries were thicker than confections and suffered from the problem of fermentation if too thin, or candying if too thick [7]. Juleps were clear, sweet liquids that were usually a pleasant vehicle for administering medicines [8].

The Arabs also used flavours such as rose water, and orange and lemon peel, to make medicines more palatable. They made advances in alchemy (chemistry) and were responsible for the design of chemical apparatus later used in Europe [9].

Medieval medicines

Following the departure of the Romans in the early 5th century AD, three main types of medicine were practised in Britain: household and herbal medicine; monastic medicine, which was based on classical texts and prayers; and that practised by Anglo-Saxon practitioners, known as leeches. Many of the latter's recipes were written in so-called leechbooks [10].

Magic was important in many treatments, and in addition to plants, animal parts and excreta were used as ingredients. The preparations found in these leechbooks included ointments, poultices, plasters, fomentations, internal preparations sweetened with honey, herbs or the burnt excreta of animals mixed with water, ale or wine, inhalations of the vapours produced by burning animal parts, and fumigations where the patient sat over a bucket containing a hot herbal decoction or burning seeds [11].

Early modern medicines

The introduction of printing in the middle of the 15th century meant that books such as pharmacopoeias became more widely available. Being printed in Latin, they could be read by scholars of most countries, and the *Pharmacopoeia Londinensis*, published in 1618, was the first such work to apply to a whole country (England) rather than a smaller area such as a city or state [12].

Few medical practitioners had a good knowledge of Latin, so the proliferation of herbals, formularies and dispensatories printed in English made medical knowledge much more accessible. For the first time the formulae and methods of preparation of many medicines could be read in English, and these were widely used. As sources of information on the dosage forms available in the 17th and 18th centuries these vernacular translations are superior to the pharmacopoeias, because they contain information drawn from many sources [13]. As well as herb simples they contain many medicines that had a large number of ingredients.

Compound medicines for internal use

Spirits and distilled waters were made by macerating drugs with spirit of wine (alcohol prepared from wine by distillation) and then collecting the liquid produced by distillation. Mixtures of oils, often ten or twelve, were distilled to produce balsams, some of which could be used externally. Quintessences were produced by distilling an essential oil in pure spirit of wine and concentrating the resulting liquor by redistilling it several times. Dry quintessences were made by dissolving an aromatic oil in spirit of wine, adding it to sugar, and allowing the product to dry by evaporation. To prepare tinctures the ingredients were digested with spirit and then strained. Elixirs were similar to tinctures, but stronger and of a thicker consistency.

Extracts were made by gently heating the constituents with spirit for approximately two days, decanting the liquor, and repeating this process several times. The accumulated liquors were then filtered through brown paper and evaporated using gentle heat until the residue was the consistency of honey. The term liquor was used for a number of liquid preparations collected from different sources and prepared in different ways. Medicated wines and vinegars were obtained by extracting the active principles of simple and compound herbs, or occasionally minerals or parts of animals (as in viper wine) using wine from Spain or the Rhine valley. Decoctions were produced by boiling drugs in water, and some of these were used externally as well as internally. To prepare infusions, herbs were bruised in a mortar, mixed with water, and allowed to stand for a variable period, sometimes with the application of heat. After standing for the prescribed time they were strained.

Sweet medicines

Sweet medicines were very popular during the 17th and 18th centuries. Herbs or their juices were heated with water, strained, and then heated with sugar to make sweet, clear preparations known as syrups. Mels or honeys were similar, but were made with honey rather than sugar. So too were oxymels, which also contained vinegar. Quiddonies or robs were also sweet preparations that were made by concentrating fruit juices and heating them with sugar.

Lohochs or eclegmata were another type of sweet preparation made using sugar and honey, to which the liquid produced by boiling herbs in water, and sometimes other powders (for example, prepared fox's lungs) were added [14]. They were thicker than syrups, and sometimes gums were included to ensure this. Used for chest or throat complaints, they were intended to be taken by licking them from the frayed end of a piece of liquorice root [15].

Electuaries remained popular. They had the same consistency as honey, or the pulp of a roasted apple, and were taken in the form of a bolus (a soft spherical mass). Tragacanth and acacia gums were used to thicken them, and most were expensive. Referring to 'Antidotus Analeptica', a restorative electuary, Culpeper remarks that by taking an ounce a day, 'you shall sooner hurt your purse than your body' [16].

Roots, stems, barks, pulps and flowers were candied and known as preserves or condita. Yet another group of preparations made with sugar were lozenges that, as they were solid, could be carried in the pocket and sucked when required.

Powdered medicines

Magistery was a chemical term applied to more than one type of substance. It was used for very fine powders made by solution and precipitation and some resins such as jalap and scammony, but could also be used for a fine powder prepared from some mineral, vegetable or animal substance. Salts were prepared from plants by bruising them in a mortar, boiling with water and straining before evaporating the solution to the thickness of honey. This was then placed in a glass or glazed vessel and allowed to crystallise.

Powders were preparations made from ingredients that were mixed together and powdered using a mortar and pestle. Such ingredients were predominantly simple or compound herbs, but sometimes included things such as coral, ivory, pearls and precious stones, gold and silver leaf, or viper jelly.

Pills were a particularly useful dosage form for medicaments with an unpleasant taste. Solid ingredients were powdered and then made into a stiff mass, frequently by mixing them with syrup of damask rose, although other syrups, balsam of Peru or oils were sometimes used. They were stored as a mass, and then formed into roughly spherical pills using the fingers. The dose was frequently 30–60 grains, and they were normally larger than 19th and 20th century pills.

Semi-solid medicines for external use

Ointments continued to be a very popular dosage form for external use. They were about the consistency of stiff honey, and were usually made by incorporating different types of medicament in a greasy base made from animal fats such as lard, butter or suet, oils, waxes, and resin. Occasionally honey was used instead. Plasters were stiffer preparations that were prepared and kept as a roughly cylindrical solid mass that could be confused with confectionery. Culpeper wrote 'I Hope no Body is so simple (as) to eat Plaster' [17]. When needed for use the required amount was cut off the roll, heated in an earthen dish and then spread on cloth or white leather and applied to the affected part.

Cerecloths or cerates were intermediate in consistency between ointments and plasters. Typically they were made using eight parts of oil, fat or juices, four of wax and one or two of powders. The softest preparations of this type were known as cataplasms or poultices. They were spread in the same way as plasters and used warm rather than hot. Simple medicated oils were made by the infusion or decoction of single drugs with olive oil, and compound oils by the infusion and decoction of a number of drugs in oil. The latter group includes oil of whelps, made from puppy dogs, earthworms, cypress turpentine and olive oil [18].

Liquid medicines for external use

Lotions were an assorted group of aqueous (water-based) medicines that were designed for external use. They included waters (to combat gout, warts, spots, eye complaints); errhines (nasal washes); epithems (embrocations); diaclysms (mouth washes); gargles; lixivia (body washes); and medicated baths.

A clyster was a 'Liquor or decoction of Medicinal things conveyed into the Guts by a Pipe' [19]. Vaginal douches were known as 'injections', and were normally administered by means of a syringe. Suppositories, which were usually made by mixing the active ingredients with honey, were about one inch long, and were rolled to the thickness of a goose quill before being inserted into the rectum. Pessaries were made for intravaginal use. John Quincy described this dosage form in the following terms: '[a] Pessary, is an oblong Form of Medicine made to thrust up into the Uterus, upon some extraordinary Occasions' [20].

Towards the end of the 18th century experimental work, notably in France, proved that many traditional remedies were of little use therapeutically. Gradually the belief in humoral medicine declined, although in folk medicine some of the simpler remedies persisted into the 20th century. However, most of the animal simples, including powdered mummies, bezoar stones (from the intestines of ruminants) and unicorn's horn (the tusk of the narwhal) were abandoned.

Modern medicines

By the beginning of the 19th century there were three pharmacopoeias in common use in Britain, published in London, Edinburgh and Dublin.

There was some variation in formulae for medicines of the same name, and this eventually led to publication of the first *British Pharmacopoeia* in 1864 [21].

The enlightenment that resulted in the decline of humoral and the rise of rational medicine was followed by the industrial revolution. This made it possible for a steadily increasing number of dosage forms to be mass produced in factories instead of being dispensed individually in pharmacies. Eventually even single products that needed to be prepared extemporaneously ceased to be made in retail pharmacies, and were obtained from specialised manufacturing laboratories. However, this was a gradual process that was not completed in Britain until the end of the 20th century.

Medicines for oral administration

The simplest dosage form was the powder, simple or compound [22]. In the latter the ingredients were finely powdered using a mortar and

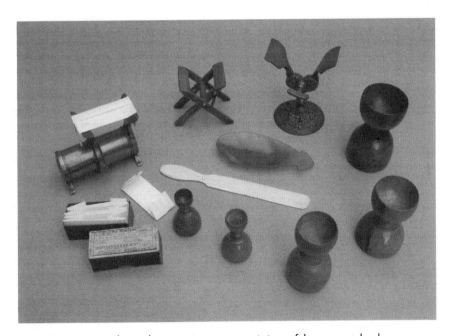

Figure 11.1 Powder-making equipment, consisting of bone spatula, horn scoop, double-ended boxwood powder measures for measuring by volume instead of weight where two types of powder were required (e.g. Seidlitz powders), three types of adjustable powder folders and powder box. Hand-wrapped powders were still being dispensed in 1990.

pestle, and finally mixed on a sheet of paper using a spatula. The amount required for a single dose was measured either by weight or volume and each powder wrapped individually in paper. Sometimes, when powders were dispensed in pairs, such as Seidlitz powders, they were measured using double-ended boxwood powder measures. The finished powders were dispensed in a box, and powder folders (often adjustable) were used to ensure that they were uniform in length and fitted accurately into the box.

The great drawback with powders was that they frequently had an unpleasant taste. To overcome this they were sometimes placed on a piece of rice paper that was moistened round the edge. Another piece of rice paper was placed on top, and the two edges were stuck together using pressure. These were known as wafers, and circular pieces of rice paper of the correct size were available commercially [23].

Cachets

An improvement on the wafer was the cachet, made from two pieces of rice paper shaped like very small soup plates. The powder was placed in the centre of the lower one, the edge moistened, and then the upper one joined to it by pressure to produce a product shaped like a flying saucer. These were known as wet seal cachets and could be dipped in water and swallowed. A French pharmacist, Stanislaus Limousin, invented a machine that made this process much easier, and this was widely employed [24]. Later dry seal cachets were developed, but these never became popular, largely because by this time most pharmacies had already acquired wet seal cachet machines [25].

Pills

Throughout the 19th and early part of the 20th centuries pills remained a popular dosage form [26]. The active ingredients were powdered and then massed, using a mortar and long-handled pestle with a narrow head, with an excipient. In the 19th century, treacle, confection of roses and soap were popular, but later syrup of glucose replaced the treacle. Solid excipients were lactose for white pills, and powdered liquorice root for coloured ones. The firm but pliable mass was rolled into an even cylinder or 'pipe' that was placed against a scale and divided into the required number of pills using a spatula. These were rounded between finger and thumb and finished by rolling on a tile using a boxwood or iron pill rounder.

The pills were varnished by rotating them in a pot containing sandarach resin, alcohol and ether. Afterwards they could be coated with silver or gold leaf by adding a little mucilage of acacia and rotating them in a spherical boxwood pill silverer. Pearl coating was achieved by using calcium carbonate and mucilage in the same way. Pill machines with brass cutters became available in Britain in the 19th century. The 'pipe' was placed on the lower cutters and then the upper ones were placed on top and pushed back and forth until the roughly rounded pills rolled into the drawer at the end of the machine. Pill machines were available for different sizes of pills from one to five grains (65–325 mg).

Tablet triturates

A new form of solid medication developed in the 19th century was originally known as 'the tablet'. The effects of glyceryl trinitrate had first been described in 1878, and it was originally incorporated in a chocolate base. Later, a base of lactose or mannitol was used to make tablet triturates. The process for making them was devised by a Dr Robert Fuller [27]. They were made using a vulcanite or metal mould that consisted of a lower plate from which projected a number of pegs (usually 50) and an upper plate with perforations, which fitted over the pegs exactly when the two plates were pressed together. Solids were finely powdered and mixed with the base. Liquids were mixed with it and evaporated to dryness, and extracts were dissolved in the minimum amount of water or spirit, then mixed and dried.

The powder produced in this way was made into a stiff paste with a liquid made from equal parts of water and alcohol, and this was forced into the perforations using a spatula, and any excess removed. The two plates were pressed together and the moist tablets forced out of the holes by the pegs and allowed to dry. The mould was lubricated using a solution of one part liquid paraffin in one hundred parts of ether. These tablets were very friable and were dissolved under the tongue. Soluble hypodermic tablets were also made in this way. Unfortunately the name 'tablet' was then applied to a solid dosage form made by compression, and the moulded ones just described became known as 'tablet triturates' or 'hypodermic tablets' when intended for use in this way.

Tablets

When the contraceptive tablet was introduced in the 1960s it was christened 'the pill' as an easy shorthand by the media. Since then the word 'pill' has become synonymous with 'tablet'. This is unfortunate because tablets and pills are different dosage forms. Pills are made by massing the ingredients, while tablets are produced by compression.

Ironically, the first real tablet was described as a 'compressed pill'. It was produced by William Brockeden, a manufacturer of Cumberland leads for pencils, who submitted his patent specification for 'shaping pills, lozenges, and Black Lead by Pressure in Dies' in June 1844 [28]. It was for a simple die and punch that consisted of three parts: a base, which had a central pillar with a concave upper surface; a collar that fitted over this; and a punch that had a concave lower surface and which fitted into the top of the collar. The ingredients to be compressed were placed in the space above the pillar. The punch was then inserted and struck with a heavy hammer.

Potassium chlorate, sodium bicarbonate and potassium bicarbonate were found to be the only drugs that could be turned into tablets without the addition of other substances. The method for producing tablets of other drugs was developed in the USA. Binding agents and disintegrants were added to the powders, which were then granulated so that they would flow freely into the tablet punches. Machines were produced for small-scale production of tablets in the dispensary, but this was very labour-intensive. Soon, virtually all tablets were produced by manufacturing chemists, initially in powered single punch machines,

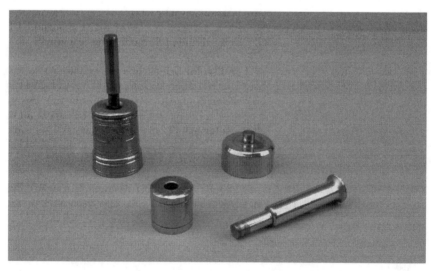

Figure 11.2 Two examples of the press patented by the artist and inventor William Brockedon, FRS (1787–1854), for which he is credited with the invention of the compressed tablet.

and later in rotary presses with multiple punches. From this time there was a steady decline in the importance of the dispensary and a corresponding increase in that of the manufacturer as a source of medicines [29]. Tablets could be sugar coated by rotating them in a copper pan, adding syrup and blowing hot air into the pan.

Capsules

Soft gelatine capsules were a good dosage form for nauseous liquids. They were initially prepared in the dispensary by dipping a collection of mounted olive-shaped moulds that had been lightly oiled into a bath of gelatine solution, allowing it to drain, and then rotating the mould until the gelatine had set. They were then cut so that each capsule had a short neck, and gently removed from the mould [30].

This was a difficult process to perform satisfactorily, and the majority of pharmacists preferred to buy pre-formed capsules. These were placed in wooden blocks that had holes drilled in them, and were filled by means of a syringe or burette. They were sealed either by touching the neck with a hot glass rod or applying a coat of thick gelatine solution to it by means of a camel-hair brush. They were mass produced using pressurised moulds and sheets of gelatine, gum and sugar.

Hard gelatine capsules consisted of two parts, one slightly smaller than the other [31]. The smaller one could be filled with powder using a small funnel and plunger, the rim coated with mucilage, and then the larger part slipped over the end to produce a cylindrical product with rounded ends.

Pastilles and lozenges

Pastilles were produced extemporaneously in the dispensary by mixing the active ingredients with a molten glycogelatin basis that had usually been flavoured and coloured. This was then poured into a tray and allowed to set before being divided with a knife into the calculated number of pastilles. Moulds designed by a Mr Bilson were available. These consisted of individual shallow tin cups soldered to a metal base. The viscosity of the mass was sufficient to allow biconvex pastilles to be made in them, but they had the disadvantage that they had to be calibrated before use.

Lozenges were made from sugar, gum, water and the active ingredient. These were mixed to a stiff paste and rolled out to the correct thickness. The paste could be divided by cutting it into rectangles, or by

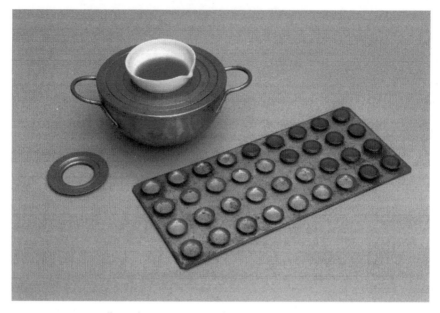

Figure 11.3 Pastille-making equipment of a type probably in use until the early 20th century.

stamping out the lozenges with metal cutters, rather like small pastry cutters. The resulting lozenges were dried using moderate heat. In the 18th century John Ching, who manufactured a famous lozenge for expelling worms, devised a roller that was thicker at the ends than the central section, so that when the paste was rolled out it produced a sheet of constant thickness [32]. Later, in the dispensary, the same end was achieved by using a lozenge board with raised sides. Lozenges were designed to be dissolved in the mouth, and were used largely for sore throats and coughs.

Liquid medicines for internal use

Mixtures, a very popular form of medication in the 20th century, were aqueous preparations for internal administration, frequently made using chloroform water, which acted both as a preservative and a sweetener. Sometimes mixtures were supplied as a single dose known as a draught.

Although not normally taken undiluted, infusions, decoctions and extracts were frequently used as ingredients in mixtures. Fresh infusions were made by pouring water (usually boiling) onto the drug, allowing it to stand for a while and then straining off the clear solution. Fresh infusions rapidly decomposed, however, so concentrated infusions were prepared using alcohol. Concentrated infusions were weakly alcoholic products prepared by maceration or percolation. One part was diluted with seven parts of distilled water immediately before use. Decoctions needed to be freshly prepared and were made by boiling the sliced or bruised drug for a specified time before straining. Soft or dry extracts were made by maceration or percolation, afterwards concentrating the resulting liquid by evaporation. In some extracts the active ingredients were soluble in water.

Tinctures were solutions of drugs in diluted alcohol. They were prepared by simple solution, or extracting the active ingredients by maceration or percolation. In maceration the drug was left in contact with the alcohol at room temperature in a closed vessel. The drug residue was then strained and pressed. The expressed liquid was mixed with earlier collections and filtered. In percolation the solid material was moistened with part of the solvent, and packed into a percolator. The remaining liquid was trickled through, and the final solution was made up to volume by the addition of alcohol. Although tinctures were usually ingredients in mixtures, they were sometimes taken alone in the form of drops. For example, one or two drops of tincture of guiacum were taken on a lump of sugar to treat rheumatism.

Emulsions consist of oily substances dispersed in water or aqueous substances in oil. Normally these would separate into two layers, but emulsification involved reducing the substance to be dispersed to very small particles and surrounding each of these with something that lowers the interfacial tension between the liquids, ensuring that the dispersed droplets remained suspended. A number of emulsifying agents were used, including gums, soaps, and proteins such as egg yolk and casein. Emulsions could be oil-in-water (such as cod liver oil emulsion), which were usually taken internally, or water-in-oil (such as oily calamine lotion), which were applied externally.

Preparations for external use

Ointments continued to be a popular form of medication but were made using several types of basis: greasy ones made from fats, waxes or hydrogenated oils; emulsifying bases that could be emulsified by water, and so were easier to wash off; oil-in-water or water-in-oil emulsion bases; and water-soluble bases. They have largely been replaced by creams that are less viscous, and can be greasy or non-greasy.

Lotions were liquid external preparations designed to be applied without friction, whereas liniments were usually intended to be rubbed into the skin. Pastes were also topical preparations and were made using starch, glycogelatin or paraffin as a basis. They were spread on lint before use or covered with lint after application.

By the 19th century plasters were usually spread on leather, calico, swansdown or other fabrics using a hot plaster iron, with the plaster mass being taken from a cylinder supplied by manufacturers. Shapes designed to be used on the breast, back, chest, shoulder, side or behind the ear were dispensed. In the 20th century machine-spread plasters obtained from manufacturing chemists were usually supplied.

Enemas continued to be used, mainly to relieve severe constipation. Powerful syringes were used to administer them in the 19th century, but a gentler technique, using a funnel and a rubber tube, was preferred in the 20th. In the second half of this century micro-enemas contained in small collapsible tubes were developed.

Suppositories are solid preparations made by mixing the active ingredient with molten theobroma oil or glycerin, gelatine and water, pouring

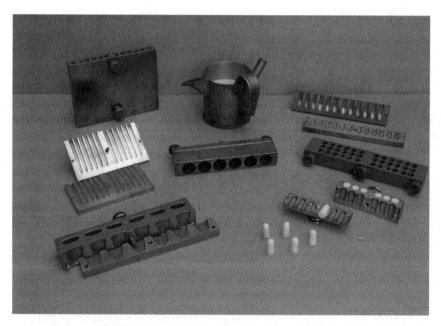

Figure 11.4 Moulds for making suppositories, pessaries and aural and nasal bougies; also shown is a suppository bath with a reservoir of hot water (like a bain-marie) to maintain the molten suppository mass at the correct temperature for pouring. Suppository and pessary moulds were still in use in the 1960s.

the resulting mass into moulds and allowing it to set. They were normally bullet-shaped to facilitate their insertion into the rectum, and melted at body temperature. Pessaries, for vaginal use, continued to be used, and bougies were medicated pencils made in the same way for urethral, aural or nasal use. As these were long and thin a hot wire was inserted into the cavity of the mould and withdrawn as the mass was poured in.

Lamellae

Lamellae were medicated discs intended for application to the eye. They were about 3 mm in diameter, and were made from glycerin, gelatine and water in which the active ingredient had been dissolved. Using a moistened camel-hair brush, the disc was placed on the inner surface of the lower eyelid where it dissolved in the lachrymal secretion, and released the drug it contained, typically atropine sulphate. A great deal of skill was necessary to prepare them, and they were normally purchased from manufacturers or wholesalers.

Inhalations

Inhalations were volatile substances that could be inhaled from a handkerchief or by using them in an oro-nasal inhaler. Others were dispersed in hot water and the resulting vapour inhaled, preferably from a ceramic inhaler such as the 'Nelson'. Powders could be blown into the nose or throat using an insufflator. Vitrellae were capsules made from thin glass that contained a volatile ingredient such as amyl nitrite and were encased in fabric. In use they were crushed between finger and thumb and the contents inhaled.

In the second half of the 20th century new types of inhaler were developed. Metered-dose inhalers deliver a measured dose of a drug in a volatile propellant directly into the respiratory tract, and breath-activated inhalers such as the spinhaler were used for finely divided powders. Liquids in the form of aerosols could be administered by nebulisers operated by rubber bulbs [33].

Injections

Injections are sterile preparations, the majority of which are made under strictly controlled conditions in manufacturing chemists. They are normally packed in single-dose glass ampoules or multi-dose rubber-capped vials, and are administered parenterally using a graduated syringe fitted with a fine needle. The commonest methods of injection are subcutaneous (just under the skin) intramuscular (larger volumes can be injected into muscular tissue) or intravenous (into a vein).

Mechanical devices that deliver a measured amount of injection at pre-set intervals from a multi-dose syringe have been in use for some time, and recently similar machines have been fitted to patients so that they can administer a dose of analgesic when they consider it necessary. Injections can be aqueous, oily, or stored as a powder or tablet to be dissolved in water for injection immediately before use.

Novel dosage forms

One important development in the second half of the 20th century was the introduction of dosage forms that either delayed the release of the drug they contained, or else released it slowly over a period of time. Tablets could be given an enteric coating to prevent their disintegration in the stomach if they would irritate the lining, or be made from combining granules that would disintegrate at different rates in the same tablet to produce sustained-release tablets.

In the same way, hard capsules could be filled with small drug pellets designed to dissolve at different rates to make a sustained-release capsule. Implants are pellets designed to be inserted under the skin where they gradually release a drug over a period of time. They have been used to administer steroids and sex hormones. Transdermal patches can now be applied to release drugs for pain relief, hormone replacement therapy or to help reduce the craving for nicotine, the drugs being absorbed gradually through the skin.

Changes in practice

In the 20th century the introduction of drugs that were much more potent than those used previously meant that accurate dosage became of greater importance. This was probably the main factor in encouraging the use of injections, tablets and capsules, which are all mass-produced dosage forms where the amount of drug to be administered can be measured accurately. In recent years not only has the number of potent drugs available increased substantially but so too has the number of excipients (diluents, lubricants and so on). Although some traditional materials are still used, most new ones are prepared synthetically [34].

The last 50 years have seen a dramatic change in the practice of pharmacy. Many traditional remedies that had survived for hundreds of

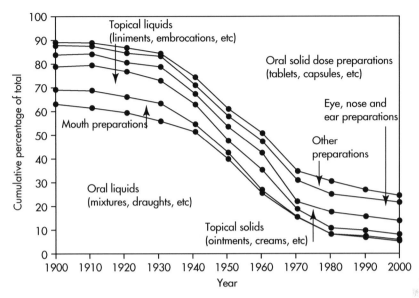

Figure 11.5 Change of dosage forms (liquid to solid), 1900–2000. Reproduced by permission from [35], p. 18.

years have disappeared, and virtually all medicines are made either in manufacturing chemists or, to a lesser extent, in hospital dispensaries. Solid dose forms such as tablets and capsules now dominate modern medicine, and have largely replaced more traditional types of medication. New drugs are invariably marketed as tablets, capsules or injections, although innovative dosage forms will undoubtedly continue to appear.

References

1. Jackson W A. A short guide to humoral medicine. *Trends in Pharmacological Sciences* 2001; 22: 487–489.
2. Cowen W H, Helfand W H. *Pharmacy: An Illustrated History*. New York: Abrams, 1991: 28.
3. Mez-Mangold L. *A History of Drugs*. Basle, Switzerland: F. Hoffmann-La Roche and Co. Ltd, 1971: 107–109.
4. Watson G. *Theriac and Mithridatium: A Study in Therapeutics*. London: The Wellcome Medical Historical Library, 1966.
5. Cowen D L, Helfand W H. *Pharmacy: An Illustrated History*. New York: Abrams, 1990: 42–45.
6. Trease G E. *Pharmacy in History*. London: Baillière, Tindall and Cox, 1964: 15.

7. Quincy J. *Lexicon Physico-Medicum: or, A New Medicinal Dictionary*, 4th edn. London: J Osborn and T Longman, 1730: 142.

8. Motherby G. *A New Medical Dictionary or, General Repository of Physic*. London: J Johnson, 1775: unpaginated, see Julap (sic).

9. Cowen D L, Helfand W H. *Pharmacy: An Illustrated History*. New York: Abrams, 1990: 45–46.

10. Cockayne O (ed.). *Leechdoms, Wortcunning, and Starcraft of Early England &c*. London: Longman Green. Three volumes published in 1864, 1865 and 1866.

11. Matthews L G. *History of Pharmacy in Britain*. Edinburgh: E & S Livingstone, 1962: 5–6.

12. Matthews L G. *History of Pharmacy in Britain*. Edinburgh: E & S Livingstone, 1962: 74.

13. Salmon W. *Pharmacopoeia Bateana, The Arcana Goddardiana, &c*. 4th edn. London: William Innys, 1713.

14. Salmon W. *Pharmacopoeia Londinensis, or, The New London Dispensatory*. London: Thomas Dawks, 1678: 622.

15. Culpeper N. *Pharmacopoeia Londinensis, or, The London Dispensatory*. London: A and J Churchill, 1695: 138.

16. Culpeper N. *Pharmacopoeia Londinensis, or, The London Dispensatory*. London: A and J Churchill, 1695: 158.

17. Culpeper N. *Pharmacopoeia Londinensis, or, The London Dispensatory*. London: A and J Churchill, 1695: 236.

18. Salmon W. *Pharmacopoeia Londinensis, or, The New London Dispensatory*. London: Thomas Dawks, 1678: 733.

19. Salmon W. *Pharmacopoeia Londinensis, or, The New London Dispensatory*. London: Thomas Dawks, 1678: 801.

20. Quincy J. *Lexicon Physico-Medicum: or, A New Medicinal Dictionary*, 4th edn. London: J Osborn and T Longman, 1730: 359.

21. Matthews L G. *History of Pharmacy in Britain*. Edinburgh: E & S Livingstone, 1962: 75–85.

22. Remington J P. *The Practice of Pharmacy*, 3rd edn. Philadelphia, PA: J B Lippincott Company, 1894: 1192–1197.

23. *Wholesale Catalogue of Surgeons' Instruments &c. &c.*, 7th edn. Manchester: James Woolley Sons & Co. Ltd, 1910: 775.

24. Remington J P. *The Practice of Pharmacy*. 3rd edn. Philadelphia: J B Lippincott Company, 1894; 1197–1200.

25. Davis H. *Bentley's Text-Book of Pharmaceutics*, 5th edn. London: Baillière, Tindall and Cox, 1949: 460–461.

26. Kirby W. The story of the pill. *Chemist & Druggist* 1939: 130: 679–682.

27. Remington J P. *The Practice of Pharmacy*, 3rd edn. Philadelphia, PA: J B Lippincott Company, 1894: 1200–1202.

28. Jackson W A. Brockeden's Press. *Pharmaceutical Historian* 1987; 17(1): 2–3.

29. Jones T M. Tablets, tabloids...and tabloids. *The Pharmaceutical Journal* 1983; 231: 301–307.

30. Mohr F, Redwood R. *Practical Pharmacy*. London: Taylor, Walton and Maberley, 1849: 358–361.

31. Jones B E. The history of the gelatin capsule. In: Ridgway K, ed. *Hard Capsules*. London: Pharmaceutical Press, 1987: 1–12.
32. Jackson W A. Ching's worm lozenges. *The Pharmaceutical Journal* 1972; 209: 164.
33. Livingstone C, Livingstone D. Inhalation therapy. *The Pharmaceutical Journal* 1988; 241: 476–478.
34. Rowe R C, Sheskey P J, Weller P J, (eds.) *Handbook of Pharmaceutical Excipients*, 4th edn. London: Pharmaceutical Press, 2003.
35. Anderson S C. The historical context of pharmacy. In: Taylor K M G, Harding G, eds. *Pharmacy Practice*. London: Taylor and Francis, 2001.

12

From secret remedies to prescription medicines: a brief history of medicine quality

Michael H Jepson

The great variety of medicines used throughout the centuries differed in many ways, not least in their quality. Not all medicines were prescribed and made by apothecaries; and not all herbs were made into medicines by trained practitioners. Indeed, in many areas the commonest medicines were home remedies, made by lay people for domestic use. There were also 'quack remedies', usually sold by itinerant peddlers, but later advertised heavily in newspapers and magazines. Other products were also available – medicines made up locally by individual chemists and druggists, proprietary medicines, and doctors' prescriptions that were extemporaneously dispensed.

The theme of this chapter reflects the growing concern about the quality of medicines in use in Britain, and the initiatives taken over several centuries to improve matters. A number of specific issues are considered: the role of stamp duty, the regulation of advertising, and the impact of the introduction of more effective drugs. The chapter explores the many types of medicine in use over the centuries and their variable quality. It reviews the changing role of chemists and druggists, and illustrates emerging concern for the safety of medicines (which is dependent upon quality), an issue that is explored further in the next chapter.

Early medicines

From earliest times humans have sought relief from the afflictions of mind and body by utilising plants and other naturally occurring materials. As the Canadian physician Sir William Osler put it: 'Man has an inborn craving for medicine. Heroic dosing for several generations has given his tissues a thirst for drugs. The desire to take medicine is one feature which distinguishes man, the animal, from his fellow creatures' [1].

The man or woman who acquired a knowledge of the use of plants, herbs and other materials for treating the sick or wounded would be in demand in their community, and could achieve a position of considerable power and influence. Human beings' natural inclination towards superstition, their curiosity about death and the 'miracle' of recovery after treatment, not surprisingly, provided the early association of religious beliefs, pharmacy and medicine. The practice of 'trepanning', used to enable 'evil spirits' to escape, and the wearing of discs of cranial bone as a treatment for migraine and epilepsy, illustrate the ingenuity of association [2].

Quack remedies and patent medicines

Quack remedies have existed from earliest times. Later they became known as 'secret remedies', a term that has tended to influence understanding of their significance. A quack was 'an ignorant pretender to skill, especially in medicine or surgery, one who offers wonderful remedies or devices' [3]. Porter notes that 'the origins of the term are obscure, but it may come from the Dutch 'quacksalver', meaning a quicksilver doctor, since mercury was widely used to treat syphilis' [4]. The term 'charlatan' also appears in the literature, and is defined as 'an imposter in medicine'.

Since the 16th century the term 'secret remedy' has been used to describe those medicines whose constituents were not disclosed on the label, and were usually advertised and promoted as proprietary medicines. The terms 'proprietary' medicine and 'patent' medicine were also frequently used. A 'proprietary' medicine was one 'the sale of which is restricted by patent' [1]. However this is not strictly true, as the term was also applied to a medicine for which the manufacturer claimed sole rights because of a secret formula.

The name of the medicine could be a 'brand' name or a 'registered trademark'. The term 'patent' implies the grant by government (or formerly the sovereign) of a sole right or exclusive privilege to make, use, or sell a new invention. A patent medicine would be a newly formulated medicine. More recently the term 'proprietary medicine' was used to describe a product prescribed by a general medical practitioner but not advertised directly to the public, while 'patent medicine' referred to those advertised to the public and available without prescription.

Patent law has evolved considerably over the centuries, and the sort of remedies formerly granted patents would today be rejected as lacking novelty and originality. Patents are intended to encourage invention by guaranteeing limited monopoly for a set time period, in return for a full disclosure of the details of the invention, sufficient to be reproducible. It is an agreement between state and inventor, to be an open disclosure of original information in return for limited protection.

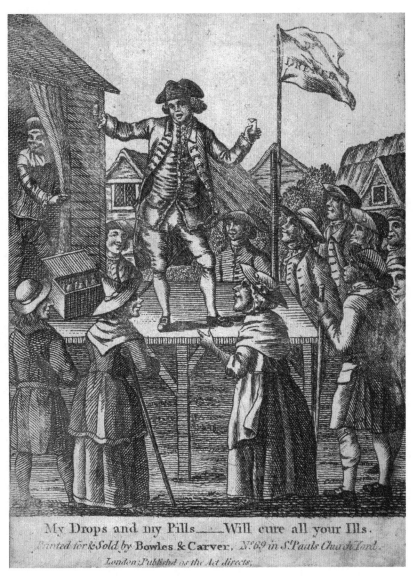

My Drops and my Pills____Will cure all your Ills.

Printed for & Sold by **Bowles & Carver**, N.º 69 in St Pauls Church Yard.

London: Published as the Act directs,

Figure 12.1   Travelling medicine seller Dr Drench claims: 'My drops and my pills will cure all your ills'. Probably 18th century.

Today, patents are issued for the production of novel drugs and systems for their delivery.

The 'quacks' that practised down the centuries were as varied as their remedies. They ranged from 'pious women with considerable skill in nursing and the use of folk remedies', to the 'rogues who duped the masses, sometimes with good humoured harmlessness but often with vicious deception and harm' [5]. Smout wrote that: 'if you wished to save yourself the expense of a physician, you could consult the apothecary directly, or you might decide to put your trust (and your life) in the hands of one of the many itinerant quacks who were usually to be found expounding their miraculous cures in the market place or at the local fair. When they had prescribed and taken your money, their chief concern would be to get out of the town with all possible speed' [6]. Their remedies were mostly of plant origin, but their content was highly variable, and there was no evidence of efficacy. Nevertheless there were some who practised in a more responsible manner.

The development of quality standards

Down the centuries there were those who endeavoured to develop controls and to apply quality standards to medicines. They have contributed to the gradually increased understanding of safety and efficacy issues, which are today enshrined in national legislation.

Medicine quality before 1860

From earliest times, when most medicines were derived from plants, the emphasis was on correct identity, collection, drying and storage. In the 16th and 17th centuries authors of herbals recorded the known facts about each of the many plants used medicinally. John Gerarde listed 'the kindes, description, place, times, names, natures and vertues, agreeing with the best received opinions' of 1,800 plants in his herbal [7]. 'Vertues' included all the medicinal properties, harmful or otherwise. Whatever the shortcomings of the preparations available, many of which had little therapeutic effect, efforts were made by those representing the physicians and apothecaries to develop and establish working standards. The 17th-century herbals formed the basis of the later pharmacopoeias [1]. Palatability also became of increasing importance [8].

Legislation also played its part. In 1456 King Henry VI gave the Grocers' Company of the City of London (which included the apothecaries) the right to 'garble' spices and drugs for the protection of the public. This involved classifying and certifying that drugs and spices were free of adulteration and substitution. Subsequently the College of Physicians, and later the Society of Apothecaries, were involved in these controls. By the reign of James I an 'Act for the well garbling of spices', gave powers to the City of London to counter 'great deceipts and abuses' associated with the sale 'of uncleane corrupt and mingled spices, drugs wares ... to the jeopardie of his Majesties person, and of his subjects'.

Parliament was clearly aware of abuses, and some legislation existed to counter an apparently growing problem. In 1511, the parliament of Henry VIII passed an Act to regulate 'medical affairs'. This meant that controls were limited to those who 'exercised' as physicians or surgeons, principally within a 7-mile radius of the City of London. Little if any control was applied across Britain before the Apothecaries Act of 1815. In this Act, the master and wardens of the Society of Apothecaries were empowered to enter the shop of apothecaries in any part of England and Wales to:

> ... examine their medicines, simple or compound, wares, drugs etc be whole-some, meet and fit for the cure, health and ease of his Majesty's subjects; and all and every such medicines etc, which they shall find false, unlawful, deceiptful, stale, unwholesome, corrupt, pernicious or hurtful, shall and may burn or otherwise destroy. [9]

Where shortcomings were found, fines were also imposed.

Adulteration of drugs

Until implementation of the Medicines Act 1968 most legislation affecting medicines in Britain relied upon the standards laid down in official, national pharmacopoeias [1]. By the 19th century, pharmacopoeias were becoming more scientifically based, but the public dangers arising from adulteration of both food and drugs led to agitation for action. In 1860 an Act for the Prevention of Adulteration of Food and Drink was passed. The first Food and Drugs Act of 1875 made it an offence for drugs to be other than of the quality demanded by the purchaser. Penalties were included for the adulteration of drugs, and public analysts were appointed to ensure effective enforcement. Later Acts in 1938 and 1955 also make reference to it being 'an offence to sell to the prejudice of the purchaser, any drug which is not of the quality demanded by the purchaser'.

Most of the medicines marketed in the 19th century as 'secret' did not fall within the scope of the legislation. Purchasers would be

Box 12.1 Major legislation concerning quality of medicines, 1450 to 1970.

Year	Legislation	Effect
1456	Grocers' Company	Given right to garble spices and drugs.
1540	College of Physicians	Empowered to search apothecary drugs and wares. Some sections only revoked in 1956.
1554	'An acte touching the incorporations of the phisitions of London'	Consolidated powers of search.
1603/4	'Act for the well garbling of spices'	Included drugs. City of London garblers began work.
1624	'Statute of Monopolies'	Basis of modern patent law and right of sole manufacture of a medicine for 14 years.
1783	Medicine tax imposed	Surgeons, apothecaries and druggists exempt.
1804	Medicines Stamp Duty Act	Duty on 'secret remedies'.
1812	Medicine Stamp Duty Act	Amending legislation.
1815	Apothecaries Act	Society of Apothecaries granted powers of search of apothecaries throughout England and Wales for 'false, deceitful, corrupt and unlawful medicines' and to burn or destroy.
1868	Pharmacy Act	Included schedule of 15 'poisons' of which sale or supply to be restricted to pharmacies. Included opium, strychnine, belladonna and mercuric chloride.
1875	Food and Drugs Act	Penalties for adulteration.
1908	Poisons and Pharmacy Act	Revised schedules of 'poisons' and 'listed sellers' of non-medicinal poisons; limited companies controlled.
1915	Medicine Stamp Duty	Doubled to contribute to cost of First World War.
1917	Venereal Diseases Act	Prohibition of advertising of medicines to treat VD.
1922	Dangerous Drugs Act	Controlled import and sale of addictive drugs, notably opium, cocaine and cannabis.

Box 12.1 (continued)

Year	Legislation	Effect
1933	Pharmacy and Poisons Act	Amendments to 'poisons' schedules and rules for labelling, packaging and selling medicines containing 'poisons'.
1938	Food and Drugs Act	Update of 1875 Act.
1939	Cancer Act	Prohibition of advertising of medicines to treat cancer.
1940	Finance (No. 2) Act	Purchase tax applied to most drugs and medicines.
1941	Pharmacy and Medicines Act	All active ingredients of medicines for sale to be disclosed on labels; list of diseases for which advertising of medicines to treat made illegal; stamp duty repealed.
1968	Medicines Act	Consolidated list of diseases for which medicine advertising to public is illegal; medicines subject to safety, quality and efficacy criteria before marketing authorisation granted; three classes of medicines established, only general sales list (GSL) allowed to be sold from any shop.

completely ignorant of what the medicine requested contained. The Arsenic Act of 1851 represented the first restriction on the sale and supply of a harmful substance. A schedule to the 1868 Pharmacy Act restricted the sale and supply of fifteen others. These were classed as 'poisons', and were to be available only from pharmacies. The list included opium, strychnine, belladonna and mercuric chloride. It was extended in 1908 by the Poisons and Pharmacy Act, and again in 1933 by the Pharmacy and Poisons Act (Box 12.1).

In spite of the professional, regulatory and legal initiatives taken to ensure that only medicines of satisfactory quality were supplied, the sale of 'quack remedies' boomed from the 17th century onwards. Outrageous and completely unsubstantiated claims were made for suspect formulas. People in desperate circumstances were exploited, succumbing to the guile of a quack. Even for the most affluent, available effective healthcare was minimal. Self-medication has always been a major factor in medicine use. Reasons range from hypochondria to a lack of trust or confidence in the medical profession linked to the inherent cost involved, whether real or imagined. Many patients were notoriously difficult to treat and were often willing to try any of the many cures on offer [10].

Patent medicines

The Statute of Monopolies of 1624 has been cited for the origin of 'patent medicines'. Under this Act, the sole right of manufacture of a new substance or article was permitted for 14 years, subject to the disclosure of the active ingredients or constituents. On 15 July 1698, the first medicine patent (number 354) was granted. It was for 'The Salt of Purging Water' and was acquired by a medical practitioner, Dr Nehemiah Grew FRS. It is now better known as Epsom Salts (magnesium sulphate) [11].

Later Richard Stoughton, a reputable apothecary in Southwark, London, patented his Great Cordial Elixir, and packaged it in a distinctively shaped bottle. This fulfilled two important purposes: the prevention of undue competition, and the creation of a distinctive brand image. Sales in America were such that a stout person was often referred to as being 'as dumpy as a Stoughton bottle' [11]. Medicines for which a patent had been granted soon became known as 'patent' medicines. This tended to give them a special status in the eyes of many, in a way that stamp duty was to do later.

Proprietary medicines, subject to trade-marking or branding only, continued as secret remedies and avoided any disclosure of ingredients. The registration and consequent protection of a product name enabled a manufacturer to profit from advertising, and minimised imitation by competitors. Some proprietary medicines were copies of the formula of the favourite prescriptions of leading physicians. Dr Gregory's Powder, for example, was heavily promoted by quacks. It contained rhubarb, magnesium carbonate and ginger, and under its official name, compound rhubarb powder, continued to appear in the *British Pharmaceutical Codex* until 1973.

The 17th and 18th centuries witnessed a high level of fraud by quacks. They were keen to take advantage of the developing technologies of the day by advertising themselves and their 'cures' in grossly exaggerated and extravagant terms on handbills and in the public press [12]. As the number of products escalated in the 18th and 19th centuries they became a matter of much concern to the more responsible members of the medical and pharmaceutical professions [13]. *The Medical and Physical Journal*, first published in 1799, stated that year:

> ... we would submit to the legislature the propriety of erecting a public board composed of the most eminent physicians for the examination, analysation and approbation of every medicine before an advertisement should be admitted into any newspaper or any other periodical publication and before it should be vended in any manner whatsoever ...

Sale of patent remedies

Most proprietary medicines and quack remedies were initially sold through booksellers rather than apothecary's shops. Chemists and druggists recognised that they were being neglected, and by the 19th century, the vast majority of pharmacies stocked and sold proprietary medicines in response to customer requests, or by recommendation to treat the symptoms described. Many pharmacies produced their own proprietary remedies, which could be very profitable, but these were mainly limited to their own locality. In these circumstances they were up against the competitive power of national advertising, which continued to grow apace. Holloway notes that chemists towards the end of the 19th century were having similar problems to those of doctors and shopkeepers. Having set up in business with small amounts of capital, they were each threatened by 'unfair competition, by undercutting and by attempts to destroy their livelihood' [14].

In the mid-19th century a number of developments contributed to improved protection of the public. These included legislation and the consolidation of the health professions, such as the foundation of the Pharmaceutical Society. However, 'at the time of the 1841 census, there were 15,000 men practising medicine in the UK, of whom some 5000 were unqualified, and even the qualified included illiterate and incompetent men' [14]. Other national, economic and social pressures, as well as military threats, contributed to the very limited progress made in controlling patent medicines and secret remedies during this period. Indeed, little occurred before publication of the Report of the Select Committee on Patent Medicines in 1914.

Many 'secret remedies' contained little more than a few vegetable extracts, but others did contain active constituents that might include opium, or heavy metals such as mercury, antimony, lead or arsenic, which were variously used for treating coughs, colds, consumption, venereal and skin diseases [15]. Only the official name and concentration of poisons included in the Pharmacy Act of 1868 were required to be declared on the label of medicines containing them. In Britain, full disclosure of all active ingredients of a substance recommended as a medicine only became obligatory with passage of the Pharmacy and Medicines Act in 1941 [16].

Secret remedies

In 1909, the British Medical Association (BMA) published a 195-page book entitled *Secret Remedies: What They Cost and What They Contain* [17]. The book presented the results of chemical analyses of a wide range of remedies, arranged in 20 disease-based chapters. These included cancer remedies, cures for inebriety, obesity cures, cure-alls, as well as cold, cough and headache cures. The preface began: 'One of the reasons for the popularity of secret remedies is their secrecy'. It was found that many people had a fascination with secrecy, and many manufacturers of proprietary medicines were happy to take advantage of this. However secrecy had a less innocuous side: cheap drugs or substitutes were used; claims about using expensive newly discovered substances were made; and claims for effectiveness were often grossly exaggerated.

These and other aspects were reported in the BMA's publication, the aim of which was to bring to an end the irresponsible marketing of medicines to safeguard a gullible public. The analytical chemist who performed the analyses was a pharmacist, Edward Frank Harrison. He is remembered today in the award by the RPSGB of its Memorial Medal to the person invited to deliver the Harrison Memorial Lecture [11].

The BMA's disclosures, and their later volume *More Secret Remedies* of 1912, had little influence on medicine sales, but they did persuade parliament that the situation needed to be addressed. However, little happened for over 30 years. The issue was not peculiar to the UK. In 1824 the Philadelphia College of Pharmacy produced a 12-page booklet detailing the formulae of eight established British patent medicines available in America. This reflected the considerable two-way trade with North America. Some states in the USA did not require the full disclosure of active constituents on proprietary medicine labels until the second half of the 20th century.

Up to the time of implementation of labelling regulations in 1976 (under the 1968 Medicines Act) all prescribed and dispensed medicines supplied to patients were devoid of the identity of the active drug, and were only labelled with the pharmaceutical form or type of medicine (for example, 'the mixture') [18]. This applied irrespective of whether they were dispensed by pharmacists, by dispensing doctors, or from hospital dispensaries. In many ways these too could be described as 'secret'. Patient trust and confidence relied heavily on the integrity of the health professionals involved.

Advertising and promotion

The names of a number of products included in *Secret Remedies* survived until the end of the 20th century, such as *Burgess's Lion Ointment*, *Beecham's Pills* and *Pink Pills for Pale People* [17]. All appeared in the chapter headed 'Cure-alls'. The wrapper around the jars of *Burgess's Lion Ointment* was headed 'amputation avoided, the knife superseded', before stating that it had become the 'most popular remedy for curing all diseases of the skin, ulcers, abscesses (including tuberculous), piles, venereal sores, tumours, toothache, gatherings in the ear, deafness', and about 30 other conditions.

The label declared it to be a vegetable preparation, but on examination it was found to contain lead oleate, beeswax, resin, olive oil, water and lard. Based on the cost of the ingredients only, the mark-up on the 3oz jar costing 3s (15p) was 1800%. None of the costs quoted in *Secret Remedies* made any allowance for the cost of formulating, manufacturing, processing, packaging, distribution or advertising, which was usually the major cost.

Beecham's Pills were advertised to be worth 'a guinea a box' (£1.05). A box of 56 pills cost, in 1909, just over 1s (5p), over 50 times the cost of the ingredients. On examination it was found to contain aloes, powdered ginger and powdered soap. The wrapper claimed that the pills were composed 'entirely of medicinal herbs' and cured well over 30 conditions, some of which came under inclusive headings such as 'all nervous affections, kidney and urinary disorders, flushings of heat and maladies of indiscretion', in addition to constipation, headache and bilious or liver complaints.

Pink Pills for Pale People were sold by the Dr Williams Medicine Company with a London address, but claimed to be manufactured in the USA. Thirty pills cost about 3s (15p), which represented a mark-up of about 360 times based on the ingredients alone. The pills were cleverly advertised for a wide range of diseases, but each advert usually focused on one disease. Four different adverts were published simultaneously in four different newspapers, covering rheumatism, eczema, sciatica and 'dark days of dyspepsia'. On examination each pill was found to contain ferrous sulphate, potassium carbonate, magnesia and powdered liquorice. It was a variation of another popular product, *Blaud's Pills* (ferrous carbonate pills).

These examples indicate how ordinary constituents in advertised medicines could be subjected to uncontrolled marketing in order to promote prices and sales. The latter half of the 19th century saw a rapid increase in sales of proprietary medicines, from £600,000 in 1860 to £3 million in 1891, and to £5 million in 1914. Fortunes were made in both Britain and the USA. *Lydia Pinkham's Vegetable Compound*, marketed as a remedy for 'female weaknesses' from 1873, made Lydia Pinkham of Massachusetts the USA's first millionairess. In England, James Morison, Thomas Beecham and Thomas Holloway all made fortunes from the sale of secret remedies. All joined the band of Victorian philanthropists. Holloway bequeathed Holloway College, which became part of the University of London [2].

Impact on retail pharmacists

The widespread availability of medicines through grocers, corner shops, emergent multiples and general stores eroded the independent chemists' share of the market. After the High Court judgement in 1880 (see Chapter 7) company pharmacy became well established, and realistic pricing was only re-established following the initiative of William Glyn-Jones in setting up the Proprietary Articles Trade Association [19]. Resale price maintenance was established to standardise prices on all proprietary medicines irrespective of outlet, and thereby control hard selling [20,21].

By the 20th century, limited legislation was introduced to prevent the most extreme advertised claims of 'cures' to the public. The 1917 Venereal Diseases Act prohibited the advertising of remedies for treating venereal diseases, but it was over 20 years later before the 1939 Cancer Act prohibited the advertising of cancer remedies. The 1941 Pharmacy and Medicines Act made it an offence to advertise any medicinal product for the treatment of several named diseases, including diabetes and tuberculosis. Exemption was given to essential scientific information in publications for health professions. The list of diseases was consolidated and extended in regulations under the Medicines Act 1968. Prohibition of advertising extended to products or items that might be used to procure abortion. These were initially included in the 1941 Pharmacy and Medicines Act [22].

Medicine Stamp Duty

The first tax, of about 8%, on the sale of patented, proprietary and recommended medicines was introduced in Britain in 1783. Vendors other than those who had served a regular apprenticeship to a surgeon, apothecary, chemist or druggist had to acquire a licence. The transition to imposing a stamp duty occurred with passage of the Medicine Stamp Duty Act of 1804 (amended in 1812), which regulated the duty on secret remedies. These were listed in a schedule to the Act: there were about

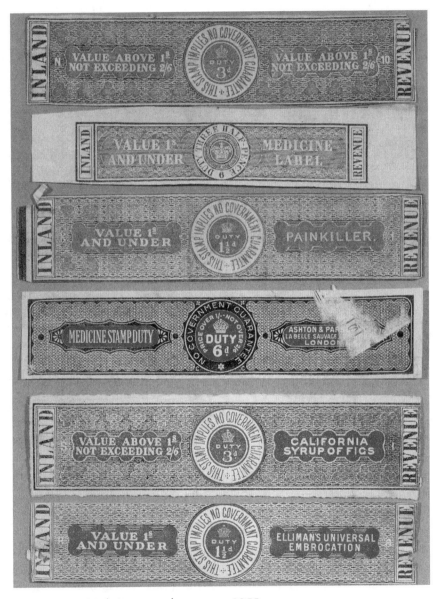

Figure 12.2 Medicine stamp duty stamps, 1855.

450 in 1804, and 550 in 1812 [17]. The 1812 Act included an important exemption for chemists and druggists when selling non-secret compound medicines which met the criterion that 'the denominations, properties etc of which are known, admitted and approved of in the prevention, cure or relief of any human ailment'.

The statutory right of chemists and druggists to sell 'known, admitted and approved' remedies unstamped remained dormant until 1903, when the case of *Farmer v. Glyn-Jones* confirmed it. The exemption was targeted at established pharmacopoeial formulations and formulae in well-known reference books [23].

One consequence of the confusion over the issue that prevailed around the turn of the 20th century was the publication of formularies by both *The Pharmaceutical Journal* and *Chemist & Druggist* [10]. Initially, the wording on medicine stamps stated 'Stamp Office: Patent Medicine', the duty paid and a space for the proprietor's name. These stamps were interpreted by some people as giving official recognition to the medicine, and by 1885 amendments were made that included the words, 'No Government Guarantee'. At first, imported medicines were exempt from duty, and many foreign manufacturers took advantage of this exemption before the loophole was closed. Medicine stamp duty was eventually repealed in September 1941 by the Pharmacy and Medicines Act [23].

Inland Revenue data from the records of duty paid under the Stamp Acts from 1804 give some indication of the scale of 'patent' medicines being sold and supplied [17]. The returns for the year ending 31 March 1899 record £266,403 10s 3d: nine years later, in the year ending 31 March 1908, the revenue raised on patent medicines had risen to £334,141 19s 2d, an increase of 25%. The number of articles stamped that year was 41,757,575, for which the public paid £3,230,401 5s 6d. Most, over 33 million, were priced at about 1 shilling (5 pence).

Counter prescribing

Like the apothecaries before them, pharmacists of the 19th and 20th centuries routinely advised members of the public about the treatment of ailments, especially minor ailments. The term 'counter prescribing' is used to describe the recommendation by a pharmacist, using his or her professional judgement, when requested to suggest treatment for one or more symptoms described by the customer. This might result in the supply of an appropriate medicine, or none, together with relevant advice, or prompt referral to a medical practitioner or other health professional, or to a hospital casualty department.

Down the centuries, as the various health professions evolved, great importance was attached to 'diagnosis', an activity that was central to defining professional boundaries. The rivalry between the College of Physicians and the Society of Apothecaries has been described in Chapter 3. Later, diagnosis was the central boundary issue when the emergent chemists, druggists and pharmacists challenged the medical apothecaries and physicians [24]. Bell and Redwood detail the arguments made at the time the Pharmaceutical Society was founded by those wishing to restrict the advisory role of chemists [25]. It was argued that it would be impossible to suppress quackery by law, and that the public should have the option of selecting such practitioners as they prefer. It was also argued that chemists and druggists should be restricted from giving advice.

Despite these attempts, chemists, druggists and pharmacists did not lose the right to give advice, and to supply, if appropriate, a medicinal product either specifically compounded or prepared to an established formula. This role of pharmacists applied not only to the treatment of human patients but also to animals, until the latter became restricted by the effects of legislation. Only in 1948 did the Veterinary Surgeons Act restrict most treatment of animals to veterinarians by placing great emphasis and consequent restriction on the word 'diagnosis'.

Dispensed medicines

'Extemporaneous dispensing' describes the practice of freshly compounding a medicinal product in response to a prescriber's specific prescription for an individual patient. Very often the prescription would not conform to a 'standard' or 'official' pharmacopoeial formulation, and required pharmacists to use their scientific knowledge and formulation skills to ensure that the preparation was physically stable. Longer term stability or efficacy could not be ensured, as such formulations were not subject to rigorous testing.

Sometimes formulae prescribed by general medical practitioners contained drugs that were incompatible, and they had to be referred back to the prescriber, but for many formulations there were no real problems: quantities supplied could be limited to short-term use, and many of the formulations paralleled established pharmacopoeial monograph formulations.

Freshly prepared medicines

In the 1970s and 1980s many official liquid formulations listed in the *British Pharmaceutical Codex* capable of being extemporaneously prepared were subject to the requirement to be 'freshly' or 'recently prepared' because of limited stability. 'Freshly prepared' meant that the formulation must be prepared within 24 hours of dispensing, and the quantity supplied was usually limited to seven days. 'Recently prepared' meant that the formulation was liable to deteriorate within a few weeks, and a 4-week limit usually applied. Dispensed medicines were labelled with a 'discard after' label. For formulations in regular use it was common practice to prepare a stock bottle (usually a 4.5 litre or 80 fluid ounce Winchester bottle) in order to facilitate dispensing. The label on the container would record when and by whom it was prepared.

After the passing of the Medicines Act in 1968, which introduced strict controls over the manufacture of medicines, many pharmacists continued to counter prescribe, necessitating the extemporaneous preparation of medicinal products. This activity was recognised and sanctioned in the exemptions detailed in the Act. It recognised that many customers seeking advice about 'minor' ailments from their local pharmacist still considered something dispensed personally for them to be preferable to a proprietary off-the-shelf medicine. Older patients in particular were used to requesting a single dose (or draught) of 'something for indigestion', for example. Under such circumstances pharmacists were able to continue to supply single doses of medicines. In some places this practice continues to this day.

A nostrum is any medicine prepared by the person who recommends it. Not surprisingly, the term was formerly used to denote a quack remedy or patent medicine, and it included counter-prescribed medicines that were extemporaneously prepared. Under the 1968 Medicines Act the term 'chemists' nostrums' was revived to refer to certain medicinal products exempted from licensing (marketing authorisations) when prepared in a registered pharmacy and which were not advertised. The *Medicines, Ethics and Practice Guide* for pharmacists states that the sale or supply must be by or under the supervision of a pharmacist, and precise labelling requirements are detailed [22].

Quality of dispensed medicines

The traditional skills of pharmacists, and their predecessors the chemists and druggists and the apothecaries, focused on the techniques required to accurately prepare medications prescribed by physicians and general medical practitioners. The range of formulations was considerable, and included individual-dose wrapped powders, bulk powders, mixtures and linctuses for oral use; lotions and liniments, ointments and creams for topical use; and suppositories, pessaries and bougies for insertion into body orifices. Descriptions of the methods for preparing these formulations were included in the various editions of the *British Pharmaceutical Codex*.

Such dispensed or counter-prescribed medicines could not be subjected to analytical checks before release, and therefore great care had to be taken in their preparation. An important part of compounding and dispensing related to the accuracy and precision of weighing and measuring liquids. Sometimes liquids such as glycerin were weighed rather than measured, where volume measurement was either not sufficiently accurate or not feasible. These techniques might introduce additional sources of error, such as the use of a less accurate balance or the reading of a calibration mark.

Packaging and labelling

Before the more stringent requirements resulting from the Medicines Act of 1968 were introduced medicines prepared in the ways outlined above would be packaged in suitable containers, predominantly made of glass, although woodchip containers and waxed cardboard skillets were also used for preparations such as ointments and powders. Boxwood was occasionally used for cased medicine bottles, and corruganza boxes were often used to hold dispensed ointments and creams.

Until the introduction of the requirements to disclose the name of the medicine prescribed, and to use only machine-produced labels, dispensed medicine labels were mainly handwritten, with bland descriptive titles indicating the form of the medicine. Such labels included 'The Liniment: To be applied as directed'; and 'The Suppositories: One to be inserted into the rectum at night'. The patient's name and the date dispensed were added, together with any standard directions such as 'For external use only' or 'Shake the bottle'. Later, a requirement to provide an expiry date where appropriate was added, such that labels saying 'discard this medicine after ... date' appeared.

Quality of medicines today

In Great Britain today medicines are subject to rigorous control in manufacture, and independent evaluation against strict criteria of safety, quality and efficacy is required before a 'marketing authorisation' (formerly known as a 'product licence') is granted. Marketing authorisations are formally granted by relevant government ministers following recommendations made by the Committee for Safety of Medicines regarding medicinal products intended for human use, and by the Veterinary Products Committee for medicinal products intended for animal use. Both these committees, and their supporting agencies, include pharmacists whose main concerns relate to quality issues.

This chapter has illustrated the fact that many factors have contributed to the evolution of measures to regulate the quality of medicines to provide adequate safeguards for the public. Considerable progress was made down the centuries, although the regulatory framework that exists today is the product of the late 20th century, and the result of the development of many new and potent drugs following the therapeutic revolution of the 1950s and 1960s.

References

1. Jepson M H. *From Dioscorides to Derrick Dunlop: Developing Quality Standards of Medicines*. Special joint lecture. London: British Society for the History of Pharmacy and the Society of Apothecaries, November 2003.
2. Jepson M H. The history and scope of pharmacy. In: Strickland-Hodge B, Jepson M H, Reid B J. *Keyguide to Information Sources in Pharmacy*. London: Mansell Publishing, 1989: 3–21.
3. *Concise Oxford Dictionary of Current English*, Fourth Edition, Oxford: Clarendon Press, 1951.
4. Porter R. *The Greatest Benefit to Mankind. A Medical History of Humanity from Antiquity to the Present*. London: Harper Collins, 1997: 284, 389, 681.
5. Wolstenholme G. Trends in regulation of the profession in the UK. In: L'Etang H (ed.) *Regulation and Restraint in Contemporary Medicine in the UK and USA*. London: RSM and Macmillan Press, 1983: 13–19.
6. Smout C F V. *The Story of the Progress of Medicine*. Bristol: John Wright & Sons, 1964: 59–78.
7. *Act for the Well Garbling of Spices*, London: James I., 1603/4.
8. Hunt S R. Sweet medicines: Sweetening agents in medieval and Tudor pharmacy. *The Pharmaceutical Journal* 1989; 243: 809–810.
9. Food and Drugs Act, 1938 abd 1955, London: HMSO.
10. Porter R. The patient in England c1660–1800. In Weir A (ed.). *Medicine in Society (historical essays)*. Cambridge: Cambridge University Press, 1992: 91–118.
11. Matthews L G. *History of Pharmacy in Britain*. Edinburgh: E & S Livingstone, 1962.
12. Jackson W A. Cancer cures and quackery. *The Pharmaceutical Journal* 1998; 261: 571.
13. Rawlings F W. Old proprietary medicines. *Pharmaceutical Historian* 1996; 26: 4–8.
14. Holloway S W F. *Royal Pharmaceutical Society of Great Britain 1841 to 1991: A Political and Social History*. London: Pharmaceutical Press, 1991.

15.   Parssinen T M. *Secret Passions, Secret Remedies: Narcotic Drugs in British Society 1820–1930*. Philadelphia: Institute for Study of Human Issues, 1983.
16.   Pharmacy and Medicines Act 1941. London: HMSO.
17.   *Secret Remedies: What They Cost and What They Contain*. London: British Medical Association, 1909.
18.   The Medicines (Labelling) Regulations 1976. SI 1726. London: HMSO.
19.   Holloway S W F. Cutting remarks: Reflections on the origins of the Proprietary Articles Trade Association. *The Pharmaceutical Journal* 1996; 256: 198–200.
20.   Holloway S W F. The origins of the Proprietary Association of Great Britain. *The Pharmaceutical Journal Supplement* 1994; 252: M2–6.
21.   Fitzsimon C. The Proprietary Association of Great Britain and the regulation of advertising. *The Pharmaceutical Journal Supplement* 1994; 252: M7–11.
22.   *Medicines, Ethics and Practice Guide for Pharmacists*. London: Royal Pharmaceutical Society of Great Britain, 2003: 27: 18.
23.   Matthews L G. *Antiques of the Pharmacy*. London: G Bell & Sons, 1971.
24.   Court W E. A history of counter-prescribing. *Pharmaceutical Historian* 1982; 12(1): 2–3.
25.   Bell J, Redwood T. *An Historical Sketch of the Progress of Pharmacy in Great Britain*. London: The Pharmaceutical Society of Great Britain, 1880.

13

From arsenic to thalidomide: a brief history of medicine safety

Gordon E Appelbe

In Great Britain concern about the dangers attached to the indiscriminate availability and use of substances can be traced to the Arsenic Act of 1851. However, over the last 30 years or so use and misuse of drugs has been brought to the public's attention as never before. More people than ever are aware of the properties of substances that, in a previous age, were surrounded by an aura of mystery. Specific controls of drugs have in most cases been thought necessary only after misuse or accident has occurred.

This chapter describes the development of the law in relation to medicines. Its focus is Great Britain during the 20th century, although developments in the USA are also considered by way of comparison. The development of such law, from the middle of the 19th century, is intimately bound up with the development of the pharmacy profession. In Britain early developments were largely a response to concerns about apparently high levels of poisoning during the early Victorian period: in the USA and Canada such developments were largely a response to concerns about high levels of adulteration of food, drink and drugs.

Medicines and safety

To define a drug comprehensively is difficult. The World Health Organization (WHO) defines it as 'a substance or product that is used or intended to be used to modify or explore physiological systems or pathological states for the benefit of the recipient' [1]. The word *control*, in its legal sense of the restrictions imposed on the distribution of substances once they are generally available, was not used in the medical literature until 1890. Only in the last 70 years or so has medical science conducted clinical trials within a recognisable framework. There must always be some patient or group of patients who will receive a new medicine for the first time, and it is clearly desirable that this should happen under careful observation by experts in hospital.

The word *safety*, when applied to medicinal products, is relative. It was the Minister of Health, Enoch Powell, who in 1963 said:

> When we use the word safety in this context we should not be understood to mean absolute safety. Safety in this field is relative whatever be the arrangements, whatever be the law. It is relative to the illness. It is relative in the sense that there is no system that can be devised which will make doctors or scientists aware of what medicine and science has not yet suspected.

Safety therefore depends on the ways in which medicinal products are applied or prescribed. Thus no case can be made for restricting the numbers of new products, although provision should be made for better follow-up of their use and the continued education of the user. A failure to take some risks may not be the way to make progress. It is argued, however, whether strict controls should be imposed merely to protect a small minority of the population [2].

In the 1960s Sir Derek Dunlop posed the question: what is the best way to achieve the safety of drugs? Is it by the adoption of tough and aggressive policies like the American Food and Drugs Administration? Is it by methods of mutual agreement and persuasion? Or is it by the more limited objectives of a Committee on Safety of Drugs, as eventually adopted in Great Britain? [3].

There is much to be said in favour of legislation to control the introduction of new medicinal products, but the law itself is poor protection against injury. It may exact penalties from those who are caught infringing its provisions, but it is usually singularly ineffective in providing remedies for those who are injured. In Britain control over the safety of drugs, particularly control of new medicinal products before their release onto the market, was largely achieved through legislation.

Development of medicines legislation in Britain

Before the middle of the 19th century there was no effective legislative control over the sale of poisons or medicines. From 1837 onwards the Registrar General's annual returns disclosed an increasing number of deaths from poisoning, more than a third of which were due to arsenic. Representations concerning its abuse, resulting from its free sale, were made to the Home Secretary jointly by the Pharmaceutical Society of Great Britain and the Provincial Medical and Surgical Association. The latter was the forerunner of the British Medical Association, and had been specifically called 'provincial' as its establishment had resulted from dissatisfaction with the London-based colleges.

Statutory control over sales of poisons was first applied to arsenic because, as the preamble to the Arsenic Act 1851 stated, 'the unrestricted sale of arsenic facilitates the commission of crime'. It was proposed that the sale of arsenic by retail should be restricted to medical practitioners and to chemists and druggists; and that it should be sold only to male adults known to the vendor personally, or on the production of a written order. This would avoid the need for the purchaser to attend the shop in person every time. The purchaser would have to state the purpose for which the poison was required, state the total quantity required, and sign and date the order. Full details of the sale would then be recorded in a book. The government accepted the proposals and the Arsenic Act received royal assent in 1851.

In 1864 the Pharmaceutical Society secured the introduction into the House of Commons of a bill containing the requirement that only pharmaceutical chemists or chemists and druggists should keep open shop for the compounding of the prescriptions of duly qualified medical practitioners. Negotiations went on for 3 years, and this ultimately led to the Pharmacy Act of 1868. However, the focus of the controls was on poisons rather than medicinal products.

Poisons legislation

The Pharmacy Act 1868 brought new developments. It introduced a Poisons List with 15 entries, including arsenic, strychnine and the heavy metals. It empowered the Society to add other substances to it, subject to the approval of the Privy Council. A 'poison' was defined as any substance included in the Poisons List. Articles and preparations containing poisons could be sold by retail only by 'pharmaceutical chemists' or by a new legal class of 'chemists and druggists'.

The registrar of the Society was required to keep registers of pharmaceutical chemists, of chemists and druggists, and of apprentices or students. The qualification of chemist and druggist (the Minor examination) became the statutory minimum for persons carrying on a business comprising the sale of poisons. The 1868 Act not only introduced the first list of poisons but also regulated the manner in which they could be sold, specifying more stringent restrictions on the sale of the more dangerous poisons. Fixed penalties were prescribed for breaches of the Act.

Around 1900, attempts were made by manufacturers of certain poisonous substances that were used in agriculture and horticulture to secure the removal of those substances from the schedule to the Pharmacy Act 1868, in order that their sale might be made by persons other than chemists and druggists. In 1901 a Departmental Committee reported in favour of a subdivision of the Poison List, and recommended that such a legislative change should permit the sale of named poisons used in agriculture and horticulture by persons other than pharmacists.

There was strong opposition from chemists and druggists, but the proposition recognised the fact that the latter were not primarily traders in poisons, but were concerned with poisons in as much as they were potent substances. Effect was not given to the recommendations until the implementation of the Poison and Pharmacy Act 1908, which extended the list of poisons and instituted a system of licensing by local authorities of dealers in certain agricultural and horticultural poisons. This Act also prescribed the conditions under which bodies corporate could carry on the business of a chemist and druggist. This system of poisons control was re-enacted in the Pharmacy and Poisons Act 1933 and, in relation to non-medicinal poisons, is now found in the Poisons Act 1972.

In 1926 another Departmental Committee was set up to consider whether any modifications or changes were necessary to the schedules in the Poisons List. The Committee, after taking 4 years to complete its enquiries, reported in 1930 that:

> Any claim savouring of monopoly in the control of poisons breaks down in the face of the facts as they exist. There is the problem of reconciling precautions against crime, carelessness and ignorance with the grant of reasonable facilities to the public in the purchase and use of poisons for the purposes of medicine, public health and industry.

The Pharmacy and Poisons Act 1933 established a Poisons Board to advise the Secretary of State on what should be included in the Poisons List. Poisons in Part I could be sold by retail only at pharmacies; poisons in Part II could be sold at pharmacies and also by traders on a local authority list. Poisons were further classified by means of Schedules to Poisons Rules made under the Act. For example, Schedule 1 poisons could only be sold by the vendor to a fit and proper person; an entry had to be made in the Poisons Register, and the entry had to be signed by the purchaser. Schedule 4 comprised a class of poisons that could be supplied to the public only on the authority of a prescription written by a doctor or dentist.

The Pharmaceutical Society was placed under a duty to enforce the Act, and was authorised to appoint inspectors for the purpose.

Proceedings under the Act were to be taken in courts of summary jurisdiction and not, as previously, in the civil courts. The Poisons Board prepared a draft Poisons List and Poisons Rules and presented them to the Home Secretary in May 1935 [4]. Pharmacy and poisons were firmly linked by statute, but the sale and manufacture of medicines was not regulated in any way except for medicines containing poisons.

Food and drugs legislation

Some control over quality was provided by a series of Food and Drugs Acts, culminating in the Food and Drugs Act 1955. Under these Acts it was an offence to sell adulterated drugs, or to sell any drug not of the nature, substance or quality demanded by the purchaser. The effectiveness of the provisions was limited by the fact that most drugs were of vegetable origin and, for many of them, there were no precise standards. Furthermore, a manufacturer of a proprietary medicine did not have to disclose its composition, provided that he paid the appropriate duty by fixing the appropriate excise stamps to each bottle or packet, as required by the Medicine Stamp Acts.

This state of affairs was changed by the Pharmacy and Medicines Act 1941, which abolished medicines stamp duty and required, instead, a disclosure of composition on each container. It also restricted the sale of medicines to shops (as distinct from temporary premises such as market stalls) and made it unlawful to advertise any article for the treatment of eight named diseases, including cancer, diabetes, epilepsy and tuberculosis. This was the first statute in which pharmacy and medicines were directly linked. The 1941 Act, however, did not apply to animal medicines.

Therapeutic substances

The first statute to control substances as medicines rather than poisons was the Therapeutic Substances Act 1925. This Act controlled by licence the manufacture (but not the sale or supply) of a limited number of products the purity or potency of which could not be tested by chemical means. These included vaccines, sera, toxins, antitoxins and certain other substances such as insulin. Six years later the law was modified as a result of the 'Lubeck Disaster'. In 1930 75 children died and 168 others were injured in Lubeck, Germany, after the oral administration of BCG vaccine to the newborn. Negligence was alleged against four people from the Lubeck Health Office that the vaccine had been prepared in a laboratory where contamination or exchange with other virulent bacilli was possible, and that the cultures had not been tested before distribution [5].

The list of therapeutic substances was greatly extended when penicillin and other antibiotics were introduced. When it first became available penicillin was controlled by lack of supplies, but it was soon recognised that there could be a real danger to patients and others of rendering strains of some organisms resistant to the drug, because of a tendency to self-medication. To curb indiscriminate use the Minister of Health was advised that the control of sale and supply of penicillin was desirable [6], and this resulted in the Penicillin Act of 1947. Similar controls were later applied to streptomycin, aureomycin and chloramphenicol. It was felt that these would help to save the public from mishap through uncontrolled use of substances where supply could not be regulated under the poisons legislation [7].

The Penicillin Act, and later the Therapeutic Substances (Prevention of Misuse) Act 1953, permitted the supply of antibiotics to the public only by practitioners, or from pharmacies, on the authority of practitioners' prescriptions. The Therapeutic Substances Act 1956 replaced these earlier Acts, bringing under the control of one statute both the manufacture and supply of therapeutic substances.

Dangerous drugs

The Dangerous Drugs Act 1920 arose directly from an international agreement about the control of narcotics that had begun with the International Opium Convention signed at the Hague in 1912. The Convention was not implemented until after the First World War. It was passed by parliament in order to give effect to the obligations into which Great Britain had entered. Certain of these provisions required the contracting powers to co-operate with one another to prevent the use of the drugs for any purpose other than 'legitimate medical purposes', and to control the import and export of the drugs. The delivery of such drugs to unauthorised persons was to be prohibited.

In Great Britain the agreement was not the outcome of public disquiet, nor the stirring of the national conscience about the abuse of drugs. The primary purpose was the suppression of the abuses connected with the trade in and the use of opium in the East. Public opinion in Britain and elsewhere was stirred by the deplorable situation there. When the League of Nations began its work in this field in 1934, Sir Malcolm Delevigne reported: 'The position in 1921 was briefly the following: enormous quantities of drugs were being manufactured and exported without any semblance even of control except in one or two countries' [8].

Development of medicines legislation in the USA

Whereas in Britain drug control was concerned with potent medicines and their potential misuse, in the USA the emphasis was on misrepresentation through advertisement or adulteration. In 1929, with new drugs being introduced with increasing frequency, the meaning and control of drug safety were further explored at a symposium held by the American Medical Association (AMA) [9]. It was argued that the introduction of worthwhile new chemicals for use in medicine required the close co-operation of three distinct types of scientific endeavour – chemistry, pharmacology and clinical studies. Clinical trials of new chemical substances should be made only after critical disinterested pharmacological studies had estimated probable toxicity and type and mode of action.

It was not considered safe to use a drug until it had found acceptability by the Council on Pharmacy and Chemistry created by the AMA [10]. Since 1919 the Council had, on its own initiative or on request, examined the evidence for new drugs not yet on the market. In these cases the Council had sought to verify the composition of the product and to determine adequate tests and standards for confirming identity. It also determined that the bacteriological or pharmacological investigations plus clinical experiments were sufficient to warrant the claims for the proposed actions and use of the medicine.

When the conditions were satisfactorily fulfilled, the Council issued its reports reviewing the evidence and indicated the conditions under which confirmatory clinical trials should be carried out. The clinician who contemplated a clinical study knew that he was working with a product of definite and disclosed composition, the probable value of which was supported by adequate preliminary investigation.

The sulfanilamide tragedy

All these procedures did not succeed, however, in averting the 'sulfanilamide tragedy' in 1938. In September that year it was reported that there had been 76 confirmed deaths from a sulfanilamide elixir containing 10% sulfanilamide in 72% diethylene glycol [11]. Apparently the manufacturer, in spite of published reports, was unaware of the possible

WINTHROP CHEMICAL COMPANY, INC.

Pharmaceuticals of merit for the physician

170 VARICK STREET — NEW YORK, N.Y.

SULFATHIAZOLE-WINTHROP

Important Notice

In the manufacture of tablets of Sulfathiazole-Winthrop, "M.P." control series (December, 1940), some of the tablets were accidentally contaminated with phenobarbital. Immediately upon discovery of this, active steps were taken by us to recover this entire series.

Our attempt to assure the return of all tablets of the "M.P." control series is being continued, in conjunction with the nationwide effort of the U. S. Food & Drug Administration and other public agencies. In the interest of public safety, your prompt cooperation with us and with these public agencies in this search will be greatly appreciated, as these contaminated tablets may be dangerous.

Please examine the mark on every package of our Sulfathiazole tablets, and return to us immediately for exchange any package marked with the letters "M.P." If you have dispensed tablets from bottles bearing these control letters, will you kindly endeavor to recover all such tablets which have not been consumed.

Needless to say, this occurrence is a matter of profound regret to us. Nothing of this nature has ever happened before in our history, and we are taking extraordinary precautions to prevent a recurrence. For more than two decades we have served the medical and pharmaceutical professions. During that period we have earned a reputation for high standards and outstanding products which we shall strive faithfully to maintain.

WINTHROP CHEMICAL COMPANY, INC.

April 3, 1941

Figure 13.1 Sulphathiazole recall notice issued by Winthrop Chemical Company, Inc., 3 April 1941. The company established in December 1940 that a batch of the drug was contaminated with phenobarbital and quickly instructed its agents to retrieve unused tablets. It did not, however, inform the FDA, whose head first learnt of the problem 3 months later. It is believed that 18 deaths had occurred before the company discovered the phenobarbital contamination and that a further 64 ensued from consumption of tablets that remained in circulation between that date and the end of March 1941, when the FDA demanded that the hazard be made public. Reproduced from [31] by permission of the History Office, US Food and Drug Administration, Rockville, Maryland.

toxicity of diethylene glycol, and distributed it freely without having tested it adequately.

The subsequent enquiry emphasised the importance of recognising that, in the examination of a drug with a view to its use in therapeutics, certain conditions needed to be fulfilled. These included the disclosure of exact composition and method of preparation, acute and chronic toxicity studies, determination of the rate of absorption and elimination, path and manner of excretion, and concentration levels in blood and tissues at varying times after administration. In addition there should be a careful examination for idiosyncrasies or side reactions.

It was recognised that these safeguards might be considered as ideal, and be regarded by some people as too rigid, but the report emphasised that 'the life and safety of the individual should not be subordinated to the competitive system of drug exploitation' [11]. As a result of this incident a new federal Food, Drugs and Cosmetic Act was introduced in the USA in 1938, and this was later claimed as a most noteworthy advance in the field of drug control [12].

Adverse reactions to drugs

In 1952 an article appeared in the *British Medical Journal* that was to be recalled some 10 years later as one of the many ignored warnings of inadequate drug testing. In the article, Dr George Discombe cited some of the tragedies seen by clinical and forensic pathologists that were due to drug idiosyncrasies [8]. The dangerous effects of amidopyrine had been well known 15 years before when it had been found to be the component of patent medicines that had killed a number of people. Between 1934 and 1937 much publicity had been given to the occurrence of agranulocytosis in subjects taking medicines containing amidopyrine.

Discombe indicated that most practitioners believed the drug had been removed from the proprietary medicines that contained it. In fact the only restriction that had been imposed was to include it in the fourth schedule of the 1933 Act, thus making it illegal to sell except on the authority of a prescription written by a doctor. The patent medicines advertised directly to the public had been withdrawn, but ethical preparations containing it and distributed under a proprietary name remained available to any medical practitioner.

Amidopyrine was not the only culprit in this respect. Cryogenine (phenylsemicarbazide) was an antipyretic popular in France, and spasmodic attempts had been made to introduce it into Great Britain. Cases of haemolytic anaemia attributed to the drug had been reported to the Academy of Medicine in France in 1950. It had been administered in suppositories advertised directly to the public, but was not on any poisons list in Britain. Discombe claimed that there seemed to be a lamentable lack of contact between clinical pathologists and the Poisons Board, and suggested the setting up of a standing committee which should have the following terms of reference:

> To collect evidence on the production of injurious effects by drugs adminis- tered for therapeutic purposes; to deduce from this and any other evidence available whether the therapeutic value of any drug is great enough to warrant its continued use; and to submit representations and recommendations to the Poisons Board on the regulations for the manufacture, sale, advertising, pack- aging, labelling or prescribing of drugs which had been shown to produce injurious effects.

Mercury in teething powders

In 1948, Warkany and Hubbard [13] had recorded several cases, and later Bivings [14] summarised others, finding mercury present in the urine of patients. Other references to the association of acrodynia with high levels of mercury in urine had been noted by Gaisford in 1949 [15]. He stated that in Manchester, where the condition was common, in almost every case there was a history of ingestion of mercury, usually as calomel in teething powders. The widespread practice of giving calomel to infants had been deprecated, and the Council of the Pharmaceutical Society advised pharmacists to warn their customers of the dangers of

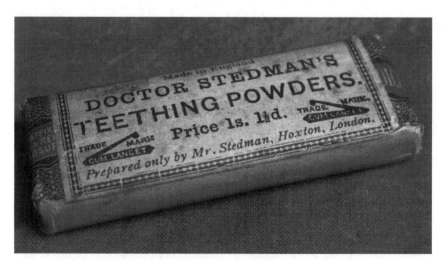

Figure 13.2 Mercury-containing product, c. 1935.

preparations containing mercury and to use great discretion in the supply of such preparations [16].

Wilson, Thomson and Holzel [17] urged that mercurial compounds should be eliminated from all teething powders, but less than a month later Holzel and James [18] described a further 176 cases of acrodynia, over 50% of which gave a history of ingestion of teething powders. Despite these warnings the House of Commons in 1952 was informed that 'enquiries are already in process at various children's hospitals. Although indiscriminate use of teething powder is clearly undesirable there is not yet definite evidence to justify general publicity'.

Twenty months later the results of those enquiries had still not been made public, resulting in a plea and report by Dathan [19] highlighting chronic mercury poisoning found in infants, the mercury being ingested in the form of teething powders. Teething powders containing mercury were eventually withdrawn in 1954, although 12 years later teething powders containing mercury were found in a grocer's shop [20].

Other incidents

In 1951 isoniazid and its derivative iproniazid were developed for the treatment of tuberculosis [21]. Because of the successful use of iproniazid in psychiatry in the treatment of both hospitalised patients with psychiatric depressions and non-hospitalised patients suffering from neurotic depression, there followed the development and clinical trial of many new compounds that also had the capacity to inhibit monoamine-oxidase.

Comparatively quickly reports were received of severe toxicity in some cases with some of these drugs, the effects involving liver, brain and the cardiovascular system. As a result, several drugs classed as monoamine-oxidase inhibitors were withdrawn in the USA. Some were subsequently reinstated on condition that they carried a warning of their side-effects not only to the medical practitioner but also to the patient.

The thalidomide disaster, 1961

By far the most notorious of the products introduced during this period is thalidomide. Thalidomide was a synthetic drug developed in Germany in 1958, and tests on animals found it had no therapeutic effect. Originally marketed for the treatment of epilepsy, it was found to be worthless for this condition, but it did induce sleep, and it was subsequently marketed as a sedative. It had prompt action, gave a natural deep sleep with no hangover and appeared to be innocuous and safe. It quickly became Germany's most popular sleeping tablet, and was widely used in hospitals and mental institutions [22]. It was sold without prescription, it was cheap, and it was an excellent sedative. In Britain and in the British Commonwealth it was marketed by Distillers as Distaval from 1958.

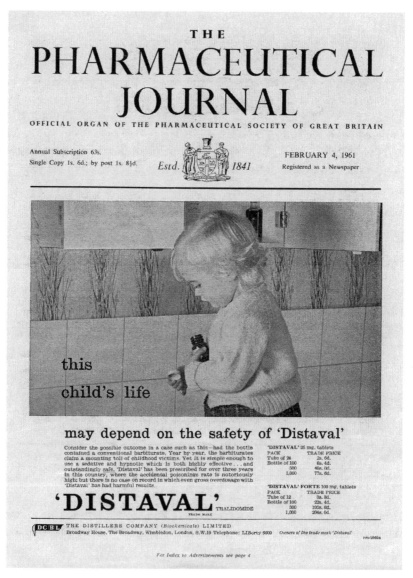

Figure 13.3 Advertisement for thalidomide on the front cover of the *Pharmaceutical Journal* in February 1961.

In 1960 an article reported neuropathic side-effects possibly implicating thalidomide, and a reply to this suggested peripheral neuritis in patients receiving it [23]. The company's literature drew attention to this potential side-effect, and in Germany the drug was reclassified as prescription-only.

Link with phocomelia

Kosenow and Pfeiffer reported several cases of phocomelia (where the limbs of the fetus fail to develop properly) but little attention was paid to them [24]. In 1961 there was a sudden increase in the incidence of phocomelia, and almost every clinic in West Germany admitted three times as many such infants than during 1960. Investigators thought that the causative factor was exogenous (such as a virus), and acted during the critical phase of development, between the third and sixth week of pregnancy. Although this was similar to that of German measles, viral infection was excluded as a possible cause because of the steady increase in the number of patients over a 2-year period, and also by the distribution of the cases.

During one of the earliest trials, conducted by Lenz, it appeared that approximately 20% of patients had taken thalidomide [25]. In November 1961 it occurred to him that the drug might be involved. He warned the company that he suspected the drug was the cause of phocomelia and that it should be withdrawn. On 26 November 1961 the drug was withdrawn from the market. Two days later the British Ministry of Health issued a firm but cautious statement that thalidomide was suspected to be the major factor in the production of phocomelia, as a result of which the drug had been withdrawn from the market: women were warned not to take any more. Between November 1961 and January 1962 circumstantial evidence rapidly accumulated in different parts of the world, which confirmed that thalidomide played an important role in the incidence of phocomelia.

The aftermath of thalidomide

These tragic events gave rise to much comment, both in the medical profession and outside, and the question was asked 'should new drugs be registered?' [26]. Dr Discombe's warning of 10 years previously was recalled. The medical profession felt that further tragedies like thalidomide could be prevented, and some acceptable scheme should be devised preventing the release of drugs until their benefits and risks had been exhaustively examined. A register of toxic reactions was called for, possibly along the lines of the register of blood dyscrasias of the AMA, or at least the submission of information on congenital defects to a central authority [27].

The role of the World Health Organization

Although the thalidomide tragedy galvanised governments around the world into action it was by no means the first time attention had been drawn to the activities of the pharmaceutical industry. A report published by the World Health Organization (WHO) in 1957 [28] had noted that in many pharmaceutical manufacturing companies good methods of examination were in effect, and it was apparent to the WHO that most countries exerted some degree of control over pharmaceutical preparations manufactured or introduced within their boundaries. However, practices varied enormously.

Some countries demanded that all pharmaceutical specialities be registered before sale. It was later claimed that this would have avoided many of the tragic consequences of the marketing of thalidomide. The report noted that, in the UK, control of pharmaceutical preparations was based on the Food and Drugs Act 1955, and the Pharmacy and Medicines Act 1941. Specific legislation for medicines existed only for the control of biological preparations in the Therapeutic Substances Act 1956.

The WHO listed certain information, disclosure of which, in their opinion, was essential before the introduction of a pharmaceutical preparation. These included declaration of the composition; details of analytical methods and methods of preparation; therapeutic indications and dosage; recommended method of selling; samples in sufficient quantity for analysis; information concerning label, package and publicity; publications or documents regarding the pharmacological action of the substance and its toxicity; and clinical reports on its therapeutic efficacy and side-effects.

Response in Britain

Following the WHO Report a subcommittee of the Standing Medical Advisory Committee was set up by the UK government in 1959 to examine the need for new controls, following an announcement by the Minister of Health, Mr. Kenneth Robinson, in the House of Commons. However little progress had been made by the time the thalidomide tragedy struck.

The response of the British government to the thalidomide tragedy was to ask the Standing Medical Advisory Committee to establish a Joint

Sub-Committee on the Safety of Drugs, in July 1962, under the chairmanship of Lord Cohen. It submitted its interim report in November 1962, containing three recommendations to Health Ministers:

- Responsibility for the experimental laboratory testing of new drugs before they are used in clinical trials should remain with the individual pharmaceutical manufacturer.
- It is neither desirable nor practicable that at this stage of their evaluation responsibility for testing drugs should be transferred to a central authority.
- There should be an expert body to review the evidence or offer advice on the toxicity of new drugs whether manufactured in Great Britain or abroad before they are used in clinical trials.

Concerns were raised in France and Italy that drugs other than thalidomide might cause congenital deformities, and this coupling of other drugs with congenital deformities had its effect on the drug companies. At the annual general meeting of British Drug Houses Ltd in 1962 the Chairman said [29]:

> The thalidomide tragedy did not directly affect your company, but one of our most widely prescribed products which contains meclozine is for use in pregnancy sickness. Inevitably since the discovery of the wholly unforeseen risks attendant on the use of thalidomide, doctors have become hesitant about prescribing any drugs during the early stages of pregnancy.

Lord Cohen's committee presented its final report in 1963. This recommended that all new drugs and preparations should be submitted to a Committee on Safety of Drugs. The report added that there should be three clearly defined stages in the testing of drugs, namely toxicity tests, clinical trials, and therapeutic efficacy and adverse reactions during general release. The pharmaceutical members of the committee felt that early legislation was the only way to safeguard the public, not a voluntary scheme. Following the recommendations a Committee on the Safety of Drugs (later of Medicines) was established in 1964 under the chairmanship of Sir Derek Dunlop.

Post-thalidomide developments

The thalidomide tragedy in 1961 represents a major watershed in the history of medicines safety, causing a complete rethink about drugs and their control. It led directly to proposals for new legislation that were published in 1967 in a White Paper entitled *Forthcoming Legislation on the Safety, Quality and Description of Drugs and Medicines*. The White Paper recommended that responsibility for control measures should be with the Health and Agricultural Ministers, and that Ministers should be advised by a Medicines Commission. The Medicines Act 1968, which was designed to replace all earlier legislation relating to medicines, was based on the proposals in the White Paper.

Between 1968 and 1978 the statutes relating to medicines, poisons and drugs were almost entirely repealed and replaced by new legislation. The Medicines Act 1968 now controls the manufacture and distribution of medicines; and the Poisons Act 1972 regulates the sale of non-medicinal poisons. As problems of drug abuse continued to increase, the law was extended and recast in the Misuse of Drugs Act 1971, which repealed the various Dangerous Drugs Acts and the Drugs (Prevention of Misuse) Act 1964.

More recently, European Community legislation has had a great impact on UK law. The Treaty of Rome and the issue of Regulations, Directives, Decisions and Recommendations by the Council of Ministers in Brussels has led to further amendments of pharmaceutical law, particularly with regard to the manufacture and distribution of medicines.

Missed opportunities

The history of drug safety in the middle of the 20th century was a history of ignored signals and a failure to learn from other countries. Dr Discombe's warning on the lack of contact between the Poisons Board and clinical pathologists where injurious effects of drugs were concerned went unheeded for 10 years, and it took the thalidomide tragedy to galvanise the country over the need for greater control. Had Great Britain simply been lucky before thalidomide in that no prior disaster had occurred?

It is also significant that 35 years elapsed between the first suggestions for a drug testing scheme made at the American Medical Symposium in 1929, and the subsequent measures taken in the USA, and the eventual creation in this country of a Committee on Safety of Drugs in 1964. Has the Medicines Act 1968 and the proliferation of committees and regulations since guaranteed that there will be no more disasters or tragedies?

In the aftermath of the thalidomide tragedy, in 1963, the Minister of Health, Mr Kenneth Robinson, addressed the House of Commons about the impact it had had. He said [30]:

> The House and the public suddenly woke up to the fact that any drug manufacturer could market any product however inadequately tested, however dangerous, without having to satisfy any independent body as to its efficacy or safety.

References

1. *Principles for Pre-Clinical Testing of Drug Safety: Report of a WHO Scientific Group. WHO Technical Report Series No. 341.* Geneva: World Health Organization, 1966.
2. Dunlop D. *Journal of Chemical Pharmacology and New Drugs* 1967; 1: 184–192.
3. Glatt H M. Carbromal intoxication. *The Lancet* 1959; 1: 887–888.
4. Linstead H. *Poisons Law.* London: Pharmaceutical Press, 1936: Chapter 1.
5. *The Extra Pharmacopoeia: Martindale,* 21st edn. London: Pharmaceutical Press, 1936.
6. Parliament: control of penicillin. *The Lancet* 1947; 1: 309.
7. Annotations. *The Lancet* 1953; 1: 280.
8. Discombe G. Agranulocytosis caused by amidopyrine: an avoidable cause of death. *British Medical Journal* 1952; 1: 1270–1273.
9. Leake C D. *Journal of the American Medical Association* 1929; 93: 1632–1634.
10. Puckner W A, Leech P N. *Journal of the American Medical Association* 1924; 93: 1627–1630.
11. Ceiling E M K, Cannon P R. *Journal of the American Medical Association* 1938; 111: 916–919.
12. Editorial. *Journal of the American Medical Association* 1938; 111: 324–326.
13. Warkany J, Hubbard D M. Mercury in the urine of children with acronydia. *The Lancet* 1948; 1: 829–830.
14. Bivings L. *Journal of Paediatrics* 1949; 34: 322–324.
15. Gaisford W. *Practitioner* 1949; 163: 282–289.
16. *The Extra Pharmacopoeia: Martindale,* 25th edn. London: Pharmaceutical Press, 1967: 763.
17. Wilson V K, Thomson M L, Holzel A. Mercury nephrosis in young children, with special reference to teething powders containing mercury. *British Medical Journal* 1952; 1: 358–360.
18. Holzel A, James T. Mercury and pink disease. *The Lancet* 1952; 1: 441–443.
19. Dathan J G. Acronydia associated with excessive intake of mercury. *British Medical Journal* 1954; 1: 247–249.
20. Harris P F. Pink disease. *British Medical Journal* 1966; 1: 977.
21. Goodman L S, Gilman A. *Pharmacological Basis of Therapeutics,* 3rd edn. London: Collier Macmillan, 1965: 191.
22. Taussig H B. A study of the German outbreak of phocomelia. *Journal of the American Medical Association* 1962; 180: 1106–1114.
23. Burley D. Is thalidomide to blame? *British Medical Journal* 1961; 1: 130.
24. Kosenov W, Pfeiffer R A. Micromelia, Haemangioma und Duodenal Stenosis Exhibit. *Kinderheilkunde,* 1961; 109: 227, quoted in Taussig H B. *Journal of the American Medical Association* 1962; 180: 1106.
25. Lenz W. Kindlicke Missbildungen nach Medikament wahrend der Graviditat. *Deutsche medizinische Wochenscrift,* 1961; quoted in Taussig H B. *Journal of the American Medical Association* 1962; 180: 1106.
26. Should new drugs be registered? [editorial]. *British Medical Journal* 1962; 2: 461.

27. Witts L J. Registry of toxic reactions. *British Medical Journal* 1962; 2: 254.
28. *Use of Specifications for Pharmaceutical Preparations: Report of a WHO Study Group. WHO Technical Report Series No. 138.* Geneva: World Health Organization, 1957.
29. *The Times.* 27 May 1963: 18.
30. *Hansard.* 8 May 1963: Column 448.
31. Swann J P. The 1941 sulfathiazole disaster and the birth of good manufacturing practices. *Pharmacy in History* 1999; 40(1): 16–25.

Part Five

Pharmacy today and tomorrow

14

Representation, regulation and recognition: pharmacy in Britain, 1986 to 2004

Nicholas Wood and Stuart Anderson

The Nuffield Report, published in 1986, was one of the defining moments for pharmacy in Great Britain. Its overall positive conclusion, 'we believe that the pharmacy profession has a distinctive and indispensable contribution to make to healthcare that is capable of still further development', [1] was to set the policy agenda for years to come. Had Nuffield reached other conclusions pharmacy today would be very different.

For the Royal Phamaceutical Society of Great Britain (the Society) the years immediately following publication of the Nuffield Report were largely occupied by the actions necessary to implement its recommendations. Two aspects came to dominate the discussion: whether a pharmacist needs to be on the premises in order to supervise activities, and the nature of the pharmacist's extended role. However in the late 1990s a range of outside events, and particularly those pointing to the need for more effective regulation of the health professions, came to dominate the agenda.

This chapter examines developments in pharmacy in Great Britain post-Nuffield, in the age of the 'new pharmacy' [2]. It is in three main sections. First, it considers both the external and internal factors that have contributed to the practice of pharmacy in Great Britain today. Secondly, it explores the impact these factors have had on the demand for pharmacists and their education. Finally, it reviews the role of the Society in the light of recent developments.

External influences

One of the most significant external influences on the practice of pharmacy in Britain in recent years has been the growth of the pharmaceutical industry, the rising costs of whose products has been a matter of increasing concern to governments around the world. Other influences have been the deregulation of medicines, and the emergence of the concept of pharmaceutical care. Together these have had a significant impact on pharmacy practice, particularly in the community, including changes in the nature of pharmacy ownership, the emergence of the extended role of the pharmacist, and alternative ways of providing pharmacy services.

The pharmaceutical industry

The pharmaceutical industry is today a global enterprise. Acquisitions and mergers were a feature of the 1990s, and have been an inevitable consequence of the need to invest huge sums in innovative research. With the increased medicines regulation that resulted largely from the thalidomide tragedy in 1961, the cost of bringing new drugs to market is now so high that only a global industry can sustain the research effort involved [3]. Nationally based research companies are usually no longer substantial enough to sustain the effort. Instead, new, smaller companies have emerged that concentrate on niche specialities such as biotechnology or the production of generics.

Perhaps inevitably, the spiralling cost of heavily researched globally branded medicines has led to a burgeoning trade in counterfeit products. Although this has been a problem in some low and middle income countries for many years, with unscrupulous manufacturers taking advantage of weak regulatory and enforcement regimes, by the early years of the 21st century the problem had begun to penetrate the well-regulated distribution chains in the developed economies, although on a much smaller scale [4].

The impact of the vast expansion of the pharmaceutical industry on the practice of pharmacy has been great. With most medicines now pre-packaged, the activity of dispensing has largely become deskilled into one that no longer requires the educational or professional input of the pharmacist. At the same time, consumer demand has meant that more information and services should be available with modern medicines, and the pharmacist's role has been shifting in response to that demand.

The deregulation of medicines

The advent of safer medicines raises some important questions: for example, should they now be more readily available than restriction to a doctor's prescription involves? Although at first slow to advocate the switch to over-the-counter (OTC) sales, the industry subsequently recognised the potential market for what were formerly prescription drugs. The drive to OTC medicines has been easier to justify in Europe than in the USA, because most European pharmacy systems restrict almost all medicine sales to pharmacies, where the intervention of the pharmacist can take place.

The same has not applied in the USA, where federal law dictates that medicines are available only either on prescription or on free sale. However, the risks associated with the widespread availability of many medicinal products such as low-dose corticosteroids, anti-ulcer drugs and emergency hormonal contraception, are well known, and are judged to be low. As a result the way has become clear for a continued expansion of the shift of medicines from 'prescription-only' to 'pharmacy only' control (POM to P deregulation). By contrast the removal of resale price maintenance on OTC medicines had little, if any, effect on the use of these medicines.

Rising prescription costs

A problem for many governments has been what to do about apparently soaring prescription medicine costs. In the American system, insurance-based Health Maintenance Organisations (HMOs) have attempted to manage the upward spiral of prescription costs, and discounted mail order dispensing has become a popular way of keeping prices affordable. In Britain, however, mail order supply of medicines has failed to take off, because price competition does not really exist in the NHS, and local pharmacies frequently offer free home delivery anyway.

Other strategies have been used in an attempt to control drug costs. In the more socialised British and European systems, for example, pharmacists have often taken the initiative by sourcing cheaper parallel-imported drugs from elsewhere in the European Union, while governments have taken positive steps to encourage generic substitution or prescribing. The results have been lower drug costs and tighter margins but, particularly in Britain, these have been largely offset by burgeoning demand and increased volumes of dispensing.

International developments

The shift in pharmacy from a focus on the product (its making and supply), to a focus on the patient (their needs for information and support in their use of medicines), has occurred largely since the 1980s.

Internationally, these developments have been highly influenced by the work of Hepler and Strand on the concept of pharmaceutical care in the USA [5]. The concept has been formally endorsed by the Fédération Internationale Pharmaceutique (FIP), and has subsequently been taken up enthusiastically by pharmaceutical associations around the world.

Pharmaceutical care promotes the idea that the pharmacist should take responsibility for the patient's use of medicines. The concept has been further developed in Europe, particularly in Scandinavian countries, and also in Britain with the institution of programmes of medicine management. Re-engineering pharmacy practice has therefore become a global necessity, and within FIP and other international organisations British pharmacists have played a crucial part in developing innovations and policies that have been acclaimed within the international pharmaceutical community.

Internal influences

Many of the factors that have shaped the practice of pharmacy in Britain are essentially within the control of the pharmacy profession, although some are the subject of statutory control. They include the changing nature of pharmacy ownership, the extended role of the pharmacist, and alternative ways of providing services.

Pharmacy ownership

The last two decades has witnessed a significant change in the pattern of pharmacy ownership. The ability to operate a retail pharmacy as a limited liability company dates from the 1880 case of *The Pharmaceutical Society v The London and Provincial Supply Association* (Chapter 6) [6]. This case opened the door to pharmacy chains, with companies such as Boots, and Timothy Whites and Taylor, emerging. Towards the end of the 20th century, this trend accelerated. Entrepreneurs such as Ralph Weston and Alan Lloyd built up significant groups, but while Boots concentrated on large stores in prime high street and shopping centre sites, rival chains focused on purchasing businesses in secondary parades.

Such pharmacies had formerly been the province of owner-managers and small local groups. Often sited close to a local doctor's surgery, these practices were for a while highly vulnerable to 'leap-frogging', the practice of finding premises closer to the local surgery than the existing pharmacy, and thus creaming off the increasingly important prescription business. Price rivalry from supermarkets on items such as toiletries and baby goods had been feeding an increasing reliance on NHS dispensing. Substantial additional loss of NHS income as a result of leapfrogging could easily result in the closure of a long-established pharmacy, with the newcomer providing no better service other than being 50 yards closer to the source of prescriptions.

By contrast, in much of continental Europe, allegiance to free trade has not been nearly so marked as in Britain. There, the prevailing culture has for many years tried to balance the establishment of an economically viable pharmacy with the needs of a local population. This has typically been achieved by a controlled licensing system, which roughly defines how many pharmacies are needed per head of population. As a result pharmacists own their own businesses in most countries.

Opening new pharmacies

By the 1980s, the free trade principles of market economics had become untenable in Britain, not least because having many small pharmacies was more costly to the NHS than having fewer larger ones. Consequently, in 1984, and after a period of fervent pharmacy openings, regulations restricting the opening of new pharmacies were introduced. Newcomers to an area would need to prove that the NHS service they proposed was 'necessary or desirable'. There was to be no restriction on the opening of a pharmacy as such, only on the granting of an NHS contract for dispensing. In almost all instances it has been the ability to secure such a contract that has defined the viability of a new venture.

For existing pharmacies, the new arrangements frequently secured their financial position. For those already situated in a good location, particularly if close to a doctor's surgery, it was no longer necessary to worry constantly that the business was insecure. With increasing reliance on NHS dispensing, coupled with a security of tenure predicated on holding an existing NHS contract, goodwill prices in the early 21st century soared. In contrast, the ability of newly qualified pharmacists to start off on their own with only modest means diminished considerably. Ownership has increasingly become restricted to those with significant funds.

Twenty years after imposition of the 'necessary or desirable' criteria, however, and following an Office of Fair Trading inquiry, the whole system is once again under review. The need for substantial funds, along with a downward pressure on margins, particularly following removal by the government of the on-cost based NHS contract, has been better suited to chain pharmacies who are able to make economies of scale. As long-established proprietors with 'good' secondary site businesses retire, it has been the chains that have offered the best pharmacy purchase prices.

Vertical integration

Over time, smaller chains have often been swallowed up by larger ones, and increasingly vertical integration has become the norm. With huge sums now involved in NHS dispensing, the attraction for a wholesale operation to own all aspects of the supply chain from factory gate to patient has become irresistible. While some pharmacy chains such as Boots have developed their own internal wholesale operations, the reverse situation, where wholesalers purchased the outlets they supplied, has seen strong growth. AAH bought and developed the Lloyds pharmacy chain, while Unichem took on E. Moss. Similarly, regional wholesalers such as Rowlands have developed their retail chains. Furthermore, wholesaling has been increasingly consolidated by means of takeovers and mergers, resulting in larger wholesale operations trading both in Britain and throughout Europe.

The resulting polarisation in pharmacy ownership (between the chains on one side and a private ownership sector that is diminishing in size on the other) has been recognised as a potential conflict, but also as a possibility for development [7]. While chain pharmacy has often developed formulaic retail solutions to maximise profitability, independents have the flexibility to find and capitalise on niche areas of practice. Indeed, it can be argued that the individual private contractor pharmacist is far better placed to respond to innovative practice at the local NHS Primary Care Trust (PCT) level than are centrally managed pharmacies. Innovative practice often needs private initiative for its development.

The need for supervision

The provision by the industry of medicines in packs ready for issue direct to patients has presented community pharmacy with a dilemma. Even if community pharmacists delegated the mechanical aspects of dispensing to suitably trained assistants, existing legislation, which requires the supervision of medicine sales including dispensing, precludes them from leaving their pharmacies [8]. If they were to be free to advise the local doctor on prescribing, then the rules on supervision had to change.

The great debate on supervision, and on the necessity for a 'final check' on dispensed prescriptions, resulted in a Special General Meeting of the Society at the National Theatre in London in 1989 [9]. Here the

Council's proposals in response to Nuffield to liberalise 'supervision' were narrowly defeated. The Council accepted the verdict of the meeting, and although small changes in the definition of supervision subsequently took place, practice has remained largely unchanged. Many have argued that an opportunity for change was lost.

One of the unintended consequences of this decision was the emergence of a new branch of pharmacy: the pharmaceutical advisor appeared as a specialist area of practice. With no liberalisation of supervision, community pharmacists remained largely tied to their dispensing benches. At the same time, the number of NHS prescriptions presented rose dramatically, fuelled by new treatments and higher public expectations. Any gaps in the workload that might have allowed community pharmacists to leave the constraints of the dispensary for a few hours in order to advise the local general medical practitioner disappeared under an avalanche of prescriptions.

The spiralling drug bill required a response from local PCTs in order to keep their drug budgets under control. Community pharmacists, who had extensive knowledge of the actions and uses of the drugs being used, as well as their costs, were ideally placed to advise doctors on rational and economic prescribing, but community pharmacists were invariably fully occupied with routine dispensing and supervision. This work would need to be done by a new breed of pharmacist, who would be employed directly by the PCT: the new breed became known as pharmaceutical advisors. Today, the function envisaged by Nuffield is fulfilled by such practitioners, rather than the local community pharmacists that had been originally envisaged.

The changing role of the pharmacist

For the world at large the 20th century was characterised by political, social and economic upheaval. For pharmacy the period witnessed no less radical change. The century witnessed the almost total replacement of extemporaneously prepared medicines by the products of the global pharmaceutical industry. The enormity of the shift that occurred in the making of medicines during this period is vividly illustrated by comparison of the 16th edition of the *Extra Pharmacopoeia* of 1915 with the 29th edition of 1989 [10,11]. The biggest change is in the number of products.

This development more than any other drove changes in pharmacy practice in the late 20th and early 21st centuries. The skills of compounding are now rarely required in either the hospital or community settings. The pharmacist in society is having to adapt to a future of adding value through services associated with the distribution and use of pharmaceutical products.

The extended role of the pharmacist

Although many factors contributed to the developing role of the pharmacist, including the changes in the industry and acceptance of the concept of pharmaceutical care, in Britain the catalyst for change was the Nuffield inquiry [12]. Despite such influences, progress towards pharmaceutical care-based remuneration systems (as opposed to ones that are dispensing-based) has been slow throughout the world.

In Britain, the government and representatives of pharmacy contractors (the Pharmaceutical Services Negotiating Committee in England and Wales and the Pharmaceutical General Council in Scotland) spent long periods at loggerheads, particularly after the government abolished the principle (based on cost enquiries) of a contractor 'on cost' profit. Repeated impositions of yearly financial settlements that ignored productivity gains further soured relations.

However, innovative new services such as medicine management require new payment initiatives, and by 2004 in Great Britain, progress was finally being made on a new NHS contract based on three service levels rather than prescription numbers. Agreement on the funding of a new community pharmacy contract in August 2004 means that implementation of the new contract has moved one step nearer [13].

Nevertheless, the main driver for change remains the need to seek a new, consumer-friendly role for the pharmacist in the light of the pharmaceutical industry's innovation and globalisation. At the same time the relationship between the industry and the profession has changed. The industry now employs individuals from almost all disciplines, and the 'special relationship' with pharmacy has effectively ended, particularly as the industry itself now employs few pharmacists. As the pharmacist medical representative and the pharmacist managing director have slowly disappeared, so too has the empathy between the industry and the dispensing pharmacist.

The changing nature of pharmacy employment

The ability to raise sufficient funds has tended to become a limiting factor in allowing the entry of younger individuals to the pharmacy ownership market. There is evidence, however, that as an alternative to ownership, many pharmacists are taking novel approaches to their careers, often seeing themselves as independent or freelance practitioners [14]. The start of the 21st century has seen many pharmacists choosing locum work rather than permanent employment, portfolio careers encompassing a variety of part-time job contracts, and the emergence of the new practice sector in primary care of pharmaceutical advisor.

New roles

The Nuffield Report provided strong support for the development of the pharmacist's advisory services to the medical profession. The report took the view that as dispensing became more mechanical, it could be safely delegated to appropriately trained staff. This would free up pharmacists' time, enabling them to utilise their knowledge and skills in an advisory capacity.

Such a development was already well on its way in hospital pharmacy, where there had been an extensive tradition of training and utilising support staff. Indeed, with a long history of pay levels lower than those in community pharmacy, the chronic shortage of NHS hospital pharmacists had made the utilisation of pharmacy technicians and other support staff an imperative.

By grasping the opportunity to move out of the dispensary and develop clinical and information services hospital pharmacists became increasingly empowered as essential practitioners in prescribing and medicines management in NHS hospitals. With by far the largest number of hospital pharmacists in Europe, the UK hospital pharmacist has increasingly become the arbiter of drug usage, leaving support staff to deal with distribution, storage and other technical tasks.

Demand for pharmacists

As a popular course with a sought-after professional qualification at its end, pharmacy student numbers have risen substantially. However, demand for pharmacists has been rising also, driven by new roles and changing work patterns. Furthermore, with large numbers of women now entering the profession, it seemed at one time that the available pool of pharmacists would need to expand considerably to account for part-time working and career breaks. However, later investigation has indicated that the effect of career breaks amongst women is less than anticipated, although there may still be significant shortages in the future, because men's working patterns also appear to be changing [15].

Early in the new millennium, and anticipating the future demand for pharmacists, new schools of pharmacy have opened or are about to open, despite a declining number of pharmacists choosing academic pharmacy as a career. The University of East Anglia and the Medway School of Pharmacy run jointly by the Universities of Kent and Greenwich have already admitted their first students, and the Universities of Kingston, Central Lancashire, Hertfordshire, Wolverhampton and Reading will do so shortly. More new schools of pharmacy are expected. The maintenance of standards has therefore taken on additional significance, and the Society's decision some years ago to reintroduce its registration examination will play an important part in doing so.

While explicitly not a device for controlling pharmacist numbers, the examination has provided a stable level of quality of entrants. Over the years that it has been running, the proportion of failures at the first attempt has been rising [16], reflecting widening access to the university sector. Hence, while the Society can only maintain partial control of graduate standards through its accreditation mechanism, it can at least ensure quality at the time of registration through its examination.

Pharmacy education

If the Nuffield Report was a philosophical milestone in the recent development of pharmacy practice, it also had much to say about the educational development of the profession. Pharmacy had been the first of the professions to adopt all graduate entry (from 1970), but with the deskilling of the dispensing process, questions were being asked about the necessity of a degree for pharmacists. It was said that the Department of Health suggested to the Nuffield inquiry that there should be a return to a diploma level qualification, at least for community pharmacists. However, the Nuffield Report instead advocated an enhanced role for pharmacists in practice, and this meant not only a retention of the educational requirements for registration but also their enhancement. In particular, Nuffield recognised the diminishing importance of chemistry, but advocated instead an increased role for communications and other sociological skills.

The four-year degree

Over the years following the Nuffield Report, the Society took the lead in implementing the recommendations, particularly in education. The case for a four-year qualifying degree was developed during the early 1990s. It was predicated on three points:

- The need for more time to teach communications skills.
- A requirement to compensate for the decreasingly rigorous A-levels required for entry to the course.
- The need to comply with the European directive on the prescribed length of the pharmacy qualifying course.

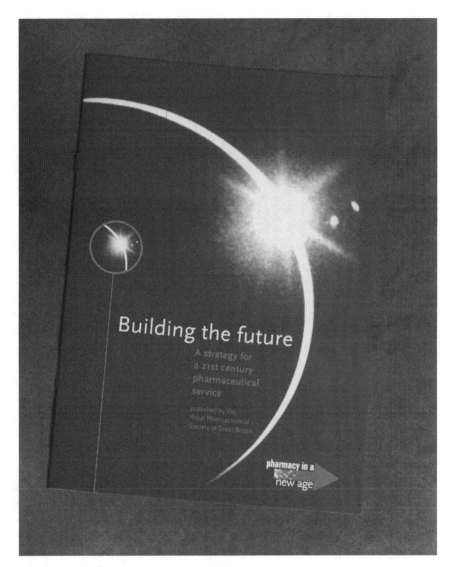

Figure 14.1 *Pharmacy in a new age, 1996.*

Scotland had run four-year degree courses for many years, because the Scottish Highers had been traditionally more generalised than the usual three A-level entries in England and Wales. While Schools of Pharmacy in all three home countries made plans to adapt to a four-year bachelors programme, the School of Pharmacy at Nottingham University insisted that its four-year programme would merit a Masters level award. Despite heavy pressure from their peers and from the Society, Nottingham maintained their stance, and all other UK schools rapidly followed suit. The degree awarded to all pharmacy students after 1997 was the MPharm (master of pharmacy).

Recognising the crucial role it plays in quality assuring entry to the pharmacy profession, the Society has revised and updated its accreditation role with Schools of Pharmacy. Because it is in the position of deciding whether or not a course is acceptable for registration, it has used its influence to ensure Schools of Pharmacy are guaranteed adequate resources in times of financial stringency.

Nuffield's examination of the state of pharmacy at the time, and its thoughts for the future, spawned further policy papers on pharmacy development. These have included joint Department of Health/Society reports [17], the Pharmacy in a New Age (PIANA) initiative [18], and the NHS Plan for Pharmacy [19], all of which have driven the new practice agenda forward.

Continuing Professional Development

Rapid technological progress has meant that the skills and knowledge gained at university can no longer be expected to last a professional lifetime. The ability to maintain fitness to practice in a rapidly changing world has become an imperative for all professions. Initially, continuing education (CE) was seen as the key to maintaining fitness to practice. In this the Americans led the way, with Britain and other western nations following closely behind. However the deficiencies of a purely CE approach rapidly became apparent, and newer concepts such as competence to practise, audit, and continuing professional development (CPD) came to be regarded as essential.

The Nuffield Report recognised the need for continued professional updating, and both the Society and the government accepted the recommendations. The Society embarked on close examination of the issues through a number of working parties, and government promoted the replacement of localised education provider initiatives with centralised committees for pharmacy postgraduate education. With support structures in place, in the early 21st century the Society is rolling out what is intended to become a compulsory system of CPD linked to the right to practise.

While initiatives such as these have become increasingly common amongst the health professions, and with the prospect of compulsory revalidation, the long-term consequences for the pharmacy workforce remain uncertain.

Role of the Royal Pharmaceutical Society of Great Britain

The Nuffield Report recognised the pivotal role of the Society in British pharmacy practice. The role of the Society in Britain differs from that in most western countries, with the notable exception of Australia and New Zealand, at least until recently. While in Europe and the USA membership of most professional associations is voluntary, and an arm of the state registers and inspects the profession, in Britain all these functions fall under the umbrella of the Society. It is a tribute to the quality of its leadership over many years that a membership organisation has not only been entrusted with such a raft of statutory and regulatory duties, but has also exercised them effectively without conflict of interest.

Ethical dilemmas

The Society has used ethical and professional dilemmas to drive forward practice developments. Legal challenges to its authority on disciplinary, educational or registration matters have been rare, and the Society has effectively promoted public interest measures such as the requirements for trained medicine counter assistants (MCAs) in community pharmacy. This particular move had been prompted by criticism of pharmacy advice by the Consumers Association, in a *Which?* report into medicine sales. The training of thousands of MCAs saw an end to the system of bell ringing and waving behind the chemist counter that had previously accompanied the so-called supervised sale of pharmacy medicines, replacing it with a far more active system of staff intervention driven by written protocols.

Incidents such as the 'Peppermint Water case' (in which a small child died following an error in extemporaneous dispensing), have led to improved record-keeping and tighter controls on dispensing processes. The regulation of dispensing assistants and pharmacy technicians, and the implementation of standard operating procedures, are other issues being developed in a continuing drive to raise professional standards.

Advertising

The Society's Code of Ethics contained strict guidelines on pharmacists advertising their services, but changes were made following the *Care Chemist* case in 1974. A complaint was made about an advertisement that appeared in the *Daily Mirror*. The advertisement had been placed by ICML, which represented a voluntary group of pharmacies known as *Care Chemists*. ICML had proceeded with the advertisement despite previous objections by the Society. The complaint was heard by the Society's Statutory Committee. It ruled that the advertisement was objectionable on three counts:

- It advertised the pharmacists' professional services and used the restricted title 'chemist'.
- The *Care Chemist* symbol implied an invidious distinction between those in the scheme and other pharmacies.
- It was considered vulgar and tended to debase the status of the pharmacist.

However, the ruling did not stop advertising; rather, it clarified for all concerned the rules with which they would have to comply. This led to a sea change in advertising, with the replacement of strict ethical control of almost any advertising, with a culture of positively encouraging the advertising and promotion of pharmacy services.

New technology

Technological innovations, particularly the use of NHS patient medication records and the use of computers, have been pioneered by pharmacy. The Society was quick to recognise that an ethical requirement for typed or printed labels would lead to the rapid computerisation of community pharmacy. Wholesalers were also quick to use the new technology. Unichem, a co-operative at the time, was the first to introduce a hand-held order terminal with its PROSPER system: it later demutualised. Computers and information technology were taken up early by pharmacy, but have been slow to develop beyond medicines ordering and labelling, although some progress has been made in computerising patient records. Pharmacy integration into the NHS network is still a long way off.

Publications

By promoting such innovations, the Society became something of a victim of its own success. Throughout the period leading up to the millennium it successfully combined the role of professional membership body and regulator. As a membership body it raised the public profile of the profession. Similarly its publications developed substantially. The *British National Formulary* remains the definitive national guide for prescribers and pharmacists. Spin-off publications include the *Nurse Prescribers' Formulary* and the *Dental Practitioner's Formulary*, and a version commissioned by the WHO.

Today, other publications of the Pharmaceutical Press (the publications department of the Society) include: *Martindale: The Complete Drug Reference* (formerly *Martindale: The Extra Pharmacopoeia*), Clarke's *Isolation and Identification of Drugs*, and Stockley's *Drug Interactions*. These books are also available on CD-ROM and on the Internet. Together they represent a significant commercial enterprise, and have helped prevent the membership fees of the Society rising faster than would otherwise be the case.

Evidence of the high regard for the Society came with the granting of the prefix 'Royal' in 1988, and with the visit of the Queen on the sesquicentenary of the granting of the Society's Charter in 1993. This event, and the years that immediately followed, represented a relative high point in the history of the Society. The Society successfully charted its way through the many changes that occurred between the 1960s and the 1990s. By the late 1990s, the Society seemed to have a secure and coveted position.

Professional regulation

However, external events, particularly questions about standards in public life, began to cast a long shadow over the self-regulating professions. During the late 1990s and early years of the 21st century, evidence began to emerge that all was not well in the regulation of the health professions. The scandals of the Bristol paediatric heart surgeons (who continued to operate on very small children despite very high death rates), and the gynaecologist-pharmacist Rodney Ledward (who continued to operate on women despite evidence of incompetence), among others, began to put the health professions under pressure [20]. Following the Kennedy Report on the inquiry into the Bristol scandal the regulatory bodies for nursing and medicine came under scrutiny, and major reforms were imposed. Far more lay input in professional regulation became the norm, and the trust previously held to be inherent in the professions began to be deemed suspect.

The Society had, however, an exemplary record in self-regulation. Unlike medicine, it was often unsparing of its own members. The

Society's structure, with the independent disciplinary machinery of its Statutory Committee, ensured the isolation of discipline from any political interference. However, the Society also exercises other regulatory functions, such as the accreditation of degree courses, and the enforcement of ethical standards. The pressure for increased lay involvement in this machinery became impossible to resist.

The basis for the Society's regulatory functions lay in a variety of Acts of Parliament. In addition, lay membership existed since 1933 with the appointment of three Privy Council nominees to the Society's Council, bringing its membership up to 24. There became an urgent need to bring greater lay involvement into the machinery. This presented problems for the Society because it is also a professional membership organisation. A Department of Health philosophy of 'one size fits all' for health regulators did not sit easily with an organisation that had members rather than registrants.

Recognising this, individuals and pressure groups such as the Young Pharmacists Group (YPG) proposed in 2002 scenarios that devolved the Society's regulatory functions to a regulatory board with substantial lay input, leaving an unchanged Council of the Society to deal with professional and membership issues. Such changes could have been implemented by Section 60 orders under the wide-ranging 1999 Health Act [21], along with suitable changes to the Society's rules and bylaws.

Proposal for a new Charter

However, advised by the government that such a proposal would be unacceptable, the Society's Council took a very different view. Proposals were made to change the composition of the Council itself to encompass the substantial lay input now expected into the whole of the Society's Council machinery. This proposal was vigorously challenged by various sectors of the membership, including the YPG and a number of past presidents. With the Society acknowledging that the changes to the composition of Council would be unlikely to receive the assent of members, the possibility of a new Royal Charter was floated [22]. The Charter model proposed changed a number of aspects of the Society's objectives and explicitly recognised its role as a regulator.

In late spring of 2003, dissatisfied with these proposals, a loose grouping of activists in the 'Save our Society' (SOS) campaign, including senior members of the profession, former Council members and YPG activists, called for a Special General Meeting. The meeting overwhelmingly carried a number of 'conservative' motions, but although some changes were subsequently made to the Society's Charter proposals, they failed to satisfy the protesters. In December 2003 the Council voted by a two-thirds majority to petition the Queen in Privy Council for a new Charter, but those who voted for the petition were immediately challenged in the Courts by legal action from four supporters of the SOS campaign.

As a consequence, the Privy Council found it necessary to put consideration of the Council's petition on hold until the outcome of the Court case had been determined. The Society thus found itself in the unenviable position of being unable to obtain the Charter that its modernisers felt it needed, while the Courts decided whether the assenting Council members had exceeded their powers and acted outside the scope of the Society's 1953 Charter. In May 2004, the High Court ruled that the Society and Council member defendants had indeed acted lawfully, and the case was dismissed.

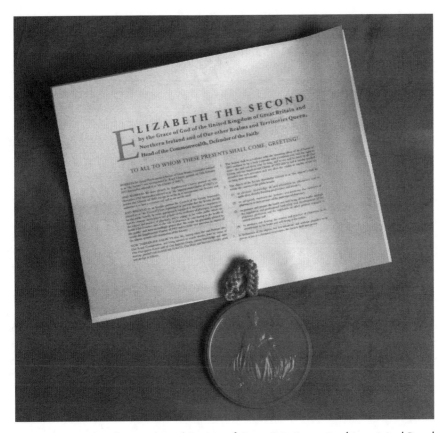

Figure 14.2 The Pharmaceutical Society of Great Britain received its original Royal Charter in 1843; the Supplemental Charter shown was granted in December 2004.

However, in June 2004 seven SOS campaigners were elected to the seven available places on the Society's Council, and a further amended version of the Charter was agreed. This changed the order and emphasis of the roles of the Society, increasing the part played by the membership while retaining the regulatory functions. The revised Charter was supported without dissent by the new Council, and put to a vote by the membership. In a low turnout of 9.3%, 84% of those voting supported the draft Charter [23]. The Council subsequently agreed by a significant majority to its further submission to the Privy Council. The Queen in Privy Council finally agreed the new Charter in October 2004. It was sealed and came into force in December 2004.

A completely new Council took office under these arrangements in May 2005. It had significantly increased lay representation as well as two pharmacy technician members. Of the former Council members who had voted in favour of the first version of the Charter, none were re-elected.

It seems that whatever other uncertainties pharmacy might face in the future, the Society itself will continue to perform both its regulatory and professional association functions for some time yet.

References

1. *Pharmacy: The Report of a Committee of Inquiry Appointed by the Nuffield Foundation*. London: Nuffield Foundation, 1986.
2. Anderson S C. The historical context of pharmacy. In: Taylor K, Harding G, eds. *Pharmacy Practice*. London: Taylor and Francis, 2001: 21.
3. Anderson S C, Huss R, Summer R, Weidenmayer K. *Managing Pharmaceuticals in International Health*. Basel, Switzerland: Birkhäuser, 2004: 71–85.
4. Anderson S C, Huss R, Summer R, Weidenmayer K. *Managing Pharmaceuticals in International Health*. Basel, Switzerland: Birkhäuser, 2004; 160–162.
5. Hepler C D, Strand L M. Opportunities and responsibilities in pharmaceutical care. *American Journal of Hospital Pharmacists* 1990; 47: 533–542.
6. Holloway S W F. *Royal Pharmaceutical Society of Great Britain 1841 to 1991: A Political and Social History*. London: Pharmaceutical Press, 1991: 274.
7. Bond C M. *Evolution and Change in Community Pharmacy*. Department of General Practice and Primary Care and Department of Management Studies, University of Aberdeen. London: Royal Pharmaceutical Society of Great Britain, 2003: 6 et seq.
8. Medicines Act 1968. London: HMSO, 1968: Section 69.
9. Narrow but clear majority for no confidence motion. *The Pharmaceutical Journal* 1989; 242: 438–444.
10. Martindale W H, Westcott W W. *The Extra Pharmacopoeia*, 16th edn. London: H K Lewis, 1915.

11. Reynolds J E F, (ed.). *Martindale: The Extra Pharmacopoeia*, 29th edn. London: Pharmaceutical Press, 1989.
12. *Pharmacy: The Report of a Committee of Inquiry Appointed by the Nuffield Foundation*. London: Nuffield Foundation, 1986.
13. PSNC agrees funding for new pharmacy contract. *The Pharmaceutical Journal* 2004; 273: 277.
14. Hassel K, Shann P. The national workforce census: (1) Locum pharmacists and the pharmacy workforce in Britain. *The Pharmaceutical Journal* 2003; 270: 658–659.
15. Hassel K, Fisher R, Nichols L, Shann P. Contemporary workforce patterns and historical trends: the pharmacy labour market over the past 40 years. *The Pharmaceutical Journal* 2002; 269: 291–296.
16. Will I. Why was the pass rate so low? *The Pharmaceutical Journal* 2003; 271: 613.
17. *Pharmaceutical Care: The Future for Community Pharmacy*. London: Royal Pharmaceutical Society of Great Britain on behalf of the Department of Health and the Pharmaceutical Profession, 1992.
18. *Pharmacy in a New Age*. London: Royal Pharmaceutical Society of Great Britain, 1996.
19. *Pharmacy in the Future – Implementing the NHS Plan*. London: Department of Health, 2000.
20. *Learning from Bristol. The Report of the Public Inquiry into Children's Heart Surgery at Bristol Royal Infirmary 1984–1995*. London: The Stationery Office, 2001.
21. Health Act 1999. London: The Stationery Office, 1999.
22. Lewis A M. All I want for Christmas. *The Pharmaceutical Journal* 2002; 269: 889.
23. Council agrees that draft Charter should go forward to the Privy Council. *The Pharmaceutical Journal* 2004; 273: 445.

15

The apothecary's return? A brief look at pharmacy's future

David Taylor

This book has demonstrated that, in the past, the role of the pharmacist centred primarily on the correct preparation and safe supply of medicines. However, during the course of the 20th century, and in particular in the 50 years since the introduction of the NHS and its counterparts in North America and Europe, the profession's part in making medicines was for the most part lost to the pharmaceutical industry. Present developments in healthcare delivery and computer technology promise change in supply processes. They offer new ways of reducing the risks and assuring the safety of medicines taking, which may or may not continue directly to involve pharmacists.

The objective of this final chapter is to look forward, in the light of national and international health and social care developments, to the future of the profession. It is based on recent reviews of the available literature on the structure and evolution of pharmacy in Britain, other countries of Europe and in North America [1,2], and also on recent research into what younger community pharmacists are seeking for tomorrow [3]. It begins with a brief outline of present and likely future trends in health and healthcare. This is followed by an overview of current pharmaceutical sector policies and service structures. The forces driving continued change are discussed, and options for the future of pharmacy as a profession assessed.

Unresolved issues

The loss of pharmacy's historic position in relation to making medicines has to a degree been offset by the emergence of clinical pharmacy in secondary care. In the community setting, however, where across Europe as a whole well over 80% of practising pharmacists work (even in the UK, where hospital pharmacy is relatively well developed, almost three-quarters of the profession's active members are community pharmacists) there has to date been less opportunity to innovate. In some respects the role of non-hospital pharmacists today is – despite the spectacular development of the pharmaceutical armamentarium since the end of the Second World War – less fulfilling than it was a century ago.

Many of the most important questions for the future of pharmacy relate to the community pharmacies and pharmacists of tomorrow, and how their clinical and/or managerial roles will evolve. In the next few decades a number of issues will need to be resolved, some of which are listed in Box 15.1. The terms of the new pharmacy contract agreed between community pharmacy contractors (pharmacy owners and their representatives) and the government at the end of 2004 will inevitably have a major impact on the development of pharmacy in Britain.

However in the longer term, and across the wider world, there is a considerable range of factors to be taken into account in looking at possible futures for pharmacy. These include the quality of the profession's leadership; the range and nature of the diagnostic and therapeutic

---

Box 15.1 Questions awaiting answers

- To what extent will public expectations of community pharmacy change?
- Will more people come to see pharmaceutical care as a gateway, or an alternative, to medical care?
- To what extent will pharmaceutical service users of all ages come to prefer using online services backed by the home delivery of medicines to the personal contact and advice offered in traditional pharmacies?
- Will young pharmacists seek increasingly to work in premises shared with medical practitioners and other professionals?
- Or will physically separate community pharmacies be preserved and be better linked by information and communications technology to other parts of the healthcare delivery system?
- Within community pharmacy, will there emerge a growing divide between specialised clinical care providers and dispensing service and basic OTC medicine providers?
- To what extent will regulatory and other policies permit or encourage the further growth of chain pharmacies and the vertical integration of the latter with wholesalers across regions such as Europe?
- Will community and hospital pharmacy merge, to work in fully integrated care providers like those pioneered by Kaiser Permanente in the USA?
- If so, will current professional boundaries remain, or will a new more unified body of health professionals evolve?

innovations that will be developed and marketed; and the willingness and ability of health service users in differing communities and social positions to extend their self-care competencies, and to take a more central role as co-producers with professionals of personal and public health.

Pharmacy in the context of the public's health

Life expectancy in Britain increased markedly during the 19th and first half of the 20th centuries, well before most modern medicines and vaccines became available. From around 1850 better drains and water supplies combined with improvements in nutrition and housing to have a major impact on the public's health. By 1900 the average British baby could expect to live to about 50 years of age, although the chance of dying in the first year of life was still greater than 1 in 10. Today the equivalent figures are approaching 80 years, and 1 in 200.

Demographic changes

The processes of demographic and epidemiological transition associated with such changes include a fall in birth rates (as parents become better assured of their children's' survival they tend to have fewer babies); the ageing of the population; and a fall in the prevalence of infectious disease and premature deaths, balanced by increased chronic illness and disability rates.

The economic and social trends associated with such progress typically include increased industrialisation; increased education and status for women relative to men; more recognition of the importance of citizen and consumer rights and personal choice; and a greater emphasis on risk reduction, audit and public service quality in society in general and the healthcare context in particular.

One corollary of smaller family sizes and a general expectation of survival to old age is that death in childhood or earlier adulthood, when sadly it occurs, is even more of a tragedy than it was in previous eras. Such changes mean that public willingness to pay for more effective care and health protection rises exponentially, even while 'objective' indicators of health-related needs may fall. At the same time the status of professionals in universally educated populations becomes normalised in 'post-transitional' societies (that is, societies that have undergone demographic transition).

In the past the majority of people worked manually, and did not earn their livings by the use of a defined body of knowledge and technical skills. Now most people are 'knowledge workers' in one way or another, and many policy-makers and members of the public appear to regard the special status of the traditional professions as increasingly anachronistic. This might help to explain why doctors, pharmacists and other healthcare providers may on occasions feel that more and more is being demanded of them, by people who treat them with less and less respect.

Worldwide, the most important health issues arguably relate to how communities that have yet to achieve average life expectancies of 70 years and over can best be helped to overcome the remaining barriers to such progress. In some sub-Saharan countries, such as Angola, a third of all children die before the end of their fifth year. This shocking figure underlines the fact that, just as the development of national health systems like the NHS was a major step in the 20th century, strengthening transnational systems of health resource transfer and provision is a key challenge for the 21st century.

This understanding has major ethical and practical implications for all the groups concerned with the supply of modern pharmaceuticals, from research-based and generic medicine manufacturers to pharmacists and other professionals responsible for their supply and appropriate use. However, there are also important opportunities for further public health gain in the 'rich world'. They relate in large part to improving the prevention and treatment of conditions most likely to affect people in later adult life.

Health improvement

Derek Wanless, in his reviews of healthcare funding and public health improvement [4,5], noted that the options for achieving further public health progress include enhancing access to effective medicines such as statins and anti-hypertensive treatments, and to interventions such as smoking cessation support. Tobacco use alone presently accounts for about half of the observed inequalities in longevity within the British community. These also include improving case management services for the minority of people with established diseases, who are at high risk of becoming unduly dependent on secondary care, and promoting self-care skills as and when this can contribute to better health outcomes for the majority of the population.

Growing governmental and professional understanding of the importance of appropriate medicines use and high quality chronic disease management has led in the UK to initiatives such as the Expert Patient Programme, and concepts such as 'concordance' and 'medicines management' in the pharmaceutical sphere. There has been a range of attempts by the NHS to learn from the experience of organisations such as Kaiser and the United Health Group of Minnesota. Studies by independent groups such as the King's Fund have specifically highlighted the potential of pharmacists in promoting self-care and contributing to better chronic condition management [6]. From an objective standpoint, the economic evidence base underpinning claims that community pharmacists can move forward from their relatively limited dispensing role to enhancing medicines use in a cost-effective manner, and also to delivering health promotion and health protection services, requires further strengthening. Nevertheless, increased interest amongst governments across the world in the potential of disease management approaches to improve healthcare outcomes and contain its costs is an important signpost to the profession's future. So too is the fact that in the 21st century, post-transitional societies, the potential for environmental and lifestyle improvements alone to further increase life expectancy and reduce mental and physical morbidity is more limited than is sometimes suggested.

During the first 50 years of the NHS, average life expectancy in the UK increased by about 10 years. Medical care enhancements can reasonably claim about half this gain, and changes in lifestyle and environmental protection the other half [7]. Problems such as smoking and obesity should be addressed by further educational and protective interventions designed to influence behaviour. However as average lifespans reach 80 years, further progress is likely to demand the informed, early use of effective medicines coupled with other specific interventions based on an improved awareness of genetically mediated health risks.

Those seeking to divine pharmacy's future need to fully appreciate the significance of this conclusion. Whatever the strengths and weaknesses of the profession's contribution today, pharmacy has an important opportunity to be at the heart of attempts to further enhance public health tomorrow through an increasingly sophisticated, socially and psychologically appropriate application of pharmaceutical science-based innovations.

A vision for pharmacy?

Since the publication of the NHS Plan in 2000 [8], a number of official documents have provided a detailed picture of current policy directions relating to pharmacy in both hospital and community settings. They include *Pharmacy in the Future* (England) [9], *The Right Medicine*

(Scotland) [10] and *Remedies for Success* (Wales) [11]. In 2003 the Department of Health also published *A Vision for Pharmacy in the New NHS* [12]. This summarised plans for pharmacy's future in England and sought to stimulate discussion about their translation into reality. Key measures designed to allow the public better, more convenient access to modern pharmaceuticals and pharmaceutical care are listed in Box 15.2.

The implementation of these measures is being facilitated by programmes such as the Medicines Management Collaborative, and the Medicines Partnership. The latter is aimed at promoting better public understanding of medicines, and supporting self-management. Extending the role of technicians and other pharmaceutical care team members as dispensers and providers of services such as smoking cessation support is also an element in the overall set of policies aimed at liberating pharmacists from their traditional dispensing activities, and

---

Box 15.2 Measures to allow better access to modern pharmaceuticals

- New repeat dispensing arrangements, which should permit pharmacists to manage long-term medication programmes better and reduce unnecessary patient visits to GP practices to consult with their doctors, or their receptionists.
- Initiatives aimed at promoting direct pharmacist treatment of NHS patients with 'minor conditions'.
- The shift of medicinal products such as proton pump inhibitors and statins to Pharmacy status. If in future there is a similar reclassification of products such as anti-hypertensive medicines in the UK this could fundamentally revise the role of OTC products in preventing serious chronic illness, as opposed to alleviating transient acute distress.
- The development of supplementary prescribing and the use of NHS Patient Group Directives (or private PGDs) to allow pharmacists to take a more proactive role in supplying NHS (or private) patients with prescription medicines.
- The introduction of independent pharmacist prescribing, consultant pharmacists and pharmacists with a special interest in given disease areas, such as type 2 diabetes.
- Improved communication and collaboration between hospital and community pharmacy, aimed at allowing higher quality and more cost-effective processes of hospital admission and discharge.
- The establishment (in or before 2008) of integrated care records for all NHS patients, using systems with the technical potential to allow appropriate access to records in community pharmacies as well as in hospitals and GP surgeries.
- The development of pharmacists and pharmacies as 'public health' resources, providing health promotion, health improvement and harm reduction services.

allowing their time and skills to be used to make other contributions to the better use of medicines and increased health gain.

In the short term it remains to be demonstrated how successful such policies will be. Many British pharmacists presently report being heavily burdened by the volume of dispensing. The practical viability of extending their clinical roles may to some seem doubtful, and at present the strength of the evidence base in areas such as 'pharmaceutical public health' is limited [13]. Understandably, some community pharmacists also fear that if they lose their substantive role as dispensers in order to take on clinical tasks and/or 'community oriented pharmaceutical care', they will risk professional redundancy should the latter fail to prove to be economically sustainable.

Glimpses of the future

A weak community pharmacy future would be one in which the profession sinks during the next decade or two into a narrowly defined drug supply management role, with competitor groups such as medicine and nursing incorporating the more clinical aspects of pharmaceutical care into their roles, while less expensively qualified technicians and dispensers' assistants supply medicines to the public. However against this negative picture there are many other more positive scenarios for the future of community and hospital pharmacy in the UK. Some brief illustrative vignettes of what these 'pharmacy tomorrows' may be are now offered.

Scenario 1: Strengthened traditional practice

In this scenario, the current distinction between community and hospital pharmacy is, together with the physical separation of community pharmacies and general practice surgeries, preserved. However, better functional integration of NHS services is achieved via good IT links and improved approaches to service management and development within PCTs and their equivalents in Wales, Northern Ireland and Scotland. Patients and other pharmacy customers use both the Internet, backed by home delivery services, and personal visits to obtain advice, medicines and other pharmacy goods and services. Community pharmacies serve as 'walk-in health centres' for NHS and private users, and act as pharmaceutical care co-ordinating points for hospital admission and discharge and specialist outreach services.

A significant part of the future NHS community pharmacy role in this scenario is about ensuring that diseases diagnosed and initially prescribed for by doctors are treated well in practice, and hence that high-quality medicines management is achieved. However, the availability of pharmacy-only (rather than prescription-only) medicines which permit the effective primary and secondary prevention of serious long-term illnesses, has also opened the way to a 'sea change' in responsible self-care.

The medical profession has welcomed strengthened traditional pharmacy practice. It is seen as reducing doctors' workloads without threatening precipitous change which could impair the delivery of 'serious medicine' and undermine medical authority. General medical practice has undergone a renaissance in this scenario. The extended commissioning powers and referral rights of general medical practitioners in an NHS economy based on primary care-supported patient choice and fixed Health Related Group payments for NHS Foundation Trusts have over time created a true primary care-led health service.

Scenario 2: Primary care (clinical) pharmacy, plus supermarket and other 'drug stores'

Primary care pharmacists work directly for or with family doctors, or in primary care organisations. Practice in this area has already been shown to be more flexible and varied than in traditional hospital and community roles [14]. In the scenario suggested here, dispensing remains located outside primary care practice. It takes place in either large high street community pharmacies, or centralised NHS dispensing units run directly by specialist medicines supply pharmacists employed by the Acute or Primary Care Trusts.

The work of primary care practice pharmacists has become almost entirely focused on their clinical role. Hospital pharmacy has also further developed its clinical and patient safety protection roles. Many younger pharmacists have welcomed this opportunity to use their skills. The public increasingly sees pharmacists as the professionals with legitimate control over the use of medicines. However, primary care pharmacists normally operate on an appointments-only basis: they are becoming almost as difficult to access as family doctors and senior nurse practitioners.

At the same time the number of independent and other pharmacies located in high street and other community settings has declined. Their business is concentrated on minimal cost dispensing and supply, based on the electronic transmission of prescriptions and increased volumes of home delivered medicines, supported by the high-volume sale of OTC medicines. Some supermarket and other pharmacies offer health checks, but it has not in the main proved economically viable for the 'shopping mall drug stores' of 21st century Britain to develop specialist clinical services.

Scenario 3: Corporate pharmacy competition

Current estimates suggest that 75% of all NHS community pharmacies will be incorporated into chains of five or more stores by about 2015. In this scenario this trend proves more rapid than expected. A few large vertically integrated 'company chemist' pharmacy chains dominate the market. Competition between them has, however, driven significant improvements. These have been achieved via a combination of centrally funded, corporate, pharmaceutical and other health service research and development programmes, coupled with a greater devolution of the authority needed to deliver locally tailored services to the professionals working 'at the coal face'.

Despite fears that care standards and professional independence would be undermined by the further corporatisation of UK pharmacy, informed NHS commissioning and sophisticated management practices (involving the franchising of company know-how, backed by good support services to individual pharmacists and pharmacy/professional partnerships with strong roots in their local communities) obviate this danger. By 2015 the integrated health companies that grew out of the pharmacy chains of the 20th century have in many instances become NHS-contracted 'alternative primary care providers', offering services to both publicly funded and private customers.

Community pharmacies are increasingly regarded as independent multi-professional health centres in a more plural healthcare system, which can be entered by several different types of 'front door'. Despite the potential for conflict with other stakeholders in primary care, inter-professional rivalries and tensions have been managed.

Scenario 4: The new apothecary model (back to the future?)

This scenario is similar to scenario 3, but competing individual practi-tioners and partnerships of pharmacists (and other health professionals) have in an increasing range of therapeutic contexts established them-selves as alternatives to NHS general practitioners, and have often been able to set up in self-employed practice. Pharmacists have moved on from medicines management to the independent provision of pharmaceutical care. Amongst some sections of the community they have become 'the people's doctors', because of the convenience and customer responsiveness of the service provided.

This has caused significant inter-professional tension. However, UK policy-makers have for over a decade committed themselves to supporting choice and competition throughout the primary care sector. As in the case of dentistry at the end of the 20th century, they encourage patterns of pharmaceutical care that are jointly funded by the public purse (which is responsible for the provision of core, essential, services) and private individuals, who are free to purchase additional services directly. By 2015 it is widely accepted as inevitable and reasonable that people who are above agreed threshold levels of death or disability risk ought to be offered free NHS protection, while the large number of other people at 'low risk' should be actively encouraged to purchase additional protection on a personal basis.

Scenario 5: Integrated pharmacy in local NHS Health Maintenance Trusts

In this model PCTs and/or their equivalents develop their mixed commissioning plus indirect primary care provider roles to become fully integrated NHS primary and secondary service providers operating in discrete geographical localities. NHS pharmacy becomes a single salaried profession in these local managed care systems. Its members have been allocated a range of managerial and clinical roles, to be undertaken in various complementary settings. The distinction between hospital and community pharmacy is widely regarded as irrelevant, and practice is managed and co-ordinated in a unified system. A continuously increasing range of dispensing and patient support work is undertaken by assistants and technicians.

Boundaries between pharmacy, nursing and medicine practice (as with those between health and social care) still exist, but have become less significant and easier to cross than in the past. Standards of care for people with chronic illnesses and complex needs are said to have improved, although there are concerns about choice. Outside the NHS primary care centres there remain a limited number of private community pharmacies/drug stores. These offer varying services to their customers. In some areas they have good links with the NHS, but in others they are more isolated. Progress in this area is 'patchy'. Many professionals in mainstream NHS pharmacy express concern about the commercialism of the pharmacists practising in the residual private sector.

Scenario 6: Integrated pharmacy in competing healthcare companies

This scenario differs from that suggested above in that, without fixed geographical boundaries and with private ownership, there is competition between the alternative independent integrated care providers. As 'for profit' organisations they are strongly motivated to combine synergistically their publicly funded and private customer offers, and to make savings and introduce innovations as and where these improve their returns on capital.

This incentivises them to encourage vigorously and effectively self-care promotion and support, in part via agreements with independent community pharmacy chains and independents operating in supermarkets and other 'high footfall' sites. Surprisingly to some commentators, this competition and plurality leads to a well integrated overall system of pharmaceutical care delivery that appears to perform relatively well. However, there is continuing political controversy as to whether or not NHS principles have been fatally undermined through private ownership of the healthcare providers. Public service commissioning remains in the hands of regional health authorities, but these in total only employ a few thousand staff in 2020.

European and North American experience

These scenarios are not necessarily mutually exclusive. In reality the future for pharmacy in Britain, and other countries in Western Europe and North America, could well involve a mix of the possibilities described. With increasing social plurality and a growing emphasis on meeting differentiated healthcare consumer preferences and needs, almost the only thing that can be predicted with confidence is that the future of pharmacy (assuming the profession has the will to respond to new challenges, and the will to adapt to survive) is likely to be much more complex and varied than its past.

However, it is worth briefly considering some of the contrasting pharmaceutical experiences of Britain's European partners, and the lessons to be learned from countries such as the USA and Canada. In the latter case, for instance, pharmacists already have extended IT-based access to medication and health records in some provinces. This has been well accepted by service users, and is an important global pointer to the future.

The USA

The USA has, like the UK, a relatively strong hospital pharmacy tradition (about a quarter of the 200,000 pharmacists in the USA work in hospitals and nursing homes) and a community pharmacy system populated by both chain and independent pharmacies [15]. Increased use of prescription medicines, combined with extensions in the roles played by pharmacists, has led to a situation in which demand for members of the profession has outpaced supply. In comparison to Europe, America also has well-developed Internet pharmacy services. There is evidence that the latter offered some service users significant advantages.

Yet there is also evidence that independent community pharmacies tend to be preferred by significant sections of the public [1]. The lack of universal 'pharmaceutical benefits' in the USA, and the expense that older persons and individuals with long-term conditions needing treatment may consequently have to face, could well be a significant factor influencing consumer behaviour. Some medicine users are forced to put cost savings before the quality of their pharmaceutical care. The collective welfare service funding traditions of Western Europe may in fact have helped to preserve patterns of pharmacy service that may not be so technically efficient in distribution terms, but offer other less easily measured benefits.

Another important difference between the USA and the UK is that whereas Britain enjoys a regulatory system with three categories of medicines (prescription-only, pharmacy and general sales products), the USA has only two available (prescription-only and general sale). The message for the future is that, despite the competitiveness of the US market and the fact that prescription medicine advertising is permitted, this has inhibited extensions in the range of medicines available from pharmacies. The UK system offers greater flexibility for progress towards a wider range of self-care options.

Europe

The fact that in much of Europe there is no general sales classification (effectively, all medicines in countries such as, say, France and Spain have to be purchased through pharmacies) arguably represents another limitation on the development of the pharmaceutical marketplace. European debate about the potential costs and benefits of 'deregulating' the pharmaceutical sector and permitting more direct pharmaceutical company promotion of medicines to the public should be understood in the light of such concerns.

There is a wide variation in the number of community pharmacies in different European countries. Greece and Spain have one pharmacy for every 500–1000 people: this contrasts sharply with the 10,000 plus people per pharmacy in the Scandinavian countries. Southern European countries allow much less delegation of dispensing and allied activities to non-technicians than is the case in Denmark and Sweden. Because of the way regulations restricting the sale of prescription medicines have been interpreted, it may also be the case that pharmacists in much of southern Europe have played more of a clinical practitioner role than the formal literature suggests. Other key points in the context of pharmacy in Europe are listed in Box 15.3.

Box 15.3 Pharmacy in Europe

- In the Netherlands, which has traditionally had large numbers of single-handed doctors in primary care, pharmacists have taken a more important part in guiding medical prescribing and managing patient care than has been the case in countries like the UK.
- At the same time they are not required to stay on their premises to supervise dispensing undertaken by qualified technicians, and when they are there they have private consulting areas in which to see clients.
- In most parts of Europe community pharmacists outnumber their hospital-based colleagues by between 10 : 1 (as in Belgium, for example) and 25 : 1 (in Spain and Germany); in the UK and Holland this ratio is in the order of 5 or 6 : 1.
- In most European countries only pharmacists can own pharmacies, and chain formation has not been allowed. This has led to major structural differences between countries such as France and the UK, which have similar-sized populations.
- France has over 50,000 community pharmacists, of whom some 27,000 are owners or co-owners; in Britain the equivalent figures are approaching 30,000, and a total of 4000 individual and corporate owners.
- The French community pharmacy system is relatively costly, but well respected.
- Volumes of medicines consumption in France are, per capita, twice or more than those in the UK.
- In countries such as Norway and Ireland, controls on pharmacy ownership and numbers have recently been lifted, along with other regulatory changes. The aim of this was to promote consumer interests by increased competition.
- Agencies such as the OFT in the UK have similarly called for deregulation.
- There is evidence from countries such as Portugal that excessive regulation can needlessly drive up overall pharmaceutical supply costs.
- However, there is a significant case for arguing in favour of healthcare systems such as the NHS being able to plan and direct their pharmacy services. Failures of markets in healthcare are the reason why public healthcare systems have been formed.

The economic incentives and powers available to pharmacists to promote the use of generic and other 'best value' medicines vary significantly across Europe, largely according to historical tradition. There is evidence that where pharmacists are appropriately supported and empowered they can play a significant part in containing medicine spending and improving the quality of pharmaceutical care, but where there are perverse financial incentives the opposite appears to be the case.

Although the structure of pharmacy has been relatively stable since the middle of the 20th century, pharmaceutical wholesaling has undergone significant change. It has become much more concentrated. If and when the rules on community pharmacy ownership are relaxed in Europe it is likely that major wholesalers such as Celesio (formerly Gehe), Phoenix and Alliance Unichem (together with internally integrated pharmacy chains like Boots) will extend their ownership of community pharmacies, and perhaps also extend offers to pharmacy service management in the hospital sector.

Choosing the future

Some historical events and trends are entirely outside the control of the individuals and institutions they affect. At a catastrophic level, wars and environmental disasters such as floods and earthquakes are often taken to fall into this category. Less dramatically, technical innovation frequently leads to redundancies, and revitalised economic and social orders. For example, the introduction of the H_2 antagonist medicines led in the 1980s to major reductions in the demand for gastric surgery. Surgeons could not prevent, and should arguably have welcomed, such progress.

Pharmacy and pharmacists are similarly in no position to turn back the tides of history. Superficially at least, the profession may be thought to be in the grip of social, technical and economic forces that make its future impossible to predict accurately, or control effectively. During the 21st century, for instance, further extensions in life expectancy and continuing changes in the incidence and prevalence of conditions such as the cancers and neurological disorders in later life should (barring unforeseen catastrophes) ultimately transform public expectations of pharmacy, medicine and nursing.

Beyond pharmacists' control

Advances in the pharmaceutical and biomedical sciences will also open up fundamentally new methods of diagnosing, preventing and treating such illnesses. For instance, near-patient testing and more personalised therapeutic regimens could well in time revolutionise approaches to the delivery of pharmaceutical care in community and other settings. Many other factors independent of the profession itself are also likely to guide the evolution of pharmacy, some of which have been touched on in this chapter. They include those listed in Box 15.4.

However, the uncertainties facing pharmacy, and the extent to which its members are unable to influence their situation, should not be overstated. From a UK policy perspective the probable direction of community and hospital pharmacy development over the next 10–20 years is relatively clearly discernible. Furthermore, if divisions within pharmacy can be overcome and its internal stakeholders in governance, education and practice development can work effectively together, there seems little reason to doubt that the profession's own choices and preferences will be a significant influence on tomorrow's decisions.

Box 15.4   Exogenous factors guiding the evolution of pharmacy

- **Further advances in the power of computers and computer-based systems**
  These will lead to new ways of informing prescribing and medicines use, and new opportunities to mechanise dispensing.
- **Revised political approaches to questions relating to safety, equity and access in the context of the medicines use**
  The desire to deregulate and widen people's freedom to purchase and use protective and other medicines is likely to a degree to be counterbalanced by perceived interests in maintaining 'high standards' of patient safety, even if in reality greater health gains could be achieved by investments elsewhere. The extent to which the state (following events such as the Bristol inquiry and the Ledward incident, Chapter 14) will seek to replace further professional bodies as guardians of the public's well-being and health service quality is similarly debatable.
- **The attitudes of other health sector stakeholders to pharmacists**
  In the UK the medical profession currently takes a relatively favourable view of proposed extensions to pharmacists' roles, and has in addition not been concerned to strongly defend GP dispensing.
  In parts of southern Europe with an excess of medical manpower this has not been the case. Perhaps even more importantly, consumer attitudes towards and requirements of pharmacy and pharmacists also remain uncertain. Reported satisfaction rates with pharmaceutical services may be reassuring, but this could be – in the UK at least – a reflection of limited expectations.

Within pharmacists' control

Research has found considerable support amongst pharmacists under 50 for the modernisation agendas being pursued by the Department of Health and Health Department in Scotland [3]. For example, nine out of ten of 450 respondents agreed that the future of pharmacy lies more in clinical practice, and the delivery of better patient care. Over 90% also said that enabling community pharmacists to access and update patient treatment records will be a vital step in extending their clinical role, and that developing informed self-care skills amongst medicine users is a central part of their professional mission. About half the respondents would like to see GP practices and health centres having co-located pharmacy dispensaries in the next 10 years.

Currently a majority of younger community pharmacists in the UK do not believe that their profession has the status it deserves, or that they have the opportunities they need to use their professional skills to the full. The workload imposed by dispensing presently seems to leave little room for role extensions. Against this, however, there is evidence that job satisfaction levels amongst primary care and hospital pharmacists are relatively high, and that the policies outlined in government documents such as *A Vision for Pharmacy* are generally in line with the majority of younger pharmacists' aspirations for the future.

Conclusion

Arguably, the most enlightened way for pharmacy to address the future would be unequivocally to put meeting the public's concerns for better health at the top of the profession's agenda. This will demand individual and collective effort aimed at adapting existing skills, services and ways of working in order to meet the highest priority requirements of the profession's customers in progressively more efficient and effective ways. In Britain up until the 2020s, a pragmatic combination of the scenarios described earlier as 'strengthened traditional practice', 'primary care pharmacy' and 'corporate pharmacy competition' can reasonably be taken to represent the most probable pharmacy future capable of delivering such an end.

Notwithstanding achievements in the more distant past, pharmacy in the second half of the 20th century was commonly seen (particularly in the community setting) as a partial, and transitional, profession, which people too often entered as a second best to medicine. Its leadership has been described as divided and weak, and pharmacy in the UK often appeared to be of lower status than pharmacy elsewhere. The opportunity for tomorrow is for pharmacy in this country to become a modernised, self-confident profession, which can offer its members greater fulfilment through maximising the health gain to be achieved through the application of existing and new medicines. In the UK the conditions needed for this progress to happen now appear to be in place. The challenge for the profession in Britain is to realise this promise, and in so doing to act as an example to the rest of the world.

References

1. Bond C M. *Evolution and Change in Community Pharmacy*. Department of General Practice and Primary Care and Department of Management Studies, University of Aberdeen. London: Royal Pharmaceutical Society of Great Britain, 2003.
2. Mossialos E, Mrazek M, Walley T. *Regulating Pharmaceuticals in Europe: Striving for Efficiency*. Maidenhead: Open University Press, 2004.
3. Taylor D G, Carter S L. *Realising the Promise. Community Pharmacy in the New NHS*. London: The School of Pharmacy, University of London, with the Social Market Foundation and the College of Health, 2002.
4. Wanless D. *Securing Our Future Health: Taking a Long-Term View*. London: The Treasury, 2002.
5. Wanless D. *Securing Good Health for the Whole Population*. London: The Treasury, 2004.
6. Lewis R, Dixon J. Rethinking management of chronic disease. *British Medical Journal* 2004; 328: 220–222.
7. Bunker J. *Medicine Matters After All*. London: The Stationery Office, 2002.
8. *The NHS Plan*. Command 4818–1. London: The Stationery Office, 2000.
9. Department of Health. *Pharmacy in the Future: Implementing the NHS Plan*. London: Department of Health, 2000.
10. Scottish Executive. *The Right Medicine: A Strategy for Pharmaceutical Care in Scotland*. Edinburgh: Scottish Executive, 2001.
11. NHS Wales. *Remedies for Success: A Strategy for Pharmacy in Wales*. Cardiff: Welsh Assembly, 2002.
12. Department of Health. *A Vision for Pharmacy in the New NHS*. London: Department of Health, 2003.
13. Royal Pharmaceutical Society of Great Britain. *The Contribution of Community Pharmacy to Improving the Public's Health – Report 1: Evidence from the Peer-reviewed Literature 1990–2001*. London: Pharmacy Health Link and the Royal Pharmaceutical Society of Great Britain, 2003.
14. Silcock J, Rayner D K, Petty D. The organisation and development of primary care pharmacy in the United Kingdom. *Health Policy* 2004; 67: 207–214.
15. Cooksey J A, Knapp K K, Walton S M, Cultace J M. Challenges to the pharmacist profession from escalating pharmaceutical demand. *Health Affairs* 2002; 21(5): 182–188.

Index

Page numbers in italics refer to figures and boxes.

A S Watson, ownership of Superdrug, 129
A Vision for Pharmacy in the New NHS
    (Department of Health), 288, 298
AAH (pharmacy wholesaler), 268
Abbott (pharmaceutical company), 166
    British factory, 167
    vitamins, 166
Abu-l-Qasim al-Zahrawi (Albucassis of Cordova),
    38
Academy (ancient Greece), 28
accident and emergency departments, 143
accreditation of pharmacy courses, 274
acetophenetidin (phenacetin), 160
acetylcholine, 184
aciclovir, *192*, 197
acquisitions and mergers, pharmaceutical industry,
    167–168, 171–172, 197
acrodynia, 252, 253
admixture of drugs, intravenous fluids, 145
adrenal cortical extracts, 187–188
    see also corticosteroids
adrenergic nerves, receptors, 183–184
adulteration
    17th century, 63
    legislation on, 227
adverse effects of drugs, 251–253
    on pharmaceutical industry, 172
advertising, *163*, *185*, 233–234, Plate 18, Plate 19
    complaint to RSPGP, 276
    Pharmacy and Medicines Act (1941), 247
    thalidomide, *254*
    USA, 294
agranulocytosis, amidopyrine, 251
agriculture, poisons, 245–246
Ahlquist, Raymond, dual receptor theory,
    183–184
AIDS, lessons of history applied, 7
Aitken Report, 142–143
Al Razi *see* Rhazes (865–925 AD)
Albucassis of Cordova, 38
alchemy, 33
Alderley Park (Cheshire), beta-receptor blockers,
    193
Alderlin (pronethalol), 194
Alemaeon of Crotone, 26
Alexander the Great (356–323 BC), 28
Alexandria
    destruction of Library, 32
    Museum, 28–29
Alexipharma (Nikander), 46
Alfred (King, 849–899 AD), 41
alizarin red, ancient Egypt, 24
alkaloids, 180

drug manufacturing, 157
    London Pharmacopoeia, 63
alkylating agents, 195
Allen & Hanburys, 118, 158, 164, 170
    salbutamol, 194
Allen, William, first president of Pharmaceutical
    Society, 74, 77
Alliance Unichem (wholesaler), 296
allopurinol, *192*, 197
al-Manuri hospital, Cairo, 39
alphabet, Phoenicians, 26
al-Qanum (Avicenna), 34–35
alternative medicine, 132
al-Zahrawi (Albucassis of Cordova), 38
amalgamations and mergers, pharmaceutical
    industry, 167–168, 171–172, 197
America *see* United States of America
American Institute for the History of Pharmacy,
    Pharmacy in History, 12
American Medical Association, safety of medicines,
    249
amidopyrine, 160
    adverse reactions, 251
ampicillin, 189, *192*
analgesics
    Hoechst, 160
    morphine, 180
    non-steroidal anti-inflammatory drugs, 193
analytical testing, hospital pharmacy quality
    control, 146–147
Anaximenes (6th century BC), 26
animal excreta, Babylonian medicine, 23
animals
    treatment by pharmacists, 237
    see also Veterinary Products Committee;
        Veterinary Surgeons Act (1948)
antagonism, competitive, 196
antibacterials *see* antibiotics; chemotherapy
    (antibacterial)
antibiotics, 168, *179*, 188–190
    legislation, 248
anti-cancer agents, 195–197
Anti-cutting Record, journal of William Glyn-
    Jones, 80–81
antidepressants, 193
    monoamine oxidase inhibitors, 253
Antidotarium (Nicolaus Salernitanus), 38
Antidotarium (Platearius), 38
antidotes, universal, 204
'Antidotus Analeptica', Culpeper on, 207
antihistamines, 190
anti-hypertensive drugs, 194, *288*
anti-malarials, 183, 187

anti-metabolites, 195–196
antipyrin, 160
Antiques of the Pharmacy (Leslie Matthews), 10
antitoxins, 182
Apotheca (ancient Rome), 32
apothecaries
  14th century, 117
  17th century, 60, 62
    physicians *vs*, 64–67
  18th century, 67–68
  Arabic, 33
  Babylonian, 22, 23
  conflict with physicians over diagnosis, 237
  future scenarios, 291–292
  modern pharmacists *vs*, 151–152
  shops, 116, 118, Plates 4–7
    18th century hospitals, 136
    American, 115–116
    Arabic, 33
    see also pharmacies (shops)
  urine examination, 59
Apothecaries Act (1815), 69–71, 227, *228*
  exemptions, 119
  on hospital pharmacy, 136
Apothecaries Bill (1748), 68–69
Apothecaries' Hall, courtyard, Plate 12
Apothecaries Oath (Basle), 40
Appointed Day, National Health Service, 92
appointments-only access, primary care pharmacy,
  290
apprenticeship, 97, Plate 14
  druggists, 68
  end of, 108
  examination requirement, 107
  Society of Apothecaries, 53–54, 64
Apuleius *see Herbal of Apuleius*
Aquitania, herb plantings, 33
Arabian civilisations, 32–36
  medicine in mediaeval Spain, 37–38
  medicines, 204–205
  pharmacy shops, 115
Archagathos the Greek, pharmacy shop (200 BC),
  115
Archimedes (287–212 BC), 29
area pharmacists, 145
Aristotle (384–322 BC), 28
arms
  Royal Pharmaceutical Society of Great Britain,
    Plate 2
  Worshipful Society of Apothecaries, Plate 9
Army, Society of Apothecaries contract, 63
arrack, medicines in, 34
arsenic, 244, 245
Arsenic Act (1851), 229, 243, 245
arsenicals, May & Baker licence, 165
arsphenamine, 162, *179*, 183
Art and Pharmacy (D A Wittop-Koning), 9
artefacts, as historical sources, 10
aseptic dispensing, 139–140, 145
  radiopharmacy, 148
Aseptic Dispensing for NHS Patients, 150
aspirin, 181, *192*
  Nyegaard & Co., 163
  Wuppertal Elberfeld, *164*
Asquith, Herbert, 84
Association of the British Pharmaceutical Industry,
  171
Assur-Bani-Pal (668–627 BC), royal libraries, 23

Assyrians, 23
Astra (pharmaceutical company), 163
  merger, 171
AstraZeneca, laboratory, Plate 24
atenolol, *192*
Athelstan (King)
  hospices, 43–44
  reign (924–939 AD), 41
atomic theories, 26–27
atropine, 184
Attorney General, Rose Case, 66
Audit Commission, on clinical pharmacy, 151
Aventis (pharmaceutical company), 171
Averroes (1149–1198), 38
Avicenna (980–1037 AD), 5, 34–35, 204, Plate 2
azathioprine, *192*, 196

Babylonian empires, 22–23, 26
Bacon, Francis (1561–1626 AD), on technology,
  26
bacteriology, 105
Baghdad, 33
Baitar, Ibn-al- (1197–1248), *Jami*, 38
balsams, 206
Banckes, Richard, *Herball*, 48
barbitone (Veronal), 162–163, *179*
barbiturates, 162–163
  phenobarbital contamination of sulphathiazole,
    250
BASF (pharmaceutical company), 169
Basle, Apothecaries Oath, 40
Bavaria, pharmacy education, 97
Bayer (pharmaceutical company), 160, 162–163,
  169
  antibacterials, 186
  British factories, 164
BCG vaccine, Lubeck Disaster,
  247–248
Beasley and Jones, trade card, *71*
Bede (673–735 AD), *De Natura Rerum*, 41
Bedlam, 135
Beecham, Thomas, patent medicine magnate, 234
Beechams
  failed bid for Glaxo, 170
  merger, 171
Beecham's Pills, 233
Behring, Emil von, diphtheria antitoxin, 182
Bell, Jacob
  on advisory role of chemists, 237
  bill referring to qualifying examination, 101
  father as unqualified chemist, 78
  *Historical Sketch of the Progress of Pharmacy in
    Great Britain*, 10–11
  on pharmacy education, 97
    chemistry, 110–111
  portrait, Plate 16
  on types of pharmacists, 118
Berridge, Virginia, on uses of history, 7
Best Buy hospital building plans, 143–144
beta-receptor blockers, 184, *192*, 193
Beveridge Report, 91
Beverley, St Giles Hospital, 43
bezoar stones, 208
Bilson, Mr, pastille moulds, 213
biotechnology
  entrepreneurs, 197–198
  origins, 193
  pharmaceutical industry, 170–171, 172, 197

Black, James
  beta-receptor blockers, 193
  Nobel Prize, 194–195
Black Death, 45–46
Black List, National Health Service, 131–132, 171
Blaud's Pills, 233
Boehringer (pharmaceutical company), 159
  mergers, 167
boluses, electuaries, 207
Boot and Company Ltd (later Boots), 121–122,
  266
  insulin advertisement, *185*
  libraries and cafes, *126*
  mergers, 128–129
  research, 164
  self-service, 125–127
  tablet production, *165*
Boot, Florence, libraries and cafes,
  126
Boot, Jesse (later Lord Trent of Nottingham), 79,
  83, 120–122
  attack on Proprietary Articles Trade Association,
  123
  Managers' Representative Council, 131
  portrait, Plate 20
Boot, John, 120–121
Boston (Mass.), apothecary shop, 116
bougies, 217
Bowen, I, pharmacy, *90*
boxwood, 239
Boyle, Robert, *Sceptical Chemist*, 62–63
Bradford Hill, Austin, streptomycin, 189
Braithwaite, J C, North London School of
  Chemistry, 103–104
branded medicines
  non-proprietary medicines *vs*, trends, *16*
  see also nostrums; proprietary medicines
Bristol, paediatric heart surgeons scandal, 277
Bristol-Myers, merger, 171
Britain
  consumption rates of medicines, France *vs*, *295*
  pharmaceutical industry, 158, 164–165
    base for foreign companies, 170
    post-war market share, 169
    Romans in, 30, 40–41, 43
    US pharmaceutical companies, 167
    see also Parke Davis (pharmaceutical
      company)
  vs USA, drug regulation, 294
British Drug Houses
  chairman on drugs in pregnancy, 257
  research, 164
British Institute for Preventive Medicine *see* Lister
  Institute
British Library, National Sound Archives, 9
British Medical Association, 84
  books on secret remedies (1909), 232, 233
  dispute over National Insurance Act, 88–89
British Medical Journal, article on adverse effects
  of drugs, 251–252
British National Formulary, 277
British Pharmaceutical Codex, 239
British Pharmaceutical Conference, 105
British Pharmaceutical Students Association,
  Future Pharmacist, Maplethorpe on pharmacy
  education, 110
British Pharmacopoeia, 63, 209
British Society for the History of Pharmacy, 8

Brockeden, William, 'compressed pills', 212
Brockwell Hall, WPRL laboratory,
  178
Bruising Apothecary, 9
bubonic plague, 45–46, 64
Buchanan, Margaret, on women hospital
  pharmacists, 136
Burgess's Lion Ointment, 233
Burroughs Wellcome (pharmaceutical company),
  161, 164
  anti-metabolites, 196
bye-laws, Pharmaceutical Society, 104, 107
Byzantium, 32

cachets, 210
caduceus, Babylonian medicine, 23
cafes, Boots, *126*
Cairo, al-Manuri hospital, 39
calomel, 252–253
Cambridge university, 35
Canada, information technology and, 293
cancer, drugs for, 195–197
Cancer Act (1939), 229, 234
Canon of Medicine (Avicenna), 34–35
capsules, 213
  Parke Davis, 161
captopril, *192*
carboys, 119
Cardwell, D L S, on individualism and education,
  105
Care Chemist case, 276
care records
  integrated, *288*
  pharmacists' view on access, 298
career breaks, 271
careers, 271
cartoons, 9, Plate 11
casualty departments, 143
cataplasms, 208
Catharanthus rosea, 195
Celesio (wholesaler), 296
Celsus, Aurelius Cornelius (20–50 AD), 29–30
central intravenous additive services, 150
Central Sterile Supply Departments, functions
  taken over from hospital pharmacies, 142
centralisation, hospital pharmacy, 146
cerates (cerecloths), 204, 208
chains *see* multiple pharmacies
charlatans, 224
  see also quacks
Charter establishing Apothecaries (1617), 53–54,
  64
Charter of Incorporation, Pharmaceutical Society
  see Royal Charter of Incorporation
Cheers, Mr (pharmacist under Jesse Boot), 121
Chelsea Polytechnic, degree course, 108
Chemical Research Laboratories (Burroughs
  Wellcome), 164
Chemist & Druggist, on Glyn-Jones anti-cutting
  scheme, 81
Chemist Examination *see* Minor Examination
chemistry
  ancient Egypt, 24
  Arab medicine, 205
  Jacob Bell on role in education, 110–111
  Paracelsus, 52
  pharmaceutical, 4
  Pharmaceutical Society school, 99

chemistry (*continued*)
  Strato (328–270/268 BC), 28
  synthetic drugs, 180–181
  see also dyestuffs
chemists
  18th century, 67–72, 117
  19th century, 77–78, 118
    advisory role, 237
    shops, 118–119
  friendly societies and, 86
  manufacturing, 158
  proprietary medicines, 231
  register, 109
  see also pharmacists
Chemists' Defence Association, 81–82
Chemists' Dental Association, 118
chemoreceptors, 183
chemotherapy (antibacterial), 182–183, 186–187, 188–190
  see also antibiotics
chemotherapy (cytotoxic), 195–197
childhood death, 285, 286
child-resistant closures, 143
China, pharmaceutical industry, 171
Chinese pharmacy, 22
Ching, John, lozenge roller, 214
chlordiazepoxide, *192*
chloroform, 181
chloroform water, 214
chloroquine, 187
chlorpromazine, 190, *192*, 193
Christianity, early and mediaeval, 32
Christie, Agatha (crime writer), 8
chronic disorders, 286–287
  research aims, 179
Chronicles of Pharmacy
  (A C Wootton), 11
Churchill, Winston, sulphapyridine and, 187
CIBA (pharmaceutical company), 160
  mergers, 171
cimetidine, *192*, 194
Circa Instans see Antidotarium (Platearius)
City of London, powers on medicine quality
  (James I), 227
Civil War, apothecaries and physicians, 64
Claudius (Emperor), expedition to Britain, 30
clay tablets, Nineveh, 23
clays, 204
clinical pharmacy, 110–111
  Audit Commission on, 151
  services, 148–149, *152*
clinical trials, 150–151
  streptomycin, 189
  USA, 249
clysters (enemas), 203, 208, 216
coatings (Cox), pill-making, 158
coats of arms
  Royal Pharmaceutical Society of Great Britain,
    Plate 2
  Worshipful Society of Apothecaries, Plate 9
cod liver oil emulsion, manufacture in hospital
  pharmacies, 137
Code of Ethics, Pharmaceutical Society, 131
Codex Aniciae Julianae (Dioscorides), 30
Cohen, Henry (Lord Cohen of Birkenhead), report
  of Joint Sub-Committee on the Safety of
  Drugs, 257
College of Physicians

conflict with Society of Apothecaries, 237
  pharmacopoeia, 51
  powers of inspection, 117, *228*
  see also Royal College of Physicians
Colleges of Advanced Technology, numbers of
  pharmacy schools, *106*
Colloquies on the Simples and Drugs of India (Da
  Orta), 51
commerce
  mediaeval, 39
  in pharmaceuticals, 115–134
Committee for Safety of Medicines, 240, 257
committee work, hospital pharmacists, 151
community pharmacy, 115–134, 283–284
  Europe, *295*
  future scenarios, 289–290
  NHS contract, 270
  pharmaceutical advisors, 269
  USA, 294
  see also pharmacies (shops)
community-oriented pharmaceutical care, 288–289
companies
  mediaeval, 42, 53
  Pharmacy Act (1908) on limited companies, 124
  see also named companies; pharmaceutical
    industry
Compendium of Medicine (Gilbertus Anglicus),
  46–48
competition
  healthcare companies (future scenario), 293
  supermarkets *vs* pharmacies, 266–267
competitive antagonism, 196
complementary medicine, 132
compound E (cortisone), 188, 191–193
compound medicines for internal use, 205–206
compound powders, 209–210
'compressed pills', 212
compulsory course, attempts to establish, 104–105
computerisation of pharmacies, 276
computerised databases, drug information, 147
concentrated infusions, 215
condita (preserves), 207
confections, 204
conserves, 204
consultant pharmacists, *288*
consumers, attitude to pharmacy, *297*
Consumers Association, report on medicine sales,
  275
consumption rates, medicines, France *vs* UK,
  295
Contagious Diseases Act, 7
continuing education, 274
continuing professional development, 274–275
contraceptive 'pill', 211
contracts, National Health Service, 270, 284
contrast media (radiological), 142
control (legislation), 243
corporate bodies
  exclusion from Pharmacy and Poisons Act
    (1868), 120
  multiple shop ownership, 79
Corpus of Simples see Jami (Ibn-al-Baitar)
corruganza boxes, 239
corticosteroids, 184, 191–193
  plant sources, 195
  see also adrenal cortical extracts
cortisone, 188, 191–193
cosmetics, as source of income, *13*

costs
  drug development, 264
  healthcare, 171
  prescriptions, 265
Council on Pharmacy and Chemistry (American
  Medical Association), 249
counter prescribing, 236–237
  see also over-the-counter sales
counterfeit products, 264
Cowen, D A, and D A Helfand, *Pharmacy: an
  Illustrated History*, 10
Cox, Arthur, pharmaceuticals manufacture, 158
'crammers', 104
Crateus, physician to Mithradates IV, 29, 46
creams, 215
Crellin, John, *Glass and British Pharmacy 1600 to
  1900*, 10
Cretan culture, 25
Crown and Anchor Tavern
  committee objecting to Hawes bill (1841), 73
  formation of Pharmaceutical Society, 74
Crown immunity
  loss, 149–151
  Rules and Guidance for Good Pharmaceutical
    Manufacture and Distribution and, 144
Crusades, 37, 38–39
cryogenine, adverse reactions, 251–252
Culpeper, Nicholas
  on 'Antidotus Analeptica', 207
  on plasters, 208
  translation of *London Pharmacopoeia*, 62
curricula, new universities, 109–110
cyclosporine, 192
cytotoxic drugs (anti-cancer agents), 195–197

Daffy's Elixir, 60–62
Dalton, John, atomic theory, 27
Dangerous Drugs Act (1922), *228*, 248–249
databases, 147
Day's Southern Drug Company, 122
  attack on Proprietary Articles Trade Association,
    123
  bought by Boots, 128
De Compositione Medicamentorum (Scribonius
  Largus), 30
De Materia Medica (Dioscorides), 30, 46
De Medicina (Celsus), 29–30
De Natura Rerum (Bede), 41
De Viribus Herbarum (Macer Floridus), 46, *47*,
  48
death in childhood, 285, 286
decoctions, 206, 215
deep fermentation, penicillin, 188–189
degrees in pharmacy, 107–108, 109
  courses (RSPGP), 272–274
  see also Master of Pharmacy
Delay, Jean (psychiatrist), 193
delayed-release preparations, 218
Delevigne, Sir Malcolm, on opium trade, 248–249
Democritus (460–370 BC), 26
demography, 285–286
Deniker, Pierre (psychiatrist), 193
dentistry
  pharmacy shops, 118
  as source of income, *13*
Department of Health
  *Pharmaceutical Care: the Future for Community
    Pharmacy*, 133

specialist advisory committees, hospital
  pharmacy, 146
A Vision for Pharmacy in the New NHS, 288,
  298
dependants, dispensing (National Insurance Act
  1911), 89
deregulation, 3, 264–265, 294, *295*, *297*
developing world, 286
diabetes mellitus, 186
  insulin, 166, *179*, 184–186
diaclysms, 208
diagnosis
  conflict between physicians and apothecaries,
    237
  present-day services, 133
diazepam, *192*
Dickson, R C M, judgement against
  Pharmaceutical Society, 128
dies, 'compressed pills', 212
diethylene glycol, sulphanilamide tragedy,
  249–251
Dioscorides (50–100 AD), 30
  De Materia Medica, 30, 46
  see also *Antidotarium* (Platearius)
diphtheria antitoxin, 182
Discombe, Dr George, on adverse effects of drugs,
  251–252
dispensaries
  1696, 64–66
  Society of Apothecaries, 63
  see also apothecaries, shops; hospital pharmacy
Dispensatory (Quincy), 62
dispensers, hospitals, 136
dispensing, 237–239
  aseptic, 139–140, 145, 148
  community practice, 129–130
  by doctors, *14*, 85–86, 87
  'extemporaneous', 237, 238
    Peppermint Water case, 275
  as income source, *13*
  mail order, 265
  National Insurance, 89–91
  present and future, 133
  radiopharmacy, 148
  rates per year, 20th Century, *15*
  workload, 289, 298
display jars, 119, Plate 9
distillation, 205–206
district pharmaceutical officers (DPhOs), 145–146
DNA, anti-metabolites from,
  195–196
Dr Gregory's Powder, 230
doctors
  dispensing prescriptions, *14*, 85–86
  see also physicians
Doctrine of Signatures, 30
Dolben, Sir William, petition for General
  Pharmaceutical Association of Great Britain,
    69
Domagk, Gabriel (research director at Bayer), 186
Domesday Book, 41
domestic products, manufacture in hospital
  pharmacies, 137
dosage forms, 203–221
douches, vaginal, 208
Dr Gregory's Powder, 230
draughts, 214
Drug and Therapeutics Committees, hospitals, 148

Drug Companies' Association, 123–124
drug information services, hospital pharmacy, 147
Drug Interactions (Stockley), 277
drug stores, America, 115–116
Drug Tariff (publication), 90–91
Drug Trade Appeal Fund, 83
Druggist Examination *see* Minor Examination
druggists
  18th century, 67–72, 117
  19th century, 77–78, 118
  proprietary medicines, 231
  shops, 118–119
    Sippara (1900 BC), 23
drugs
  20th-century discoveries, 177–201
  categories, USA *vs* UK, 294
  definition, 243
  term, 5
dry quintessences, 206
dry seal cachets, 210
dual receptor theory (Ahlquist), 183–184
Dublin Pharmacopoeia, 62
Duchy of Lancaster, 42
Dunlop, Sir Derek, on safety of medicines, 244
Durham College of Science, practical chemistry, 103
dyestuffs, 181
  ancient Egypt, 24
  origins of pharmaceutical industry, 160

E Merck *see* Merck (pharmaceutical company)
E Moss, wholesaler take-over, 268
East India Company, Society of Apothecaries contract, 63
Ebers, Georg *see Papyrus Ebers*
eclegmata (lohochs), 206
Economic and Social Research Council, use of history, 7
Edict of Palermo (1231 AD), 39–40, Plate 3
Edinburgh Pharmacopoeia, 62
education
  medication error prevention, 142–143
  pharmacists, 3, 97–113
    clinical pharmacy, 149
    present day, 272–274
Education Act (1944), 108
Edward I (King), 39
Edward III (King), 39
Egyptian civilisations, 23–25, 26, 115
Ehrlich, Paul, 183
elaboratories, 136
electuaries, 204, 207
elements (Greek philosophy), 26
  scheme of Galen, 30–31
Elements of Materia Medica and Therapeutics (Pereira), 99
Elion, Gertrude
  anti-cancer agents, 196
  Nobel Prize, 194–195
Elixir Salutis (Daffy's Elixir), 60–62
elixirs, 206
Elizabeth II (Queen), visit to Royal Pharmaceutical Society, 277, Plate 23
emetine, 180
Empedocles (490–430 BC), 26
employment, in pharmacy, 270–272
emulsions, 215
enemas (clysters), 203, 208, 216

Eno's Fruit Salt, advertisement, Plate 18
enteric-coated tablets, 218
entrepreneurs, biotechnology, 197–198
epidemics, plague, 45–46
epithems, 208
Epsom salts, 230
ergotism, 44
errhines, 208
errors, medication, 139, 142–143
ethical medicines, 156
  amidopyrine in, 251
Ethics, Code of, Pharmaceutical Society, 131
Europe, 294–296
  early universities, 35
  herbals, 33
  licencing of pharmacies, 267
  over-the-counter sales, 265
  pharmacists, 78
    medical profession and, 297
  pharmacy education, 97
  pharmacy shops, 115
European Community, drugs legislation, 258
Evolution of Pharmacy in Britain (Poynter), 11
examinations, 103
  failure rates, 104, 105, 272
  Licentiate of Society of Apothecaries, 136
  Pharmaceutical Society, 99, 101–103, 107, 245
  private teaching tailored to, 104
  Royal Pharmaceutical Society of Great Britain, registration, 272
  Society of Apothecaries, 53–54
excipients, 218
  pills, 210
expiry dates, 239
ex-servicemen, pharmacy training, 107
'extemporaneous dispensing', 237, 238
  Peppermint Water case, 275
Extra Pharmacopoeia, 269
extracts, 206, 215

failure rates, examinations, 104, 105, 272
fairs (mediaeval), 42
Farmer v. Glyn-Jones (1903), 83, 236
Fédération Internationale Pharmaceutique, 266
Fellows of the Pharmaceutical Society of Great Britain, 109
fermentation
  Egyptian medicines, 24
  penicillin, 188–189
finance *see* costs
Finance (No. 2) Act (1940), *229*
fixtures, hospital pharmacies, 138
flavours, Arab medicine, 204–205
Fleming, Alexander, penicillin, 188
Flixton, mediaeval hospice, 44
Florey, Howard, penicillin, 188
fomentations, hot, 203–204
Food and Drugs Acts, 227, 228, 229, 247
Food, Drugs and Cosmetic Act (USA, 1938), 251
formularies
  17th century, 62–63
  British National Formulary, 277
  National Insurance, 91
  Pharmaceutical Journal Formulary, 129
Forthcoming Legislation on the Safety ... of Drugs and Medicines (White Paper), 257–258

Four Thousand Years of Pharmacy
(La Wall), 11
Fourneau, Ernest, sulphanilamide, 186–187
Fownes, George, chemistry at Pharmaceutical
Society school, 99
fox's lungs, 206
France
community pharmacy, *295*
dyestuffs and pharmaceuticals, 160
pharmacy education, 97
pharmacy shops, 115
World War II, drug discovery, 190
franchising, 291
fraudulent miracles (Greek temples),
28
Frederick II of Hohenstaufen (emperor), 39–40
free trade, 67, 267
freelance pharmacists, 271
freshly prepared medicines, 237–238
friendly societies, 85, 86–87
Frith Guilds, 41
Fuller, Dr Robert, tablet triturates, 211
Funk, Casimir, vitamins, 184
furniture, hospital pharmacies, 138
Future Pharmacist, Maplethorpe on pharmacy
education, 110

Galen, Persian *see* Rhazes (865–925 AD)
Galen (129–199 AD), 5, 30–31, Plate 2
galenicals, 31
garbling, 63, 226–227
gases, medical, 144
Geber ibn Hayyan *see* Jabir ibn Hayyan (b. 776
AD)
Geigy (pharmaceutical company), 160
mergers, 171
gelatine, capsules, 213
gene therapy, *192*
General Medical Council, on dispensing laws, 88
General Pharmaceutical Association of Great
Britain, 69
General Rules of Medicine (Averroes), 38
generic medicines, 148–149, 156, 265
Europe, 296
Gerarde, John (herbalist, 1545–1612), 48, 226
German Herbarius, 48
Germany
pharmaceutical industry
development, 167–168
origins, 159–160, 162–163, 181
post-war market share, 169
World War II, 190
pharmacy, 115
education, 97
Gilbert the Englishman (Gilbertus Anglicus,
d. 1250), 38
Compendium of Medicine, 46–48
Gilds (mediaeval), 41–42, 51–52
Gilds-Merchant, 41–42
Gillray, James, *Taking Physic* (cartoon), Plate 11
Glasgow University, degree in pharmacy, 108
glass
shop windows, 118–119
tax on, 70
Glass and British Pharmacy 1600 to 1900 (John
Crellin), 10
Glaxo (pharmaceutical company), 170
mergers, 171

research, 164
vitamins, 166, 184
globalisation, pharmaceutical industry, 157,
169–170, 264
Globoid (aspirin tablet), 163
glycerine, weighing, 239
glyceryl trinitrate, 211
glycol, sulphanilamide tragedy, 249–251
Glyn-Jones, William (later Sir William), 79–83,
234
action on dispensing laws, 87–88
Farmer v. (1903), 83, 236
as MP, 84
undercut by pharmacy multiples, 122–123
glysters (enemas), 203, 208, 216
Good, John Mason, *History of Medicine, so far as
it relates to the Profession of the Apothecary*,
10
goodwill prices, pharmacies, 267
Goose Gate, Nottingham, shop of Jesse Boot,
120–121
gout, 197
Graeco-Roman era, 29
grants, higher education, 108
Gray, Samuel F, *Supplement to the
Pharmacopoeia*, 62
Great Cordial Elixir (Richard Stoughton), 230
Great Fire of London, apothecaries and physicians,
64
Great Moments in Pharmacy (Thom), Plate 3
Greece, number of pharmacies, 294
Greek civilisations, 25–29, 203–204
Green, Charles, painting, Plate 17
Green, J A, on post-war expansion of
pharmaceutical industry, 168
green cross, 119
Greenhough case, 72
Grete Herball, 48
Greux, Gustave-Marie, engraving of Dutch
pharmacy, *116*
Grew, Dr Nehemiah, patent on Epsom salts, 230
Grocers' Company, 53, 117, 226–227, *228*
group pharmacists, hospitals, 141–142
growth hormone, *192*
guiacum, tincture of, 215
Guild of Public Pharmacists, 137
Guilds (mediaeval), 41–42, 51–52
Guy's Hospital, pharmaceutical department, 138
gymnasia (ancient Greece), 27

H B Pare (pharmacy), 122
H₂ receptor antagonists, 296
haemolytic anaemia, cryogenine, 251–252
Hall, Dr John, of Stratford, 59–60
Hall, Sir Noel *see* Noel Hall Report
halothane, 144
Hammurabi (1795–1750 BC), 22
Hanckwitz, A G, laboratory, *155*
Hanseatic League, 42
Harrison, Edward Frank, analysis of secret
remedies, 232
Harrison, John, of London, Elixir Salutis, 60–62
Hawse, Benjamin, MP, parliamentary bill, 72–73
Hayyan, Geber ibn *see* Jabir ibn Hayyan
(b. 776 AD)
Health Act (1999), 278
health centres, community pharmacies and, 133,
291

health improvement, 286–287
Health Maintenance Organizations (USA), 265
Health Maintenance Trusts (NHS), pharmacy
  integrated, 292
healthcare companies, competition (future
  scenario), 293
healthcare costs, 171
Heatley, Norman, penicillin, 188
Henry VI (King), grant of right to Grocers'
  Company, 226–227
Henry VIII (King), legislation on medicines, 227
Hepler, C D, and L M Strand, on pharmaceutical
  care, 266
Heppell & Co., shop interior, *124*
Heraclitus of Ephesus, 26
Herbal of Apuleius, 46
herbalism, 17th century, 60
Herball (Banckes), 48
Herball (Gerarde), 49
herbals, 46–51, 226
  ancient Chinese, 22
  Codex Aniciae Julianae (Dioscorides), 30
  early European, 33
herbergia, Oxford, 44
heresy, 32
heritage, history as, 7
Hernandez, Francis, *Rerum Medicarum*, 51
Herophilus (335–280 BC), 28–29
higher education, 108
Hippocratean Corpus, 27
Hippocrates (460–377 BC), 27
histamine H$_2$ receptor antagonists, 296
*Historical Sketch of the Progress of Pharmacy in
  Great Britain* (Jacob Bell), 10–11
History of Drugs (Mez-Mangold), 10
*History of Medicine, so far as it relates to the
  Profession of the Apothecary* (John Mason
  Good), 10
history of pharmacy, 4–13
  purposes, 6–7
  sources, 8–10
History of Pharmacy in Britain (Leslie Matthews),
  11
Hitchings, George
  anti-metabolites, 196
  Nobel Prize, 194–195
Hittites, 25
Hodders Ltd, 122
Hodgkin, Dorothy, insulin structure, 186
Hoechst (pharmaceutical company), 160, 162, 169
  British factories, 164
  merger, 171
Hoffman-La Roche (pharmaceutical company),
  160
  vitamins, 166
Hohenheim, Theophrastus von (Paracelsus), 5, 52
Hohenheim, Wilhelm von (father of Paracelsus), 52
Holloway, Sydney, *Royal Pharmaceutical Society
  of Great Britain 1841 to 1991*, 11
Holloway, Thomas, patent medicine magnate, 234
Holy Trinity, Salisbury, lying-in hospital, 44
home-delivered medicines, 290
honeys, 206
honours degree, University of London, 108
hormonal products, 166, 184–186
horticulture, poisons, 245–246
Hortus Sanitatis, 48
  apothecary shops, Plate 6, Plate 7

hospices, mediaeval, 43–44
hospital manufacturing, 146–147, 149–151
hospital pharmacy, 135–154
  service responsibilities, *150*, 271
  USA, 293–294
hospitals
  al-Manuri hospital, Cairo, 39
  Department of Health standard plans, 143–144
  mediaeval, 43–46
hot fomentations, 203–204
House of Commons, mercury in teething powders,
  253
House of Lords
  corporate bodies and Pharmacy and Poisons Act
    (1868), 120
  Rose Case, 66
Howard, Luke (pharmacist), 158
human growth hormone, *192*
human insulin (Humulin), recombinant, 186, *192*
humours (Hippocratean), 27
  17th-century medicine, 58
  scheme of Galen, 30–31
hypertension, drugs for, 194, *288*
hypodermic tablets, 211

iatreion (ancient Rome), 32
Ibn Rushed *see* Averroes (1149–1198)
Ibn Sina *see* Avicenna (980–1037 AD)
Ibn-al-Baitar (1197–1248), *Jami*, 38
ibuprofen, *192*
ICI *see* Imperial Chemical Industries
ICML, *Care Chemist* case, 276
idiosyncratic drug reactions, 251–252
IG Farben, 167, 169, 190
illustrations, 9–10
  mediaeval herbals, 48
immunosuppressants, 197
Imperial Chemical Industries, 167, 168, 189
  sulphadimidine, 187
  see also Zeneca
implants, 218
Imuran (azathioprine), *192*, 196
Ince, Joseph, *Latin Grammar of Pharmacy*, 99
income of pharmacists, sources compared, *13*
income tax, income base level (1911), 85
incunabulae, 48
independent pharmacies
  freelance, 271
  private contractors, 268
India, pharmaceutical industry, 171, 179
indigo blue, ancient Egypt, 24
industrial drug manufacture, 155–174
industrial relations, judgement against
  Pharmaceutical Society, 130–131
infirmarians, monasteries, 135
information services, hospital pharmacy, 147
information society, knowledge workers, 285–286
information technology
  Canada, 293
  Internet pharmacy, USA, 294
infusions, 206, 214–215
inhalations, 217
inhalers, 217
injections, 217
inspections
  hospital pharmacy, 146–147
  powers, College of Physicians, 117, *228*

instrument repair, hospital pharmacies, 137
insufflators, 217
insulin, 166, *179*, 184–186
integrated care records, *288*
integrated pharmacy, Health Maintenance Trusts (NHS), 292
interferon beta-1b, *192*
internal use, compound medicines for, 205–206
International Opium Convention, 248
Internet pharmacy, USA, 294
inter-regional sample testing, hospital pharmacy, 146
intravenous fluids, 144–145
    admixture of drugs, 145
    central intravenous additive services, 150
inventors, biotechnology, 197–198
Investigation into the Provision of Pharmaceuticals to Health Authorities (Modern Materials Management Group), 149
Ionia, philosophers, 26
iproniazid, adverse reactions, 253
Ireland, deregulation, *295*
Islam, 38
Isolation and Identification of Drugs (Clarke), 277
isolation of French pharmaceutical industry, 190
IT *see* information technology
Italy, pharmacy shops, 115

Jabir ibn Hayyan (b. 776 AD), 33
Jack, David, salbutamol, 194
Jackson, Bill, *Victorian Chemist and Druggist*, 10
James I (King)
    Act for well garbling of spices, 227
    Charter establishing Apothecaries, 53–54
Jami (Ibn-al-Baitar), 38
Japan, pharmaceutical industry, 169
Jenner, Edward, 182
John Bell & Co., laboratory, *157*
John Bell and Croyden, 118
John of Arderne of Newark (1306–1390), 38
Joint Sub-Committee on the Safety of Drugs, 256–257
juleps, 204
Jundi-Shapur, Byzantine scholars, 32

Kennedy Report, Bristol heart surgeon scandal, 277
Kingfisher Plc, dealings, 129
King's Bench, Greenhough case, 72
King's Fund, on promotion of self-care, 287
Kitasato, Shibasabuto, diphtheria antitoxin, 182
Knights' Guilds, 41
Knoll (pharmaceutical company), mergers, 167
knowledge workers, 285–286
Koch, Robert, 182
Krateus, physician to Mithradates IV, 29, 46
Kremers and Urdang's History of Pharmacy, 11

La pharmacie Rustique, 59
La Wall, C H, *Four Thousand Years of Pharmacy*, 11
labelling, 143, 232–233, 239
laboratories
    Hanckwitz's, *155*
    John Bell & Co., *157*
    pharmaceutical industry, 164, 178, Plate 24
lamellae, 217
Lancaster, Duchy of, 42

Lancet
    on doctors and dispensing, 87
    on poisons legislation (1911), 79
Landseer, Sir Edwin, portrait of Jacob Bell, Plate 16
Largactil (chlorpromazine), 190, *192*, 193
Latin, pharmacy education, 99
Latin Grammar of Pharmacy (Ince), 99
Latin Herbarius, 48
Latin names, *London Pharmacopoeia*, 63
'laudanum' (Paracelsus), 52
Laune, Gideon de, 53, Plate 8
lay involvement, professional regulation, 278
lazar houses, 45
leapfrogging, pharmacies, 266, 267
Ledward, Rodney (gynaecologist-pharmacist), 277
Leech Book of Bald, 41
leech jars, Plate 10
    see also specie jars
leeches (Anglo-Saxon practitioners), 205
legislation
    mediaeval, 226–227
    quality of medicines, 223–241
    sexually transmitted diseases and, 7
    see also safety of medicines; *specific Acts*
Leicester, Gild-Merchant, 41–42
lend-lease agreements, 187
Lenz, W, on thalidomide, 255
Leonard's pharmacy, *125*
leprosy hospitals, mediaeval, 45
leukaemia, mercaptopurine, 196
levodopa, *192*
Lewis & Burrows Drug Stores Ltd, 122
Liber Servitoris (Albucassis of Cordova), 38
libraries, Boots, *126*
licencing
    pharmacies, 267
    products, 239–240
Licenciate of Society of Apothecaries, 136
life expectancy, 285, 287
Lilly (pharmaceutical company)
    British operation, 167
    insulin, 166
limited companies, Pharmacy Act (1908) on, 124
Limousin, Stanislaus, cachet-making machine, 210
liniments, 216
Linstead, Sir Hugh
    on academic pharmacy, 110
    Report on hospital pharmacy, 140–142
liquid medicines, *219*
    dispensing, 237–238
    see also specific dosage forms
liquors, 206
Lister Institute (formerly British Institute for Preventive Medicine), 182
    vitamins, 184
lixivia, 208
Lloyd George, David, 84
    on Glyn-Jones, 82
Lloyds Pharmacy, 129, 266, 268
loans, for Crusades, 39
logos (Heraclitus of Ephesus), 26
lohochs, 206
London
    City, powers on medicine quality (James I), 227
    first pharmacy shop, 115
    Great Fire, apothecaries and physicians, 64

London (*continued*)
  mediaeval gilds, 42
  pharmacists' mass meeting (1911), 88
London and Provincial Supply Association, 120, 266
London Directory, druggists (18th century), 67
London Dispensatory (Thomson), 62
London Pharmacopoeia, 50, 51, 62, 63
London polytechnics, 107
London University
  Bachelor of Pharmacy degree, 107–108
  honours degree, 108
  School of Pharmacy (formerly Pharmaceutical Society school), 100, 105
  degree courses, 108
lotions, 208, 216
Louis the Pious, 33
lozenges, 207, 213–214
Lubeck Disaster, 247–248
Lyceum (ancient Greece), 28
Lydia Pinkham's Vegetable Compound, 234
lying-in hospitals, mediaeval, 44

Macer Floridus, *De Viribus Herbarum*, 46, 47, 48
maceration, 215
Mackness, Mr, London and Provincial Supply Association, 120
Madagascar periwinkle, 195
magic
  ancient Egypt, 25
  mediaeval medicine, 205
magisteries, 207
Mago Ltd, 122
mail order dispensing, 265
Major Examination, Pharmaceutical Society, 99, 101
management structures, hospital pharmacy, 145–146
Managers' Representative Council (Jesse Boot), 131
Manchester
  acrodynia, 252
  masters course in clinical pharmacy, 149
  pharmacy education, 100
  University, degree in pharmacy, 108
Manual of Chemistry (Fownes), 99
manufacturing
  in hospitals, 146–147, 149–151
  industrial, 155–174
manufacturing chemists, 158
Maplethorpe, C W, on pharmacy education, 110
marketing authorisations, 239–240
Martin, N H, on chemists and education, 103
Martindale: the Complete Drug Reference, 277
Martindales (wholesaler), 118
mass production, 161
Master of Pharmacy, 111–112, 274
  courses
    Manchester, 149
    Nottingham, 274
Materia Medica (Dioscorides), 30, 46
Matthews, Leslie
  Antiques of the Pharmacy, 10
  History of Pharmacy in Britain, 11
Maul, Mr Justice, Greenhough case, 72
May & Baker, 158, 160, 164
  sulphapyridine, 167, 187
  World War I, 165

measurement, 239
mechanical injection devices, 218
Medical and Physical Journal, proposal for medicines legislation, 230–231
medical gases, 144
medical officers, resident, apothecaries as, 136
medical profession *see* medicine
medical records
  integrated care records, *288*
  patient treatment records, pharmacists' view on access, 298
Medical Research Council
  vitamins, 184
  World War I, 165–166
medical schools, mediaeval, 37–38
medication errors, 139, 142–143
medicine
  17th century, 58–62
  pharmacy and, 4, 21
    College of Physicians conflict with Society of Apothecaries, 237
    future relationships, *297, 298*
    present relationships, 290
    separation, 39–40, 78
Medicine Act (1802), 69–70
Medicine Control Agency, licences, 150
medicine counter assistants, training, 275
medicine men, 21–22
Medicine Stamp Duty Acts, 83, 234–236, 247
  on medicine sellers, 68
Medicine Tax (1783), *228*
medicine trolleys (hospital wards), 139, 142
medicines, 5
  consumption rates, France *vs* UK, *295*
  NHS Black List, 131–132
Medicines Act (1968), 144–145, *229*, 234, 258
  'extemporaneous dispensing', 238
  nostrums, 238
Medicines, Ethics and Practice (RPSGB), 131
Medicines, Ethics and Practice Guide for Pharmacists (RPSGB), 238
medicines information service, national, 147
Medicines Partnership, 288
Medicines (Labelling) Regulations (1976), 143
mels, 206
Memorial Sloan-Kettering Cancer Institute (formerly Sloan-Kettering Institute), 196
mepaquine, 183, 187
mercaptopurine, *192*, 196–197
merchants, mediaeval, 42
Merck (pharmaceutical company), 159, 169
  American subsidiary becomes company, 166
  barbiturates, 163
  globalisation, 170
  mergers, 167
Merck, George, 163
mercury
  and quacks, 224
  teething powders, 252–253
mergers, pharmaceutical industry, 167–168, 171–172, 197
Mesue, Johann, the Senior (777–857 AD), 33
metered-dose inhalers, 217
Meydenbach, Jacob, *Hortus Sanitatis*, 48
Mez-Mangold, L, *History of Drugs*, 10
micro-enemas, 216
micro-organisms, drug production from, 193
middle ages, 37–56, 205

Minor Examination
   failure rate (1900), 105
   Pharmaceutical Society, 99, 101, 245
miracles, fraudulent (Greek temples), 28
Misuse of Drugs Act (1971), 258
Mithradates IV, King of Pontus (115–63 BC), 29
mixtures, 214
Modern Materials Management Group (3M),
   Investigation into the Provision of
   Pharmaceuticals to Health Authorities, 149
Mohammed (570–632 AD), 32–33
Mohr, Francis, *Practical Pharmacy* (with
   Theophilus Redwood), *98*, *99*
monasteries
   illustrations, 9
   libraries, 41
   medicine, 35, 135
Mongols, plague, 45
monoamine oxidase inhibitors, adverse reactions,
   253
Monsanto, merger, 171
Montpellier, medical school, 38
More Secret Remedies (BMA), 232
Morison, James, patent medicine magnate, 234
morphine, 180
Morson *see* Thomas Morson
mountebanks, 17th century, 60
Mulford company, merger with Sharpe and
   Dohme, 166
multinational corporations, 155, 157
multiple pharmacies, 119–127, 266, 267–268
   corporate bodies, 79
   future scenarios, 291
   mergers, 128–129
mummies, powdered, 208
Museum of Alexandria, 28–29
mustard gas *see* nitrogen mustards
Mycobacterium leprae, 45
Mystery and Art of the Apothecary (Thomson), 11

Names of Herbs in Greke ... (William Turner), 48
narcotics *see* opium
National Formulary, 91
National Health Service, 91–92, 131–132
   Appointed Day, 92
   Black List, 131–132, 171
   effect on dispensing, 130
   hospital pharmacy, 140–152
   on pharmaceutical industry, 169
   pharmacists, 92
      contracts, 270, 284
National Health Service Act (1946), 91–92,
   131–132
National Insurance Act (1911), 84–91
   on dispensing, 130
   on hospital pharmacy, 137–138
   on pharmacy education, 107
national medicines information service, 147
National Pharmaceutical Association (formerly
   Retail Pharmacists Union), 131
National Pharmaceutical Union (formerly Retail
   Pharmacists Union), 131
National Sound Archives, British Library, 9
National Theatre, RSPGB meeting on supervision,
   268–269
Nebuchanezzar (605–562 BC), 23
nebulisers, 217
Needhams Ltd, 122

Neo-Salvarsan, 183
Nestorians, Jundi-Shapur, 32
Netherlands, pharmacy, 116, *295*
New Hospital for Women, dispensary, *138*
New London Dispensary (Salmon), 62
Newcastle, pharmacy education, 103
nicotine, 184
Nikander, *Alexipharma*, 46
Nineveh, libraries, 23
nitrogen mustards, 195
Nobel Prize, 194–195
Noel Hall Report, 145, 146
non-proprietary medicines
   vs branded medicines, trends, *16*
   as source of income, *13*
non-steroidal anti-inflammatory drugs, 193
norethisterone, *192*
Norman conquest, 40, 41
North London School of Chemistry, 103–104
North of England Pharmaceutical Association,
   lectures, 103
Norway
   deregulation, *295*
   pharmaceutical industry, 163
nostrums, 238
   see also proprietary medicines
Notions of the Agreeable no. 21 (cartoon), Plate 13
Nottingham University, degree course, 108, 274
Novartis (merged pharmaceutical company), 171
Novocain (procaine hydrochloride), 162
nucleic acids *see* anti-metabolites
nucleus hospital plans, 144
Nuffield papers, 273, 274
Nuffield Report (1986), 111, 132–133, 263, 272
Nuovo Receptario (pharmacopoeia), 51
Nyegaard & Co. (pharmaceutical company), 163

Office of Fair Trading, enquiry into pharmacies,
   267
Office of Scientific Research and Development
   (USA), nitrogen mustards, 195
oils, 208
ointments, 207, 215
on-call pharmacy services, 148
opium
   alkaloids, 180
   trade, 248–249
opticians, 118
oral examinations, 102–103
oral history, 8–9
Orange Guide, 144
Orta, Garcia Da, *Colloquies on the Simples and*
   Drugs of India, 51
orthoclone, *192*
Osler, Sir William, on desire for medicines,
   223–224
OTC sales *see* over-the-counter sales
'outlandish herbals', 51
outpatients, prescriptions, 143
over-the-counter sales (OTC sales),
   265
   Nuffield Report (1986), 132
Oxford
   herbergia, 44
   University, 35
oxymels, 206

packaging, 239

paclitaxel (Taxol), *192*, 195
paediatric heart surgeons, Bristol, 277
Palermo *see* Edict of Palermo (1231 AD)
pamaquine, 183, 187
p-aminobenzoic acid, antagonists, 196
Papyrus Ebers, 24–25, Plate 1
papyrus scrolls, 23–24
Paracelsus, 5, 52
Paradisi in Sole Paradisus Terrestris (Parkinson),
  51
parallel-imported drugs, 265
Parke Davis (pharmaceutical company), 182
  British operations, 164
  capsules, 161
  hormonal products, 166
Parkinson, John (1567–1640), herbals, 51
partisanship, early histories, 11
pastes, 216
Pasteur, Louis, 182
Pasteur Institute, 182
  sulphanilamide, 186–187
pastilles, 213, *214*
pastophors, ancient Egypt, 25
PATA (Proprietary Articles Trade Association), 81,
  123, 234
patent medicines, 224–226, 230–234
  tax revenue raised, 236
  see also nostrums; proprietary medicines
patents, 224–226
  German, abolition in World War I, 183
pathologists, observation of drug reactions,
  251–252
pathology services, functions taken
  over from hospital pharmacies, 142
Patient Group Directives, *288*
patient treatment records, pharmacists' view on
  access, 298
patient-centred pharmacy *see* pharmaceutical care
patrons, mediaeval hospitals, 44–45
pay
  hospital pharmacists, 140
  present-day, 270
pearl coating, pills, 211
Penbritin (ampicillin), 189, *192*
penicillin, 139–140, 168, *179*, 188–189
  drug resistance and, 248
Penicillin Act (1947), 248
Pentothal (thiopentone sodium), 167
pepperers, 115, 117
Pepperers, Guild of, 41
Peppermint Water case, 275
percolation, 215
Pereira, Jonathan (professor of materia medica), 99
perfumers, Babylonian, 23
peripheral neuritis, thalidomide, 255
periwinkle (*Catharanthus rosea*), 195
Perkin, William Henry (chemist), 181
Persian empire, 26
Persian Galen *see* Rhazes (865–925 AD)
pessaries, 208, 217
pest houses, 46
Peters, Hermann, *Pictorial History of Ancient
  Pharmacy*, 9
Peterson, Durey, on biosynthesis of drugs, 193
petition, General Pharmaceutical Association of
  Great Britain, 69
Pfizer, 170
  merger, 171

penicillin, 168
pharmaceutical advisors, 269, 271
pharmaceutical care, 265–266
  community-oriented, 288–289
  future scenarios, 291–292
  view of pharmacists, 298
*Pharmaceutical Care: the Future for Community
  Pharmacy* (Department of Health), 133
pharmaceutical chemistry, 4
Pharmaceutical Formulas (publication), 129
Pharmaceutical Historian (journal), 12
pharmaceutical industry, 155–174, 263–264
  development
    origins, 157–161, 209
    early 20th century, 162–165
    World War I, 165–166
    interwar years, 166–167
    World War II, 168
    1950s, 168–169
    late 20th century, 170
  biotechnology, 170–171, 172, 197
  drug discovery, 177–180
  France, wartime isolation, 190
  laboratories, *157*, 164, 178, Plate 24
  mergers, 167–168, 171–172, 197
  product range, 5
Pharmaceutical Journal
  on Chemists' Defence Association, 81–82
  on friendly societies, 86
  on Glyn-Jones anti-cutting scheme, 80–81
  on National Insurance Act (1911), 89
Pharmaceutical Journal Formulary, 129
Pharmaceutical Press, publications, 277
Pharmaceutical Society
  arsenic, representations on, 244
  building, Plate 15
  bye-laws, 104, 107
  examinations, 99, 101–103, 107, 245
  formation, 72–75, 237
  hospital pharmacy, enquiry (1939), 139
  judgement on industrial relations, 130–131
  limited companies, attempted bill against,
    123–124
  Pharmacy and Poisons Act (1933), 246
  pharmacy school, 99
  professional standards, committee on (1955),
    127–128
  registration of practitioners, 245
  Royal visit, 277
  on self-service stores, 127
  Special General Meeting (1965), Royal Albert
    Hall, *127*, 128
  on staff shortages, 143
  *v. the London and Provincial Supply
    Association*, 120, 266
  after World War II, 109
    educational policy, 108
  see also Royal Pharmaceutical Society of Great
    Britain
pharmaceuticals, 5
pharmaceutics, 4
Pharmacia (pharmaceutical company), mergers,
  171
pharmacies (dispensaries) *see* dispensaries
pharmacies (shops), *90*, Plate 22
  18th century, 136
  dentistry, 118
  future scenarios, 292

future walk-in health centres, 289
health checks, 291
mediaeval, Plate 4
origins, 115
ownership patterns, recent changes, 266–267
see also apothecaries, shops; druggists, shops;
     multiple pharmacies
pharmacists, 271, *288*
19th century, 78
ancient Egypt, 25
community pharmacy, 132–133
dispensing prescriptions, *14*
education, 3, 97–113
     clinical pharmacy, 149
     present day, 272–274
hospital
     19th century, 136
     committee work, 151
Jacob Bell on, 118
London mass meeting (1911), 88
National Health Service, 92
     contracts, 270, 284
prescription rates (1913), 89–91
promotion of self-care, 287
view of pharmaceutical care, 298
see also hospital pharmacy; supervision of
     pharmacies
pharmacobotanists (*rhizotomoi*), 28
pharmacognosy, 4
pharmacology, 4
experimental, 105
Pharmacopoeia Londinensis, 205
pharmacopoeias
17th century, 62–63
19th century, 208–209
basis for legislation, 227
mediaeval, 51, 205
see also named works
pharmacopolae (ancient Rome), 31
pharmacy
origin of term, 25
'practice' as academic subject, 111
status as profession, 298–299
see also medicine, pharmacy and
Pharmacy: an Illustrated History (Cowen and
     Helfand), 10
Pharmacy Act (1852), 78–79, 119
bill to amend for compulsory education,
     104–105
Pharmacy Act (1868), 79, *228*, 245
pharmacy education, 101–103
poisons, 79, 229
Pharmacy Act (1908), 107, 124
Pharmacy and Medicines Act (1941), *229*, 232,
     234, 247
Pharmacy and Poisons Act (1868), 120
Pharmacy and Poisons Act (1933), 131, *229*, 246
on hospital pharmacy, 138–139
Pharmacy in a New Age, 273
Pharmacy in History (American Institute for the
     History of Pharmacy), 12
Pharmacy in History (George Trease), 11
Pharmacy in the Future, 287–288
Pharmline, 147
phenacetin, 160
Phenergan (promethazine), 190
phenobarbital, contamination of sulphathiazole,
     250

phenothiazine amines, 190
chlorpromazine, 190, *192*, 193
phenylsemicarbazide, adverse reactions, 251–252
Philadelphia
College of Pharmacy, on patent medicines, 232
pharmacy education, 97
philosophers, ancient Greece, 26–29
phocomelia, thalidomide, 255
Phoenicians, 25–26
Phoenix (wholesaler), 296
photographic services, as source of income, *13*
photographs, as historical sources, 9
physicians
17th century, *59–60*
     apothecaries *vs*, 64–67
ancient Egypt, 25
dispensing prescriptions, *14*, 85–86
prosecution by Society of Apothecaries, 72
Physiological Research Laboratories (Burroughs
     Wellcome), 164
Pictorial History of Ancient Pharmacy (Hermann
     Peters), 9
pilgrimages, mediaeval England, 44
pill machines, 211
pills, 7, 210–211
coatings, 211
     Arthur Cox, 158
     Avicenna, 204
confusion with tablets, 211–212
hand making, Plate 21
mass production, 161
pre-19th century, 207
Pink Pills for Pale People, 233
plague
1665 epidemic, apothecaries and physicians, 64
Black Death, 45–46
plasters, 207–208, 216
Platearius, Matthaeus, *Antidotarium*, 38
Plato (427–347 BC), 28
Pliny the Elder (23–79 AD), 30
poisons
early legislation, 243, 244–247
hospital pharmacists and, 138–139
Pharmaceutical Society opposition to restrictions
     (1852), 101
Pharmacy Act (1868), 79, 229
Pharmacy and Poisons Act (1868), 120
Poisons Act (1972), 246, 258
Poisons and Pharmacy Act (1908), 83–84, *228*,
     246
Poisons Board, 246, 247
drug reactions and, 252
Poisons List, 245, 246
polio vaccine, *192*
Pontefract, St Nicholas Hospital, 43
Poor Law Dispensers' Association,
     137
Porter, R,
AIDS and lessons of history, 7
on quacks, 224
portfolio careers, 271
Portugal, regulation, *295*
Post Office Directory, druggists (18th century), 67
potassium bicarbonate, 212
potassium chlorate, 212
poultices, 208
poverty, 17th century, 57–58
powders, 207, 209–210

Powell, Enoch (Minister of Health), on safety of medicines, 244
Powers-Weightman-Rosengarten (pharmaceutical company), 166
Poynter, F N L, *Evolution of Pharmacy in Britain*, 11
Practical Pharmacy, title page, *98*
pregnancy, drugs in, 257
prescribing
  community pharmacists, *288*
  cost control, 171
    NHS Black List, 131–132, 171
  hospital pharmacists, 271
  repeat, 133, *288*
  supplementary, 133
  see also counter prescribing
prescription records books, as historical sources, 8
prescription sheets (hospitals), 142
preserves, 207
preventive medicine, health improvement, 286–287
price schedule, *Pharmaceutical Journal* on friendly societies, 86
primary care pharmacy, *vs* community pharmacy, 289
Primary Care Trusts
  future pharmaceutical services, 289
  pharmaceutical advisors, 269
primitive medicine, 203
printing, mediaeval, 48, 205
private care, *vs* NHS care, 292
private contractors, pharmacies, 268
private pharmacy schools, 103–104
  end of, 108
  numbers of, *106*
Privy Council
  nominees on RSPGB Council, 278
  objection to altering examination bye-laws, 104
  petition for new RSPGB Charter, 279
  Pharmaceutical Society examinations, 102
procaine hydrochloride, 162
product licences, 239–240
product specifications, standard, 147
production units, hospital manufacturing, 146–147
professions, loss of status, 286
professors, 105
profit-making healthcare companies (future), 293
proguanil, 187
promethazine, 190
pronethalol, 194
Prontosil rubrum, *179*, 186
propranolol, 184, *192*, 194
Proprietary Articles Trade Association, 81, 123, 234
proprietary medicines, 129, 224, 230, 231
  Food and Drugs Acts and, 247
proprietary schools *see* private pharmacy schools
proton pump inhibitors, *288*
Provincial Medical and Surgical Association, representations on arsenic, 244–245
provincial schools of pharmacy, 99–100
  degree courses, 108
psychotropic drugs, 193
  chlorpromazine, 190, *192*, 193
Ptolemys, 28–29
public health, 285
Public Pharmacist and Dispensers' Association (formerly Poor Law Dispensers' Association), 137

publications, Pharmaceutical Press, 277
pumps (mechanical injection devices), 218
pupilage *see* apprenticeship
purges, *58*
purine analogues, 196–197
Puri-Nethol (mercaptopurine), *192*, 196–197
Pythagoras, 26
  elements, scheme of Galen, 30–31

quacks, 60, 224, 226, 229, 230
quality control, hospital pharmacy, 146–147, 149–151
quality of medicines, 223–241
quiddonies, 206
Quincy, John
  Dispensatory, 62
  on pessaries, 208
quinine, 180–181
  World War II, 187
quintessences, 206

R J Mellowes' pharmacy shop, Plate 22
rabies vaccine, 182
radiology
  functions taken over from hospital pharmacies, 142
  silver recovery, 139
radiopharmacy, 147–148
Rauwolfia serpentina, 195
Razi, Al *see* Rhazes (865–925 AD)
recall notice, sulphathiazole, Winthrop Chemical Company Inc., *250*
recently prepared medicines, 237–238
receptors, 183–184
  drugs affecting, 193–195
    beta-receptor blockers, 184, *192*, 194
    H$_2$ receptor antagonists, 296
recombinant human insulin (Humulin), 186, *192*
records
  integrated care records, *288*
  patient treatment records, pharmacists' view on access, 298
Redwood, Theophilus, 99
  on advisory role of chemists, 237
  Historical Sketch of the Progress of Pharmacy in Great Britain (with Jacob Bell), 11
  Practical Pharmacy (with Francis Mohr), *98*, 99
Regional Pharmaceutical Officers Committees, hospital building plans, 143–144
regional pharmacists, 145
regional quality control pharmacists, 146
registration
  drug reactions, 255–256
  of practitioners, Pharmaceutical Society, 245
  RPSGB examination, 272
regulation
  pharmaceutical industry, 170
  pharmacy profession, 277–280
  see also legislation
  UK *vs* USA, 294
religion, medicine and, 224
Remedies for Success, 288
remuneration
  hospital pharmacists, 140
  present-day, 270
repeat prescribing, 133, *288*
replacement therapy, 184–186

Rerum Medicarum (Hernandez), 51
research, 109, 111
  ancient Greece, 28
  chronic disorders, 179
  pharmaceutical industry, 162–163, 164, 167, 178
    regulation and, 170
  use of history, 7
  see also laboratories
residency schemes, hospital pharmacy, 148
resident medical officers, apothecaries as, 136
restraint of trade, Pharmaceutical Society, 128
restructuring of services, Noel Hall Report, 145
Retail Pharmacists Union, 130–131
retail price maintenance, 81, 234
Rhazes (865–925 AD), 33–34
rheumatoid arthritis, 191
rhizotomi (ancient Rome), 31
rhizotomoi (ancient Greece), 28
Rhône-Poulenc (pharmaceutical company)
  chlorpromazine, 193
  merger, 171
  sulpha-drugs, 167
  sulphanilamide, 186
rice paper, 210
Richard I (King), 39
Riedel, 'Schweizerapotheke', 159
Right Medicine, The, 287–288
Robert E Price, shop front, *123*
Robinson, Kenneth (Minister of Health), on thalidomide tragedy, 258
robs (quiddonies), 206
Roche (pharmaceutical company), biotechnology investment, 170
rod and serpents (*caduceus*), 23
Roman civilisations, 29–32, 203–204
  Britain, 40–41
  valetudinaria, 43
Rose Case, 66–67, 117
Royal Albert Hall, Pharmaceutical Society Special General Meeting (1965), *127*, 128
Royal Charter of Incorporation, Pharmaceutical Society, 74
  Supplemental Charter, 278–280
Royal College of Physicians
  17th century, 64
  charter, on druggists, 67
  Rose Case, 66–67
  see also College of Physicians
Royal Navy, Society of Apothecaries contract, 63
Royal Pharmaceutical Society of Great Britain
  coat of arms, Plate 2
  education, 272–274
  historical sources, 8–9
  histories of, 10–11
  Medicines, Ethics and Practice, 131
  Medicines, Ethics and Practice Guide for Pharmacists, 238
  photographs, 9
  present-day role, 275–277
  professional regulation, 277–280
  registration examination, 272
  supervision of pharmacies, 132–133, 268–269, 275
Royal Pharmaceutical Society of Great Britain 1841 to 1991 (Sydney Holloway), 11
RP 3276, precursor of chlorpromazine, 190
RPM (retail price maintenance), 81, 234

Rules and Guidance for Good Pharmaceutical Manufacture and Distribution, 144
rural areas, dispensing (National Insurance Act 1911), 89
Rushed, Ibn *see* Averroes (1149–1198)

safety of medicines, 243–260, *297*
  Committee for, 240, 257
sagae (ancient Rome), 32
salbutamol, *192*, 194
Salernitanus, Nicolaus, *Antidotarium*, 38
Salerno, medical school, 37–38
sales, pharmaceutical industry, 156
sales assistants, Nuffield Report (1986), 132
salesmen, pharmaceutical industry, 168–169
Salisbury, Holy Trinity (lying-in hospital), 44
Salmon, William, *New London Dispensary*, 62
salts, from plants, 207
Salvarsan (arsphenamine), 162, *179*, 183
sample testing, inter-regional, hospital pharmacy, 146
sanatoria, National Insurance Act (1911), 86
Sandoz (pharmaceutical company), 160
  merger, 171
Sanger, Fred, insulin sequencing, 186
'Save Our Society' group, 278–280
Sceptical Chemist (Boyle), 62–63
Schedules, poisons, 246
Schering (pharmaceutical company), 159, 162, 169
  hormonal products, 166
Schoffer, herbals, 48
School of Pharmacy, University of London (formerly Pharmaceutical Society school), 100, 105
  degree courses, 108
schools of medicine, mediaeval, 37–38
schools of pharmacy
  numbers of, *106*
  Pharmaceutical Society, 99
  present day, 272
  provincial, 99–100
    degree courses, 108
  after World War I, 107
  see also private pharmacy schools
Schuppach, Michel (apothecary), *59*
'Schweizerapotheke' (Riedel), 159
science, role in pharmacy education, 109–110, 111–112
Scotland
  degree courses, 274
  herbalism, 17th century, 60
  pharmacists, 78
Scribonius Largus (1–50 AD), 30, 204
Searle, merger, 171
secret remedies, 224, 227–229, 231–233
  Medicine Stamp Duty Act (1804), 235–236
  National Insurance and, 90–91
Secret Remedies (BMA), 232, 233
Seidlitz powders, 210
Selecta a Praescriptis (Pereira), 99
self-care, 286–287
  view of pharmacists, 298
self-medication, 229–230
self-service, 125–127
Septuagint, 29
serpents, *caduceus*, 23
servi medici, 31
service restructuring, Noel Hall Report, 145

sexually transmitted diseases, learning from history, 7
Shakespeare, William, 8
Sharpe and Dohme, 166
Shen Nung (emperor), 22
shops
   sales assistants, Nuffield Report (1986), 132
   see also apothecaries, shops; pharmacies (shops)
'short-line stores', hospital pharmacy, 149
Sicily, Edict of Palermo, 39–40
sick pay, National Insurance Act (1911), 85
Signatures, Doctrine of, 30
silver recovery, 139
silvering of pills, 211
Simmonds, John, John Bell & Co. laboratory man, 157
simvastatin, *192*
Sina, Ibn *see* Avicenna (980–1037 AD)
Sippara (1900 BC), druggists shops, 23
sleeping tablet, thalidomide as, 254
Sloan-Kettering Institute, 196
Smith, Adam, on apothecaries, 67
Smith Kline & French, 159, 162
   British connections, 165
   globalisation, 170
Smith Whitaker, Dr (BMA medical secretary), 88–89
SmithKline Beckman, merger, 171
SmithKline Beecham, merger, 171
smoking, 286
Smout, C F V, on quacks, 226
soap solution, manufacture in hospital pharmacies, 137
social history, 6
Society of Apothecaries, 53–54, 97
   17th century, 63–67
   Apothecaries Bill 1748, 68
   conflict with College of Physicians, 237
   Licentiates, 136
   powers under Apothecaries Act (1815), 227
   prosecution of physicians, 72
Society of Chemist Opticians, 118
Socrates (469–399 BC), 27
sodium bicarbonate, 212
solid medicines, *219*
   see also specific dosage forms
South London School of Chemistry and Pharmacy, 104
South Western Polytechnic, 107
Spain
   mediaeval medicine, 38
   number of pharmacies, 294
specialisms, ancient Egypt, 25
specialist advisory committees, hospital pharmacy, 146
specialist pharmacists, *288*
specie jars, 119
   see also leech jars
spice trade, mediaeval, 39
spicers, 115, 117
Spicers, Guild of, 41
spinhalers, 217
spirits, 205–206
Squibb (pharmaceutical company), 159
   merger, 171
St Anthony's fire, 44

St Bartholomew's Hospital, Smithfield, 44, 135
   dispensary, *140*
St Giles Hospital, Beverley, 43
St Nicholas Hospital, Pontefract, 43
St Thomas's Hospital, 135
   staff shortages, 142, 143
Stamford, mediaeval hospitals, abuse by wardens, 45
stamps
   Medicine Stamp Duty Acts, *235*, *236*
      see also Medicine Stamp Duty Acts
   National Insurance Act (1911), 86
standard product specifications, 147
Standards for Pharmaceutical Services in Health Authorities in England and Wales, 149
standards of service, clinical pharmacy, 149
Standing Advisory Committees, admixture of drugs to intravenous fluids, 145
Standing Committee of chemists and druggists (1802), 70
Standing Medical Advisory Committee, thalidomide tragedy and, 256–257
state
   role, *297*
   see also Department of Health; National Health Service
statins, *288*
Statute of Labourers (1350), 44
Statute of Monopolies (1624), *228*, 230
Statutory Committee, Pharmaceutical Society, 131
Steedman's powders, advertisement, Plate 19
sterile dispensing *see* aseptic dispensing
sterile water, 144–145
steroid hormones *see* adrenal cortical extracts; corticosteroids
stock bottles, 238
Stoughton, Richard, Great Cordial Elixir, 230
Strato (328–270/268 BC), 28
streptomycin, *179*, 189
substitutions, generic, 148–149
sugar
   Arab medicine, 204
   sweet medicines, 206–207
   tablet coating, 213
sulphadimidine, Imperial Chemical Industries, 187
sulpha-drugs, 167, 186–187
sulphanilamide, *179*, 186–187
   competitive antagonism, 196
   tragedy, 249–251
sulphapyridine, 186
   May & Baker, 167, 187
sulphathiazole, recall notice, Winthrop Chemical Company Inc., *250*
sulphonal, 160
sulphonethylmethane, 160
Sumerians, 22
Superdrug (store chain), 129
supermarkets
   competition with pharmacies, 266–267
   health checks, 291
   pharmacies, 129
   self-service pharmaceuticals, 127
supervision of pharmacies
   Netherlands, *295*
   Royal Pharmaceutical Society of Great Britain and, 132–133, 268–269, 275
Supplement to the Pharmacopoeia (Gray), 62
Supplemental Charter (RPSGB), 278–280

supplementary prescribing, 133
Supplies Departments, functions taken over from
    hospital pharmacies, 142
suppositories, 208, 216–217
suramin, 183
Sussex Drug Co., 122
sustained-release tablets, 218
sweet medicines, 206–207
Switzerland, pharmaceutical industry
    origins, 160
    post-war market share, 169
syringe pumps (injection devices), 218
syrups, 204, 206

tablet triturates, 211
tablets, 211–213
    enteric-coated, 218
    production machinery, 161, *165*
Tabloid (Burroughs Wellcome trademark), 161
Tacuinum Sanitatis, apothecary shop, Plate 5
Tagamet (cimetidine), *192*, 194
take-overs and mergers, pharmaceutical industry,
    167–168, 171–172, 197
Taking Physic (Gillray cartoon), Plate 11
tamoxifen, *192*
taxes
    on glass, 70
    on medicines, 234–236
    see also Medicine Stamp Duty Acts
Taxol (paclitaxel), *192*, 195
Taylors Drug Company, 122
    merger with Timothy Whites, 128–129
teaching hospitals, 141
    clinical pharmacy services, 148
    clinical trials, 150–151
technical colleges, numbers of pharmacy schools,
    106
Technical Instructions Act (1889), 106–107
technicians, hospital pharmacy, 148, 151
teething powders, calomel, 252–253
temperaments (Galen), 31
teratogenic drugs, thalidomide disaster, 170, 172,
    253–257
terra sigillata, 204
thalidomide disaster, 170, 172, 253–257
Thatcher, Margaret, financial strictures, 111
The Right Medicine, 287–288
Theatrum Botanicum (Parkinson), 51
Theophrastus (372–287 BC), 28
'therapeutic revolution', 177
Therapeutic Substances Act (1925),
    247
Therapeutic Substances Act (1956), 248
Therapeutic Substances (Prevention of Misuse) Act
    (1953), 248
theriacs, 204, Plate 5, Plate 6
    preparation, *43*
thiopentone sodium, 167
Thom, Robert A, *Great Moments in Pharmacy*,
    Plate 3
Thomas Morson (manufacturer), 118
    factory, 158
Thomson, *London Dispensatory*, 62
Thomson, C J S, *Mystery and Art of the
    Apothecary*, 11
thyroxine, *179*, 184
Timothy White (pharmacy multiple), 122
    merger with Taylors Drug Company, 128–129

tinctures, 206, 215
tobacco use, 286
Todd Thomson, Dr Anthony, botany teacher, 99
toiletries, as source of income, *13*
trade *see* commerce
trademarks, 161
training *see* education
transdermal patches, 218
transnational health resource transfer, 286
treacles *see* theriacs
Trease, George, *Pharmacy in History*, 11
trional, 160
tuberculosis, sanatoria, National Insurance Act
    (1911), 86
Turner, William (1500–1568), *Names of Herbs in
    Greke ...*, 48
twenty-four-hour pharmacy services, 148
Tyndall, John, *Penicillium notatum*, 188
Tyrer, Thomas, on Bayer (pharmaceutical
    company), 160

UK *see* Britain
undercutting, by multiple pharmacies, 122–123
undergraduate courses, clinical pharmacy, 149
Underwoods, taken over by Boots, 129
unguentarii (ancient Rome), 32
Unichem (pharmacy wholesaler), 268
    PROSPER system, 276
    see also Alliance Unichem (wholesaler)
unicorn's horn, 208
unit-dose packs, 142
United Kingdom *see* Britain
United Nations Industrial Development
    Organization, on pharmaceutical industry,
    157
United Society of Chemists and Druggists,
    opposition to Pharmaceutical Society
    examinations, 102
United States of America, 293–296
    legislation, 249–251
    nitrogen mustards, 195
    over-the-counter sales, 265
    patent medicines, 232
    pharmaceutical industry
        British operations, 164–165
        globalisation, 169–170
        Merck, 163
        origins, 159, 162
        post-war market share, 169
        salesmen, 168
        World War I, 166
    pharmacy shops, 115–116
    vitamins, 166–167
    World War II
        drug discovery, 187–188
        penicillin, 188–189
universal antidotes, 204
universities, *35*
    new technological (1963), 109
    pharmacy schools
        numbers of, *106*
        present day, 272
    see also specific universities e.g. London
        University
university status, pharmacy, 109–110
Upjohn (pharmaceutical company), mergers, 171
Urban II (Pope), 38–39
urine examination, *59*

USA *see* United States of America
use rates, medicines, France *vs* UK, 295
Usines de Rhône, 160

vaccines, 181–182
  BCG, Lubeck Disaster, 247–248
  polio, *192*
vagrancy, mediaeval England, 44
valetudinaria, 43, 135
variolation, 181–182
varnishing, pills, 211
Venerable Bede (673–735 AD), *De Natura Rerum*, 41
Venereal Diseases Act (1917), *228*, 234
Ventolin (salbutamol), *192*, 194
Veronal (barbitone), 162–163, *179*
vertical integration, 268
Veterinary Products Committee, 240
Veterinary Surgeons Act (1948), 237
Viaud, Pierre, on isolation of French pharmaceutical industry, 190
Victorian Chemist and Druggist (Bill Jackson), 10
vinegar, medicated, 206
viper wine, 206
Vision for Pharmacy in the New NHS, A (Department of Health), 288, 298
vitamins, 166–167, *179*, 184
vitrellae, 217
Voluntary Hospital Officers' Association, merger with Public Pharmacist and Dispensers' Association, 137

W T Warhurst (multiple pharmacy), 122
wafers, 210
Wallis, Patrick, on 18th and 19th century histories of pharmacy, 11
Wands (multiple pharmacy), 122
Warburton, Henry, MP, Committee of enquiry into medical profession, 72
wardens, mediaeval hospitals, 44–45
wards (hospital)
  medication on, 139, 142–143
  pharmacists on, 138–139, 147, 148
Waring, Edwin (pharmacist under Jesse Boot), 121
Warner-Lambert, merger, 171
water, sterile, 144–145
waters, 208
weighing, 239
welfare state, 84–91
Wellcome (pharmaceutical company), mergers, 171
Wellcome Library, historical sources, 8
Westminster College of Pharmacy, 104
Weston, Ralph (entrepreneur), 266
wet seal cachets, 210
whelps, oil of, 208
Which? (Consumers Association), report on medicine sales, 275
Whiffens (pharmaceutical company), 158
wholesalers, 268, 296

William Warner (pharmaceutical company), pill production, 161
willow bark, 181
Wills, G S V
  on training courses, 105
  Westminster College of Pharmacy, 104
windows
  Boot's, *121*
  chemists' shops, 118–119
wine
  distillation, 205–206
  medicated, 206
Winfrey, Richard, MP, 83
Winthrop Chemical Company Inc., sulphathiazole recall notice, *250*
wise women, 21–22
witch doctors, 21–22
withdrawal notices, sulphathiazole, Winthrop Chemical Company Inc., *250*
Wittop-Koning, D A, *Art and Pharmacy*, 9
women
  chemists, 103
  hospital pharmacists, 136
  pharmacists (present-day), 271
woodcuts, 48
Wootton, A C, *Chronicles of Pharmacy*, 11
working conditions
  hospital pharmacy, 140–142
  multiple pharmacies, 122
World Health Organization
  drug definition, 243
  on introduction of new drugs, 256
World War I, 183
  on pharmaceutical industry, 165–166
  schools of pharmacy after, 107
World War II
  drug discovery, 187–190
  nitrogen mustards, 195
  pharmaceutical industry, 168
Worshipful Society of Apothecaries, 117
  coat of arms, Plate 9
WPRL, laboratory, Brockwell Hall, *178*
Wuppertal Elberfeld, aspirin, *164*

xanthine oxidase, 196
X-rays
  functions taken over from hospital pharmacies, 142
  silver recovery, 139

Yale University, nitrogen mustards, 195
Yersinia pestis, 45
York, mediaeval hospice, 43–44
Young Pharmacists Group (YPG), 278

Zahrawi, Abu-l-Qasim al- (Albucassis of Cordova), 38
Zeneca (pharmaceutical company), merger, 171
zidovudine, *192*
Zovirax (aciclovir), *192*, 197
Zyloric (allopurinol), *192*, 197